The Rural Efficiency Guide
A Guide To Health

by R.W. Correll and R.L. Warner
U.S. Dept. of Agriculture

with an introduction by Roger Chambers

This work contains material that was originally published by
the Us Department of Agriculture in 1917.

This publication was created and published for the public benefit,
utilizing public funding and is within the Public Domain.

This edition is reprinted for educational purposes
and in accordance with all applicable Federal Laws.

Self Reliance Books

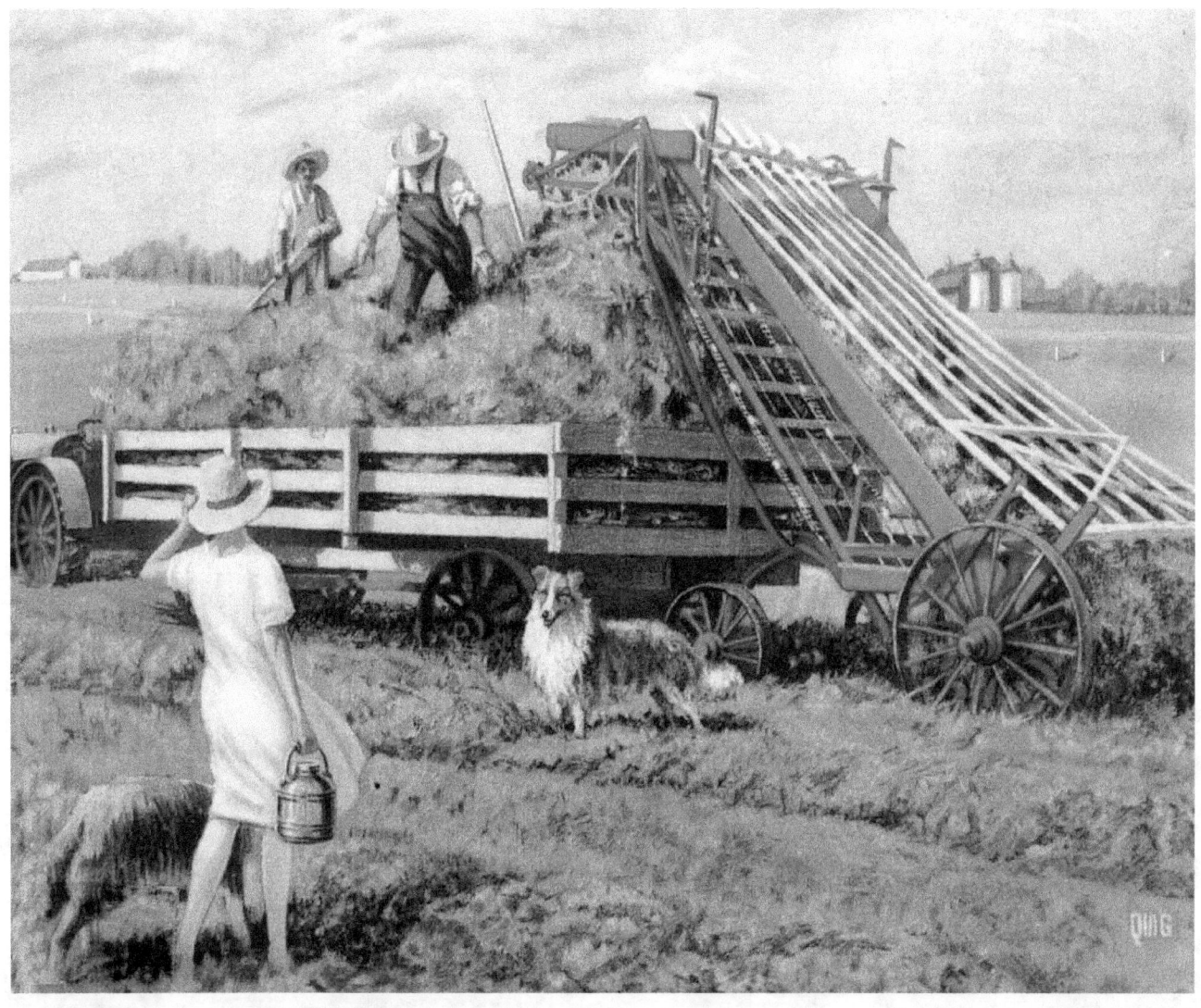

Get more historic titles on animal and stock breeding, gardening and old fashioned skills by visiting us at:

Introduction

I am pleased to present yet another title in the *U.S. Department of Agriculture's "Rural Efficiency"* book series. These incredible books, now a century old, give us an insight into life in rural America in a bygone age. A great read for anybody interested in homesteading, long-term survival situations, or in rural American history.

The work is in the Public Domain and is re-printed here in accordance with Federal Laws.

As with all reprinted books of this age that are intended to perfectly reproduce the original edition, considerable pains and effort had to be undertaken to correct fading and sometimes outright damage to existing proofs of this title. At times, this task is quite monumental, requiring an almost total "rebuilding" of some pages from digital proofs of multiple copies. Despite this, imperfections still sometimes exist in the final proof and may detract from the visual appearance of the text.

I hope you enjoy reading this book as much as I enjoyed making it available to readers again.

~ Roger Chambers
PNW, 2017

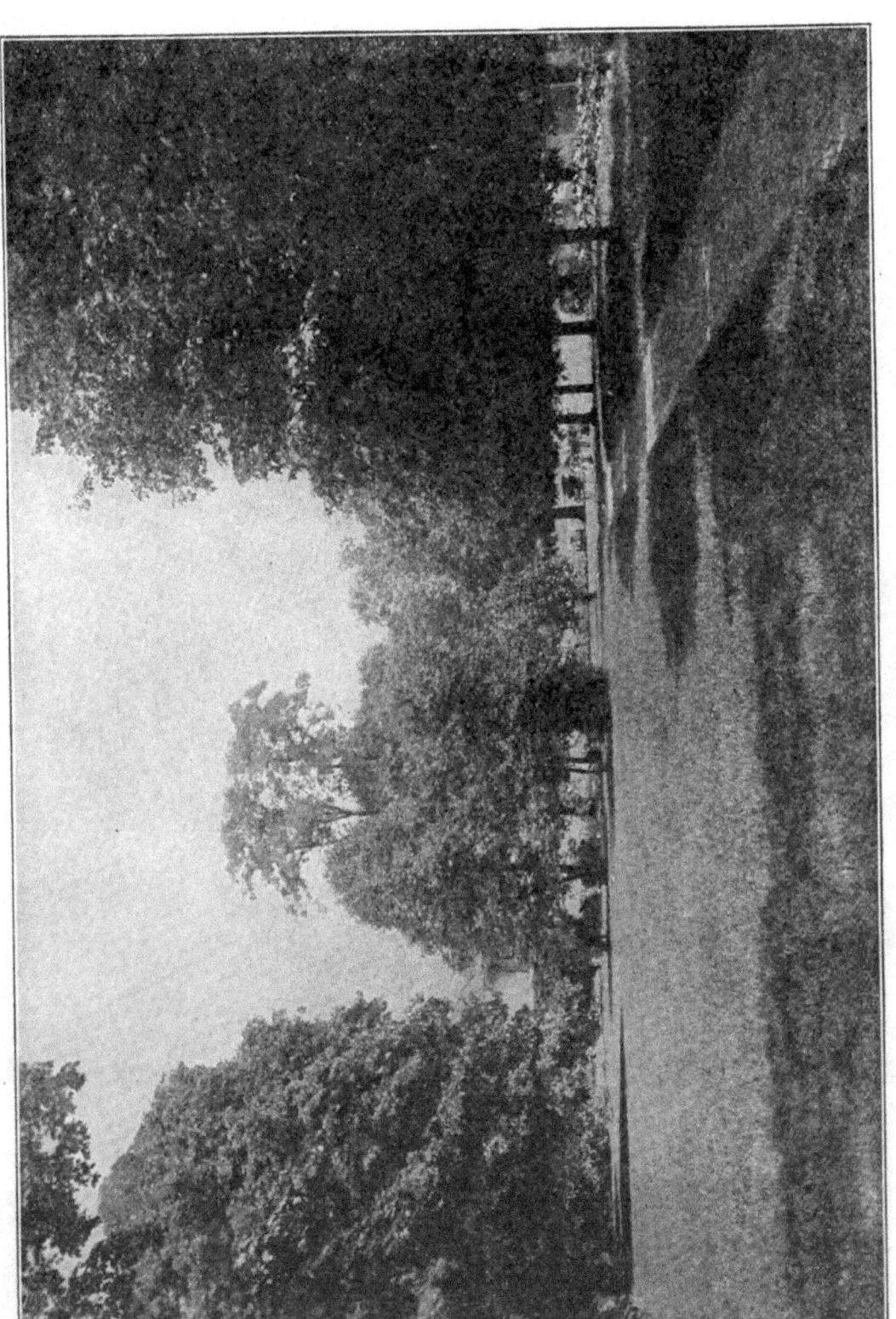

A RURAL HOME SCENE.

The Compilers' Preface

The name of this set of books, "The Rural Efficiency Guide," conveys to some extent the purpose of the compilers in getting this material together. There never has been a time in the history of the world when it was so important that the Farmer, the Agriculturist, the Stockman, be efficient in his work as at the present time. He is required to produce a greater amount of produce, a better quality of produce, and the work must be done in less time than ever before. The idea of this set of books is to point the way, to be a guide to greater efficiency in all the lines taken up. It is also of the greatest importance that the farmer be efficient in caring for his health and that of his family. He must be physically and mentally fit in order to accomplish his work in an efficient way and thus carry out his obligations to the other workers of the world.

The work is the result of many years of experience and study in the rural sections. The compilers were not only born and reared on the farm, but have spent over 20 years studying the conditions and needs of the rural sections. The four books have been compiled with one purpose in view—to render the people a true service, "The Service for Others Efficiency." We have endeavored to eliminate all that is impractical, to give only what can be used and will prove of real value in the home and on the farm and to give it in plain, simple language which may be understood by all.

Every one of the authors connected with the work is an authority of the highest standing in his or her line and of the widest practical experience. They are all actively engaged at the present time in their respective lines of work and have endeavored to give to the people just the information they need. They are also of irreproachable character, commanding the highest respect and confidence of the people in their respective communities and throughout the country wherever known.

It is the firm belief of the compilers that this set of books will prove a true guide to efficiency in the lines taken up, a source of very valuable information in every home and an investment which will bring large returns on the capital invested. May they fulfill in a large way the purpose for which they were written.

Sincerely,

THE COMPILERS.

TABLE OF CONTENTS

HEALTH

Pages

How To Keep Well 1-53
  Body Hygiene, Drugs and Drugging, Home Hygiene, Germs and Their
  Carriers, Disinfectants, Special Exercises, How to Prevent Colds, Pneu-
  monia, Tuberculosis and Typhoid, How To Keep The Baby Well, "Who
  Am I," "Safety First," "Don'ts," "Get The Habit."

General Nursing 54-98
  Home Nursing, The Nurse, Provision for the Care of the Sick, Care of
  Sick Room Supplies, Choice and Preparation of the Bed, Care and Treat-
  ment of Patient, Diet, Diets for Special Diseases, Methods of Giving
  Baths and Treatments for Therapeutic or Curative Effects, General
  Treatments, Antiseptics, Mouth Washes, Gargles, Common Laxatives,
  Doses, Puberty, Menopause, Pregnancy and Emergency Care.

Baby Department 99-140
  Instruction to Mothers, Birth Registration, Baby's Room, Bed, Other
  Equipment, Clothing, Baths and Bathing, Certain Cases When Bath
  Should be Omitted, How to Lift the Baby, Care of the Special Organs,
  Feeding, Exercise, Sleep, Bathing, Amusement and Recreation, Tech-
  nique of Nursing, Regularity in Nursing, When to Feed, Artificial Feed-
  ing, Milk, How to Feed the Baby, Preparation of the Food, How to Give
  the Baby the Bottle, Normal Feeding, Drinking Water, Infant Stools,
  Development, Teeth, Weaning, Sleep, General Care, Medicines, Habits,
  Training and Discipline, Bad Habits, Punishment, Early Training,
  Vehicles, Caution, Toys, Common Ailments.

Emergency Department 141-188
  Apoplexy, Bandaging, Roller Bandage, Triangular Bandage, Bites,
  Bruises, Bullet Wounds, Burns, Choking, Collapse, Compress, Com-
  pression of the Brain, Concussion of the Brain, Convulsions, Cramps,
  Cuts and Lacerations, Cold Compresses, Death, Dislocations, Drowning,
  Drugs, and Poisons, Electrical Burns, Electrical Injuries, Epilepsy,
  Fainting, Fire, Fish Bones in the Throat, Fish Hooks, Fits, Foreign
  Bodies in the Throat, Ear, Eye and Nose, Fractures, Freezing, Gas
  Poisoning, Gunshot Wounds, Heat Exhaustion, Hemorrhage, Hysteria,
  Shock, Snake Bites, Splinters, Splints, Sunstroke, Tourniquets, Wounds.

Nursing and First Aid Treatment of Special Diseases 189-271
  Abscess, Adenoids, Appendicitis, Asthma, Biliousness, Inflammation of
  the Bladder, Boils, Brights Disease, Bronchitis, Bunions, Cancer, Car-
  buncles, Catarrh, Chapping, Chicken Pox, Chilblains and Frost Bites,
  Colds, Colic, Conjunctivitis, Constipation, Corns, Croup—Spasmodic,
  Diabetes, Diarrhea, Diphtheria, Dysentery, Earache, Eczema, Erysipelas,
  Eyes—Weak or Diseased, Feet, Felons, Gallstones, Gangrene, Goitre,
  Gout, Grippe, Granular Eyelids, Hay Fever, Headaches, Hernia, Hives,
  Hydrophobia, Indigestion or Dyspepsia, Infantile Paralysis, Inflamma-
  tion of Large Intestine, Inflammation of Small Intestine, Inflammation
  of Stomach, Ingrown Toe Nails, Insomnia, Itch, Ivy Poison, Jaundice,
  Kidneys—Congestion of, Lice, Malaria Fever, Measles, Measles—Ger-

TABLE OF CONTENTS

Pages

man, Mumps, Neuralgia, Peritonitis—Acute, Piles, Pimples and Blackheads, Pleurisy, Pneumonia, Ptomaine Poisoning, Rheumatism, Ringworm, Scarlet Fever, Septicemia, Smallpox, Sore Mouth, Sore Throat,
Coughs and Hoarseness, Stye, Suppression of the Urine, Tetanus,
Tonsils—Enlarged, Tonsilitis, Toothache, Tuberculosis, Tumors, Typhoid, Ulcers, Varicose Veins, Warts, Wens, Whooping Cough, Worms.

FOR YOUNG MEN 272-273

PRESCRIPTION DEPARTMENT 274-291
Cautions, How to Reckon a Child's Dose, Way to Take Oils, Liniments,
Ointments and Salves, Plasters and Poultices, Patent Prescriptions.

BEAUTY HINTS 292-299
Hands, Feet, Face, Hair, Scalp.

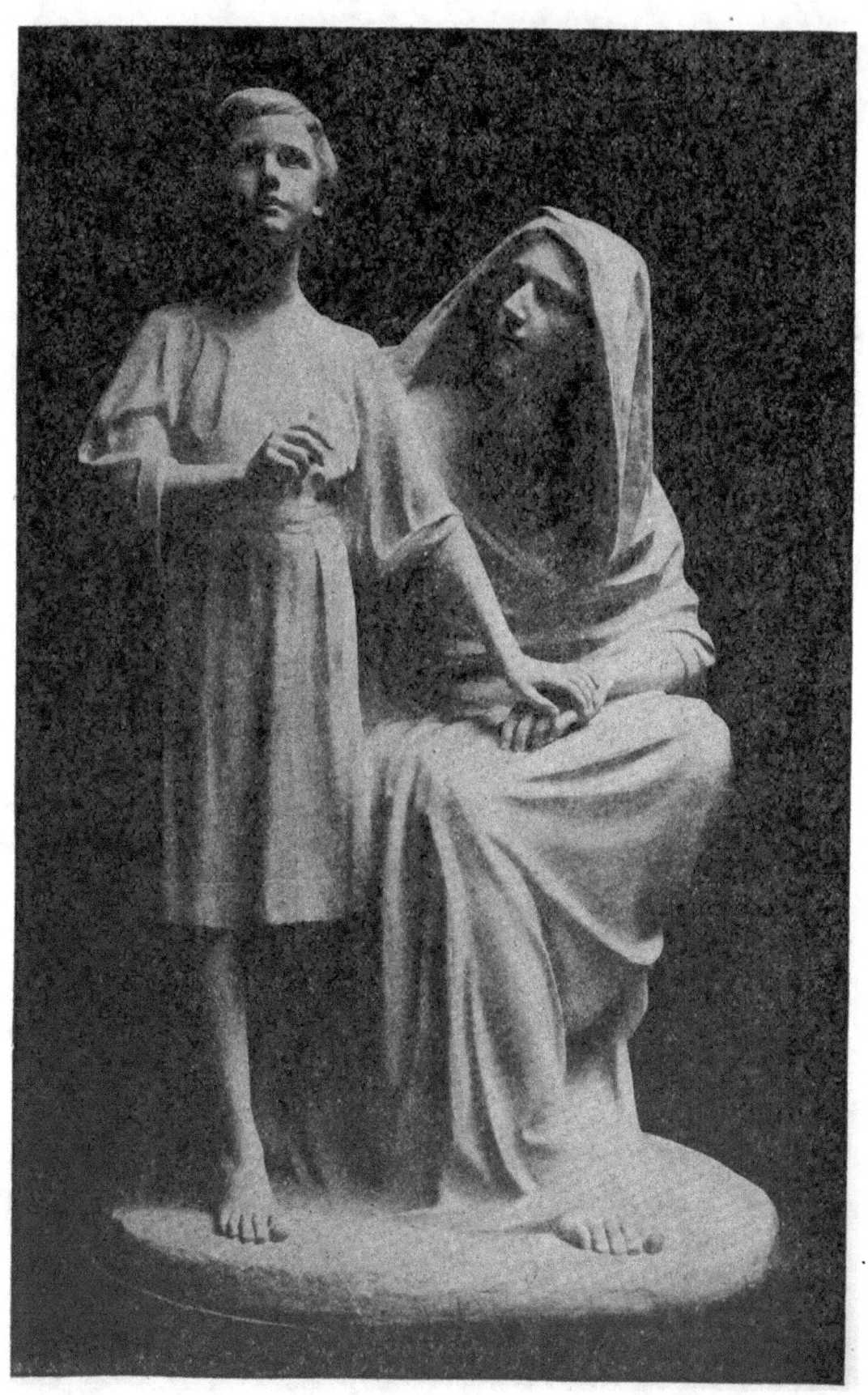

HOW TO KEEP WELL.

Body Hygiene—Home Hygiene—Prevention of Disease.

Introduction.—The great idea of human welfare societies, the science and art of hygiene and of the future medical profession, is and will be, not only to cure the sick and nurse them back to health, but to develop strong healthy bodies, to increase the power, vitality and endurance of the human body. To make it immune to disease. To develop in it a vital surplus which has been called "the balance in the savings bank of life". The future doctor will be employed to keep us well and strong and be paid for the time he keeps us so and not for the time it takes him to bring us back to health after we are sick. Dr. Woods Hutchinson, one of the world's foremost writers on medical subjects, says: "A feature of special interest and importance to the public stands out in the proposed scheme of the new National Medical School. It is that particular, if not chief, attention is to be paid to and the broadest and fullest facilities furnished for, the training and equipment of the new doctor, the real doctor, the preventer rather than the curer, the builder-up instead of the patcher up, the sanitarian, the school hygienist, the health officer. This is in line with the best and broadest thought of the medical profession today. Preventive medicine is unmistakably the medicine of the future. The public is rapidly and increasingly coming to demand the preventer instead of the curer, and we hope the former will one day catch up with the latter and largely put him out of business." The old saying "an ounce of prevention is worth a pound of cure" is an idea that is taking possession of the minds of the people and should be one of the ruling principles in our lives. Below we give a few of the simple laws of health and rules of hygiene which should be followed. If these are practiced day after day until they become habit and a part of our life, we will soon have a keen sense of enjoyment in all of life's activities. Simply to live, breathe and move, will be a delight.

BODY HYGIENE.

Value of Oxygen.—This is one of the main elements of air and the very basis of life. The vital importance of this element to the health and life of the individual is demonstrated by the fact that if the supply of air is cut off, one dies in a few minutes. Important as is the quantity and quality of food and drink, one can live for days without either, but only for a few minutes without oxygen. It purifies the blood in the lungs, gives the body warmth and energy, makes it possible for the food we eat to be transformed into bone, muscle and tissue. It is said that diseases of the lungs are the cause of four-fifths of all indispositions, ill health and actual diseases among all civilized

1

people. Good development of the chest and lungs and thorough systematic ventilation of the lungs, are essential to a strong heart, a vigorous circulation and power of the tissues to resist disease. One-third of the whole volume of the blood is always circulating in the lungs and each particle passes through them 8,000 times per day. It is there that it unloads the poisonous waste matter which it has gathered up through the body and gets the required amount of oxygen. If by superficial and improper breathing, the needed amount of oxygen is not there, the blood must return to the tissues carrying part of the poisonous waste matter with it, instead of the much-needed supply of oxygen. The healthy strong body must throw off these impurities of the blood and have a bountiful supply of the life-giving oxygen.

Very few people realize that they don't know how to breathe, and that if they did, they would live longer and better. They would add many years to their life and get more joy out of living. If it were not that our breathing is involuntary, we would die. Few know the value of practicing that deep, forceful, dynamic breathing which brings into action all the vital organs of the body. They do not know the peace and force resulting from such breathing. Every such inhalation means added youth, and the exhalation carries old age with it. We must have the life-giving oxygen spoken of above as it is the fuel that keeps up the steam in the body machine and which burns up the waste matter.

When you arise in the morning, forcefully expel the used air from the lungs. Drive out every particle it is possible to expel. Contract the muscles of the abdomen so as to drive it out of the lower part of the lungs. When you have done this, stand before the open window or go into the open air and slowly fill the lungs full of fresh air. When they feel full, stop inhaling and expand the muscles of the abdomen so as to allow the lower part of the lungs to fill, now forcefully expel the air and refill the lungs. Repeat this at least five or six times, filling the lungs fuller each time if possible, till you feel as though the veins and arteries would burst. Next, hold your breath 10 or 12 seconds, then forcefully expel the air. If this exercise is repeated each morning before beginning the day's work and each night before retiring, it will soon add health and vigor to the body and mind, making the life more efficient.

Ventilation.—Because of the great importance of fresh air to the human system, ventilation becomes one of the first and most important rules of hygiene. The ventilating system of the home is of prime importance to the health of the family. Again, it makes no difference how perfect the ventilating system is, unless it is used, the family will not be benefited thereby.

There should be a good source from which to draw an abundance of fresh air. The air should be kept in motion and should not be too warm. These are the prime requisites of proper ventilation.

In the average home, the best ventilation is to be had through the windows. They should always be kept open in the summer and very often in the winter. Where it is possible, the windows should be opened at opposite sides of the room, so that the air may be kept in motion. If this is not possible, somewhat of the same result may be obtained by opening the window at the top and also at the bottom. The foul air escapes at the top and the fresh air enters at the bottom. A window board may be used which will deflect the cold air upwards so that it will not flow right to the floor and make the feet cold. This can be done by fitting a board, five or six inches wide and as long as the window is wide, so that it rests on the window-sill and is tight in the frame at either side. The open grate fire is also a good means of ventilation.

The temperature of the living room, should never be above 70 degrees F., and for the healthy vigorous body 65 degrees F., is better. People do not catch cold by being in the cold air, but by going from ill-ventilated, stuffy, overheated rooms into the cool fresh air.

The air of the house should not be allowed to become vitiated by poisonous gases from coal stoves or by lighting and heating with gas, neither from tobacco smoke or germ-laden dust. Keep the air of the living-room pure and fresh.

The sleeping-room should be thoroughly ventilated as two-thirds of the oxygen absorbed by the body during the twenty-four hours is absorbed between six o'clock in the evening and six o'clock in the morning. Therefore the vitality of the individual depends largely on the air of the bedroom. The air should be perfectly fresh on retiring. The temperature of the room should not be above sixty dgrees F. The windows should be wide open. In the coldest part of the winter and in stormy weather a screen can be made by stretching some porous cloth such as cheese-cloth over a frame which fits the window space and placing this in the window so as to prevent too much of a draft on the sleeper.

It has been found by those who have slept out-of-doors, that the best ventilated sleeping room is much inferior to the sleeping porch or the open tent. This idea has long been recommended to the person with weak lungs or one suffering from tuberculosis, however, since the nursing and medical profession have come to realize the great value of fresh air to the vigorous, strong body, it is highly recommended to persons of all classes, by the best authorities, for infants and children as well as adults. Of course in severe cold weather there must be a good heavy mattress, plenty of covers and the head may be protected by a hood which comes well down around the neck. Out door sleeping is far easier than most people suppose and greatly increases the power of the body to resist cold and disease, and greatly promotes the vigor, vitality and endurance. On retiring at night, every particle of clothing worn during the day should be removed and thrown over a chair to air. The bed clothes should also be thoroughly aired every day.

Cultivate the fresh air habit; walk in it, sleep in it, work in it, live in it, and when you ride, ride this hobby; it is cheaper than a jitney and has no tire troubles. It will put bloom in your cheek, fire in your eye, and sharpen your wits; it will put spring in your step, laughter in your heart and money in your pocket. Be known as a fresh air crank and turn your crankiness to good purpose.

Light and Sunshine.—Live out of doors as much as possible. Sunlit air is best. Light and sunshine are absolutely necessary for a healthy body. This is proven by the fact that a plant placed in a dark place will become pale and sickly. It is the same with people. It is hard to explain just how the sun influences health, but it is a well known fact that it does. Many of the disease germs will not live long in the sunlight, as it is a great disinfectant and purifier. Every hospital has its sun-room and every house should have one. Open up the windows, take down the heavy blinds and draperies, let the sunshine in. Children, like young plants, need much sunshine. They should also take their recreation and exercise in the open air. The air in the best of homes is far inferior to that out of doors. Do not be afraid of damp, foggy air as even this as a rule is far better than that found in the most of houses. The evils of damp, foggy air are greatly exaggerated.

Exercise and Recreation.—Even though one is doing physical work in the open, it is not always that all the muscles of the body receive proper exercise. In order to have a well developed, healthy body every muscle must have the proper regular exercise. The part that does not receive it will become weak and subject to disease and decay. The part of the body which is weak and undeveloped can be made strong and healthy just through giving it the proper exercise. Nothing can take the place of out door or physical exercise. It is the automatic regulation of digestion, respiration and circulation. Especially should those who work much indoors have at least one hour a day of vigorous exercise in the open.

Learn to swim. It is the one perfect exercise in the world for developing all the muscles of the body. It produces symmetry as well as perfection.

Sleep and Rest.—The bed is the most important piece of furniture in the house. It should be plenty large; it should have a thick, hard, sanitary, smooth mattress, good springs, coverlets long enough to tuck in well at the bottom and a thin pillow. A loose porous night garment should also be worn. There should be plenty of fresh air as before suggested. The great principle is to keep the feet warm and the head cool, as good sound sleep is proportional to the departure of the blood from the head. One's best sleep is with the stomach empty. A full stomach will divert the blood from the head, but disturbs the sleep later. Water and fruit may be taken without injury before going to bed. Good natural sleep is one of the greatest means to health and the health-seeker should avail himself of it to the full. Adults should have at least eight hours of sleep out of every twenty-four. Children need much more. Good sleep depends to quite an extent on the state of the mind before going to bed. Forget your work, don't worry, think pleasant thoughts, get in a restful state of mind, absolutely relax. Begin at the great toe and relax every muscle before going to sleep. Don't try to hold the bed up. Imagine you weigh a ton. Learn to "let go." Learn to rest as well as to exercise. While we sleep nature restores and rebuilds the body, therefore, in order to have strong, healthy bodies we must have deep, full, restful sleep.

Care of Skin.—The skin is one of the most important parts of the whole body. It has three distinct functions; it is the organ of the sense of touch, an organ of excretion and an organ of heat regulation. Therefore, to have good health we must keep the skin in the "pink of condition." As the organ of the sense of touch, the little nerve endings in the skin stand guarding the body from external harm.

As an organ of excretion its importance is shown by the fact that there are about two pints of perspiration produced daily. In this way there is a great deal of oily, poisonous waste matter thrown out on the skin every day. It throws off double the amount of moisture that is thrown off through the lungs. It is one of the most important aids to the kidneys and the fact that the perspiration and urine are to a certain extent alike, has been proven. In the course of a day the skin, especially those parts which are covered, become infested with impurities which when allowed to remain become thicker every day and may produce injurious effects by obstructing the excretory openings and affording lodging for disease germs. This will not only be injurious to the skin itself but to the entire system.

Every action of the body produces heat. When we work hard or exercise, we get "warmed up." A certain amount of this heat is necessary to our bodily health, too much is dangerous. The blood carries this internal heat to the surface and through the wonderful network of blood vessels in the skin it is radiated from the body. In this way the surplus heat is thrown off. When we exercise much in the hot sun, the body becomes so hot that we would soon be overcome by the heat, if it were not for this heat radiation through the skin. When we feel cold just the opposite action takes place. The little blood vessels contract and drive the warm blood as much as possible to the deeper parts of the body, thus preventing the loss of heat. In this way the skin as a heat regulator keeps the body most of the time at an even temperature.

Because of the great importance of the skin as shown by the functions mentioned above it must be kept clean and in a healthy condition. Every adult, man or woman, should have at least two or three warm cleansing baths every week. Children may be bathed more frequently with good results. In addition to the cleansing baths, tonic baths such as cold water baths, saline or salt water baths, alkaline or soda water baths, are very beneficial. By means of these tonic baths the network of blood vessels in the skin is kept toned up, invigorated, elastic and full of red blood. They are also invigorating to the nervous system and beneficial to the body as a whole. One of these tonic baths as described below, may be taken every morning.

Cleansing Bath.—The purpose of the cleansing bath is to clean the skin. The water should be about 90 degrees F. or slightly below the temperature of the body. Good soap should be used and the body scrubbed. A person should not stay in the water longer than 15 or 20 minutes and the bath is best taken just before retiring. No bath should be taken less than an hour before or after meals.

Cold Bath.—This bath should be taken on arising in the morning while the body is warm. It should not be taken when the body, or any part of it, is cold. Neither should it be taken during the menstrual period or by people of very weak constitutions. The water should be about 60 degrees F. and the duration of the bath from a few seconds to two minutes. It should be followed by brisk rubbing with a coarse towel until the skin is red and the body tingling all over. The strong full-blooded person will find the daily cold plunge very invigorating. It will also strengthen the body to resist colds.

Salt or Saline Bath.—Dissolve a teacupful of salt in half a tub of water at 70 degrees F. Rub the body vigorously during and after the bath. This will be found very refreshing and excellent for the skin.

Soda or Alkaline Bath.—This bath is generally used to allay an itching or burning condition of the skin. Use two tablespoonfuls of baking soda to each gallon of water. More soda may be used if desired, however, as it requires so much soda to the amount of water used, it is better to use little water and sponge the body all over.

Hot Bath.—The hot bath is used to induce free perspiration and thus open up the pores of the skin. A cold can often be broken up if the hot bath is used early. The temperature of the water should be about 99 or 100 degrees F. and the duration of the bath should be very short as it is very weakening.

The skin must have breathing space, especially at night when relaxed. All cosmetics, pore plugging powders and rouges should be removed. The clothing should be light and loose so as to allow free circulation of air. Water drinking is one of the best means of improving a bad skin and keeping it in good condition. Every one should drink several glasses of water before breakfast and also before retiring as well as much during the day. This encourages perspiration, cleaning out the pores of the skin and inducing free skin breathing. Cleanliness inside and out.

Care of Scalp.—In order for the hair to grow and be healthy, the scalp must be as well taken care of as any other part of the skin. Although the scalp does not perspire as much as the rest of the body, there is an oily waste matter thrown off and the surface of the skin scales off as does the rest of the body. If this accumulation of tiny scales and oily matter is not properly removed by brushing and shampooing, an itchy condition of the scalp results known as dandruff. If short hair is shampooed at least once a week and long hair at least once or twice a month, the scalp being kept thoroughly clean and in a healthy condition, most of the dangers of dandruff and other infections will be avoided. The scalp should also be massaged well every day with the tips of the fingers and the hair brushed well night and morning with a good bristle brush. The wire hair brush should not be used neither should the scalp be scratched by the finger nails as this is liable to cause serious irritation and scalp trouble. Men and boys may wet their hair with cold water as often as they wish providing it is rubbed dry. It should not be wet and smoothed down as the moisture sets up a sort of fermentation in the natural oil of the scalp and gives it a sour odor. Keep the scalp healthy and clean if you want nice hair. There is no drug known to medicine which will cause hair to grow or make it thicker or curlier. All hair tonics claiming to do this are frauds. The scalp should be massaged often with the fingers wet in a strong solution of common table salt and water. Men can do this every morning with excellent results. The hair should always be rubbed dry afterwards. This will keep the scalp in a good healthy condition and thus promote the growth of the hair.

Care of the Eyes.—The eye, being the organ of the sense of sight, most important of the five senses, should be well cared for. This care should begin the minute the child is born as it is claimed on good authority that one-sixth of all blindness is caused by a little germ which gets into the baby's eye at birth. This first cleansing, however, should be done by the physician or nurse attending the case. The eyes also often become diseased by getting infectious germs in them from dust or by touching them with dirty fingers. Styes are known to be nothing more or less than little boils on the eyelids, and it is now known that boils are due to external infection. We therefore know that styes are due largely to rubbing the eyes with dirty fingers and to germ-laden dust. Children should not be allowed to rub their eyes to any extent but should be taught how to care for them in a sanitary way. Styes are also caused by a weakened condition of the eyes due to eye strain. Such diseases as measles, smallpox, tuberculosis or rheumatism often affect the eyes, leaving them weak or diseased. By preventing these diseases we will greatly lessen the amount of blindness. However, the eyes should have special care at such times and these serious after effects guarded against.

Eye strain, often due to defects in the structure of the eyes, poor illumination or over-work, is the cause of many reflex evils such as headaches, nausea, dizziness, etc., which are sometimes ascribed to entirely different causes. If these symptoms appear it is well to have the eyes examined by a reliable eye doctor in order to determine if eye strain is the cause, and if so, remedy the defect by carefully fitted glasses. Great care should also be taken not to read in too bright a light, as the glare of the sun, or in waning light. Neither should one read on moving trains or during constant motion as this is extremely hard on the eyes. The indirect effects of the eye strain are far more serious than most people think and should be remedied just as soon as detected.

Care of Ears.—The ear, the organ of hearing, is very delicately formed, consisting of three parts, the external, middle and internal ears. It is closely connected with the brain and so delicate that unwise, rough handling of the external ear often seriously injures the hearing. The ear needs very little care during health. In fact more harm is done by too much care than not enough. Nature has provided the ear with little glands which secrete the ear wax which carries out all dust and dirt entering the ear. Of course if large foreign bodies get into the ear such as a bean, button, stone or insect it should be removed, but this should be done by a physician. It is an exceedingly dangerous habit for mothers to use a hair pin, tooth pick, or anything of that sort to clean the child's ear. It is pretty good policy to follow the German saying "Pick the ear with nothing smaller than the elbow." During infectious diseases, especially those that affect the throat, the ear should be carefully looked after as they often affect the ears and frequently bring on deafness.

The ear should never be slapped or allowed to be pulled as such treatment is liable to cause inflammation of the middle ear. It is also a dangerous policy in cases of colds or catarrh to snuff fluids up the nose as they often cause inflammation of the little tube leading from the mouth to the ear, called the eustachian tube. Because of its importance and delicate nature, the ear should be handled with the greatest care.

Care of Nose.—The nose performs the following important functions: it serves as a passageway for the air in breathing; warms, moistens, and filters the inspired air; it is the organ of the sense of smell; it aids in phonation; it affords ventilation for the ears. By far the most important function is in respiration. It prepares the air for the lungs by heating it, moistening it and cleaning it of the little particles of dust and dirt. The passages are lined with a soft moist skin or mucous membrane which is covered with tiny little hairs. The purpose of these is to catch the dust, dirt and disease germs and keep them from going into the lungs. When we breathe much hot, stuffy, foul air containing dust and disease germs this mucous membrane of the nose becomes inflamed and we say we "catch cold". Catarrh is the result of a succession of neglected colds. Mouth breathing is the result of allowing the passages of the nose to become obstructed by adenoids, dirt, etc., then all the dirt and disease germs which would otherwise be taken out of the air go directly into the tender air passages of the lungs and cause very serious trouble. Mouth breathing often causes sore throat or serious throat trouble and it is said that a great amount of deafness comes from diseases of the throat. The proper treatment of deafness is prevention. Neglect of nose and throat troubles in early life causes much deafness in middle life. The presence of adenoids can be detected from the way a child breathes and a physician should be consulted at once. Keep the passages of the nose free from obstruction and in a good healthy condition as by so doing you add greatly to the general health of the body.

Tonsils and Adenoids.—Enlarged tonsils and adenoids have such a marked effect upon the health of a child that the parents should know how to detect their presence and what to do in case their child has them.

The tonsils are little glands, one of which can be seen on either side of the throat. They can be seen by having the child open its mouth wide and by pressing the tongue down with the handle of a spoon. They can very easily be seen if they are enlarged. Adenoids are little growths which appear in the back part of the throat where the nose and the throat join. They are like little white heads of cauliflower which hang down in such a way as to stop up the back part of nose so that the child cannot breathe through it. This causes the child to breathe through the mouth, which is one of the most important symptoms of enlarged tonsils and adenoids. If a child takes cold easily, has sore throat often, complains of earache, has red eyes and sore nose; if it breathes through the mouth, sleeps with the mouth open, snores, appears dull, snuffles a great deal, it undoubtedly has adenoids and enlarged tonsils. The child most always stands with the mouth open and the upper lip and jaw extended over the lower.

If these symptoms appear, take your child to a good physician and have him carefully examined. The adenoids should be removed at once, and if the tonsils are in bad condition they should also be removed. They may affect the child very seriously in a short time. Mouth breathing is a serious matter as it allows dust and disease germs to be taken directly into the throat and lungs which otherwise would be taken out of the air in passing through the nose. A child with adenoids and diseased tonsils has a much greater chance of getting such diseases as diphtheria, measles, scarlet fever and whooping cough. They also predispose the child to rheumatism and heart disease. Bad teeth, diseased tonsils and adenoids are good places for the development of disease germs, which, with their very dangerous poisons, are carried directly into the stomach, bowels and lungs. They also disfigure the face and hinder the growth of the body.

They should be detected as early as possible and removed at once by a good surgeon. The operation is not a serious one and may be performed at any time of the year or age of the child. Do not neglect this matter as it is very serious. Every father and mother who have the best interests of their child at heart, will not neglect these deformities which can so easily be removed and which so seriously affect the health of their child. Give the child the best start in life possible. The child's entire future may depend upon this little thing.

Mouth and Teeth.—The proper care of the mouth and teeth are of utmost importance to the health of the body. In the first place if there is faulty development or if there are any irregularities of the teeth, if the upper and lower

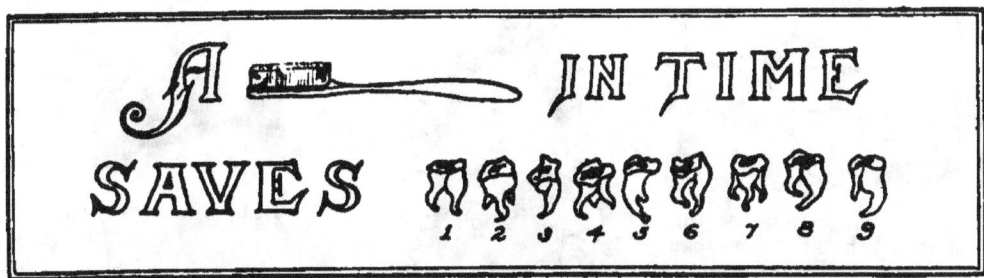

teeth do not fit well together, they should be carefully examined by both a dentist and a doctor. These deformities which interfere with the proper mastication of food can often be corrected if taken in time. Even an adult may have crooked teeth straightened. Often the whole appearance of the face can be changed, and the health greatly improved. It is well to begin with the child as early as possible. The earlier it is done the easier it will be to straighten the teeth. In the next place the teeth, gums and jaws must have the proper exercise as well as the other parts of the body. As soon as a child has all of its first teeth it should be given the proper foods and taught how to chew them. Soft pasty foods which may be swallowed with little chewing do not give the exercise the teeth need to make them strong and healthy. The child as well as the adult should have plenty of hard crusty foods, foods which require a great deal of chewing. In the chewing of hard food the teeth act as a force pump. Pressure drives the blood out. Release of pressure permits blood and lymph vessels to fill. This will give the gums, teeth and jaws good exercise, arousing the circulation and causing healthy conditions.

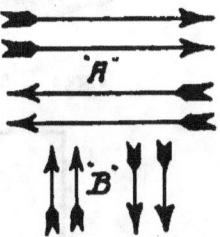

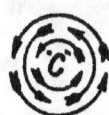

"A"—Usual method of brushing teeth. "B"—Up and down movement. Better method than indicated by A. "C"—Rotary movement. Correct method of brushing teeth.

The teeth should be cleaned night and morning and after each meal. The choice of a brush is important. In early childhood as a rule a small narrow soft bristle brush should be used, the size of the brush and the stiffness of the

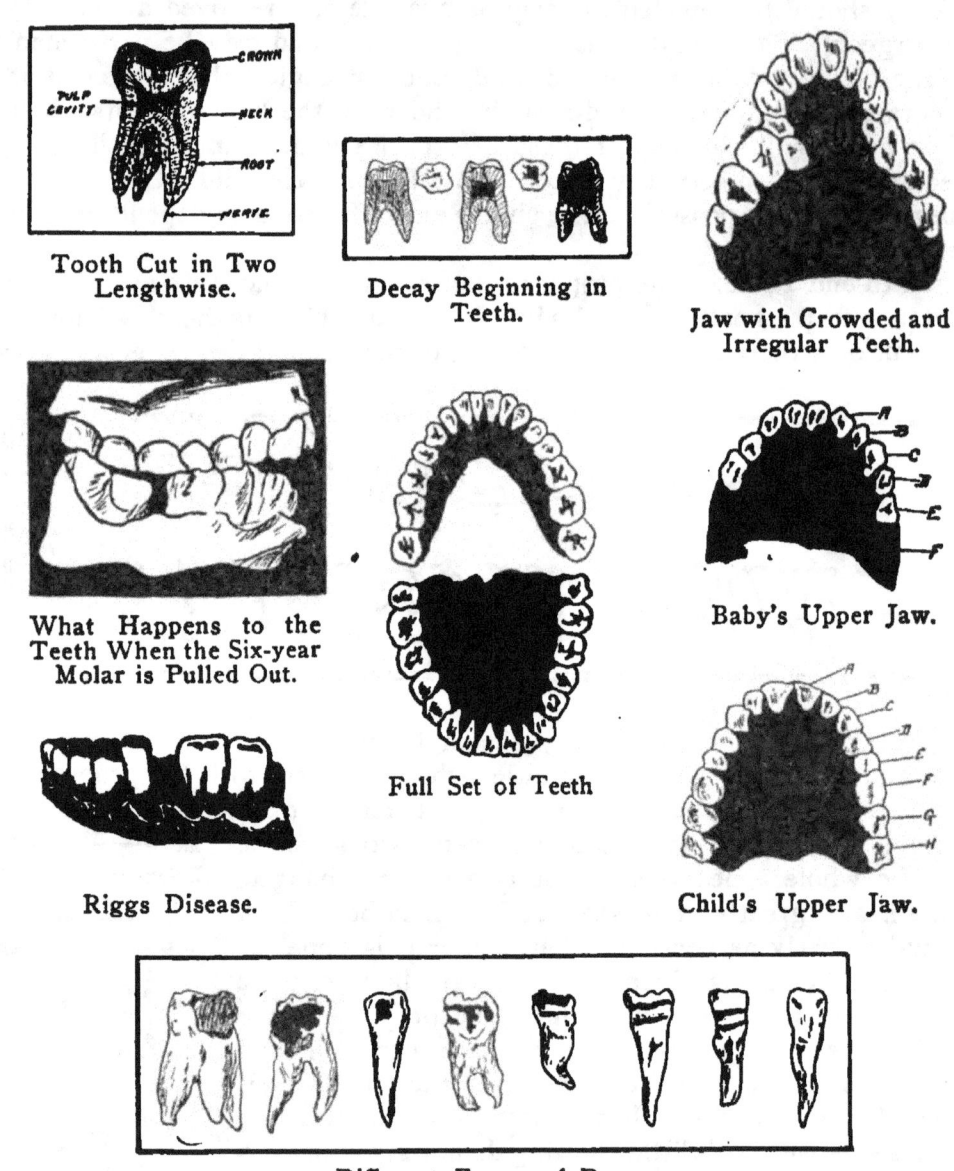

Tooth Cut in Two Lengthwise.

Decay Beginning in Teeth.

Jaw with Crowded and Irregular Teeth.

What Happens to the Teeth When the Six-year Molar is Pulled Out.

Full Set of Teeth

Baby's Upper Jaw.

Child's Upper Jaw.

Riggs Disease.

Different Forms of Decay.

bristles increasing with the age of the patient. The way the teeth should be brushed is indicated by the accompanying figures. In most cases the movement used is indicated by figure A; however the up and down movement indicated by figure B is better, and the rotary movement as shown in figure C obtains by far the best results. The last method cleans the teeth far better than either of the other methods. The bristles of the brush should be placed firmly against the teeth and the rotary or scrubbing movement used. It is also well to have a brush the bristles of which are uneven in length so that the innermost crevices of the teeth may be reached as well as the outer. All surfaces of the teeth should be gone over carefully in this way. Remember a thoroughly clean tooth never decays. A dentist should be consulted once or twice a year. Never lose a tooth if art can save it.

The temporary teeth of children should be solid and enduring in order that they may remain in place until the permanent teeth are ready to come through. Otherwise the permanent teeth may be extremely irregular and deformed. Every time you pull a tooth, you throw more work on the rest. Get a small looking-glass which you can put into the mouth and examine the teeth carefully. Examine the teeth of the children often. If there are any spots coming on them or any cavities, go to the best dentist you can find, have them filled and cleaned at once.

Good teeth are worth more to a child than much gold or many jewels. Take the best of care of them. You may not be able to save much money for your child but you can save its teeth and they are worth more than much money. Good teeth will do much to keep the child in good health, and health is far better than wealth.

Children's teeth are often caused to decay by the diseases of childhood, such as whooping-cough, measles, scarlet fever, etc. Another cause of decay is uncleanliness. There is an acid, formed by the decomposing food particles, which eats away the enamel, thus starting the decay. Another cause is the biting of hard substance such as nuts, thread, etc., which cracks the enamel. All these causes should be carefully avoided.

The accompanying cuts illustrate dental decay, ulceration of the teeth, pyorrhea, etc., the results of improper care. These dreadful conditions result not only in the loss of the teeth, improper mastication of food with its attendant evils, but also in the manufacture of poisons which affect the whole system. Diseased, ill kept teeth are also the breeding place for the germs of the most serious infectious diseases. The average unclean mouth will be found to contain regularly more than thirty different species of germs each numbering its millions. The mouth is the gateway to the body and should be kept in a thoroughly sanitary condition.

Throat.—The membranes of the throat are very tender and many of the infectious diseases affect them seriously. The throat must therefore be well taken care of. The tonsils becoming diseased and enlarged not only hinder breathing through the nose and ventilation of the ears but predispose the owner to tonsilitis and other serious diseases. It is well especially when contagious and infectious diseases are prevalent to spray the throat with some good mild antiseptic solution such as a teaspoonful of baking soda dissolved in a tumbler of water. Much serious trouble can be prevented by keeping the throat free from germs and in a good healthy condition.

Hands.—As the hands are constantly ministering to the wants of the body, coming in contact with the food we eat, etc., it is necessary that they be kept clean, free from dirt and contamination. Under the ends of the nails is a convenient place for disease germs to lodge and as they often come in contact with the parts of the body where delicate membranes are exposed or where the skin is broken, if not kept clean, may cause serious infection.

It has been said that "death lurks under the finger nails." Children should not be allowed to suck their fingers or put them in their mouths as such serious diseases as infantile paralysis may result. Their little hands gather up the deadly germs and plant them on the delicate membranes of the nose and mouth where they multiply with frightful rapidity. The germs do little harm on the outside of the body but will destroy health and threaten life when planted inside. The mother should wash the child's hands often and keep them free from dirt as much as possible. She should always wash her own hands before preparing or handling the child's food.

The condition of the hands is often indicative of the state of health. The fingers covered with hang nails show lowered vitality. Brittle, seamed nails show digestive disorders. A rosy tint on the finger ends indicates health.

Feet.—A pair of healthy, strong feet are most essential to the enjoyment of life. Yet how often we abuse them by wearing the wrong kind of shoes and stockings, by not bathing them as frequently as they should be bathed and by neglecting them in various other ways. Few realize the complex structure of the foot and especially of the arch. It is the arch which receives and transmits the weight of the body to the earth and the health of the foot depends largely on keeping this in good condition.

The palms of the hands and the soles of the feet are the most porous parts of the body. They not only absorb moisture rapidly but also throw off a great deal of waste matter. This is especially true of the feet. If they are not kept clean, this poisonous matter will be reabsorbed and taken back into the system. They should be washed at least once a day, kept warm and dry. Lack of proper care of the feet causes not only a great deal of trouble through injury to the feet themselves, but also affects the rest of the body. Pains and suffering in the feet, such as corns, etc., usually tell quickly on the health, causing lines in the face. Many of the most serious troubles the human system is heir to are caused by cold, wet, unclean feet. They should be bathed often and thoroughly massaged now and then. Proper exercise will strengthen the arches and proper shoes will prevent corns, callouses and much trouble. Don't neglect the feet, take as good care of them as any other part of the body.

Care of Bowels, Constipation.—The body must be freed of waste matter thoroughly and regularly. Constipation if allowed to continue long becomes dangerous to the whole system. This poisonous waste matter left in the body is a common cause not only of headache but also lowers the vitality of the system, making it subject to colds and more serious ailments. Although constipation is often constitutional, it can be greatly remedied by observing rules of diet and exercise. Drink plenty of water when the stomach is empty; a glass or two just before going to bed and before breakfast in the morning is especially beneficial. The food should contain sufficient bulk to promote action of the intestines and also contain the proper amount of laxative elements. Most all fruits, especially figs, prunes, apples, dates, etc., are laxative. Also fresh vegetables and greens of all sorts. Breakfast foods of whole grain cereals, bran, graham bread, etc., also oils and fats. Foods which tend to constipate are white of egg, bread made of fine wheat flour, cornstarch, rice, boiled milk, etc. Buttermilk which contains lactic acid is good for the bowels as it prevents poisoning caused by the decomposition of protein in the intestines. An enema may be taken occasionally but not habitually. Avoid the habitual use of drugs as the more one uses these the more he becomes dependent upon them. They should only be used under medical supervision. Follow strictly the rules of hygiene as to diet, exercise, fresh air and cleanliness. Obey the calls of nature promptly, establish proper habits and you will do much to avoid constipation.

Posture.—Correct posture is of extreme importance to the development of strong, vigorous bodies and to the maintenance of health. Sit, stand and walk erect. Throw the shoulders back and square them evenly, keep the chest high and well arched forward, stomach in, neck straight, chin in and feet well directed forward. By sitting, standing or walking in a stooped-over, slouchy manner the vital organs of the body are crowded and it is impossible for them to function freely. The blood becomes stagnated in the liver and digestive organs, the digestion is impaired, the lungs are crowded and deep, full breathing is impossible. It will also bring on curvature of the spine which will affect the whole nervous system. Don't have the "consumptive stoop" or the walk of the "slouch." "Brace up," it will not only add greatly to the health, strength, vigor and beauty of your body but you will have more self-respect and self-confidence.

Foods.—In order that the body may be strong and healthy, able to resist disease and accomplish its work, it must be well nourished. The mother can do much in this way by the careful, wise selection of food for the family. In the selection of food, three objects must be kept in view, the obtaining of foods which contain the elements necessary to build up the body, furnish it with heat and strength and repair its tissues. To build up the body and repair the worn out tissues, an element known as protein is necessary. This is found in all foods but in large quantities in such foods as meat, milk, fish, eggs and cheese. Also to repair the bones and to keep the body clean we need many different kinds of minerals such as lime, iron and sulphur. These are chiefly obtained from water, fruits and vegetables although such foods as milk and eggs contain valuable minerals also. The best and cheapest foods for the production of heat and energy for the body are such as contain starch, sugar and fat. Starch is supplied chiefly in such foods as cereals, flour, meals, beans, peas, lentils, also such vegetables as potatoes. Sugar is obtained from fruits and such vegetables as beets and carrots, however, most of it taken into the body is in the pure form obtained from the sugar beet and sugar cane. Fats are obtained chiefly from the fat of meats, butter, cream, cheese, oils and nuts A well balanced diet is one which furnishes the body with these elements in the proper amount. It is rather difficult to get these in the proper amount needed for all ages in the daily diet, however, it should contain some high protein foods such as meats, milk, eggs, cheese, etc., for building and repairing; the foods which contain sugar, starch and fats for fuel and energy and the vegetables and fruits which contain the minerals, iron, lime and sulphur. Also plenty of good pure water should be taken each day.

Children should be given foods which contain plenty of the element protein for the growth and building up of the body. Milk and eggs are especially strong in protein and also contain great amounts of minerals for the growth and strengthening of the bones of the child. Even skimmed milk is good. Although it does not contain fats, it contains much protein. Young children should have very little meat. Old people should also eat sparingly of meat and more of fruits.

The diet should also consist of plenty of hard, bulky and uncooked foods, such as crusts of bread, toast, hard biscuits, hard fruits, fibrous vegetables, nuts, etc. These are an important feature of the hygienic diet. Hard foods require a lot of mastication which promotes the flow of saliva, develops healthy teeth and is generally beneficial. As a rule our foods are too concentrated and do not contain the bulk which promotes good digestion and action of the bowels. The food should contain so much "woody fiber" which is obtained from fruits, and such vegetables as lettuce, celery, spinach, asparagus, cabbage, cauliflower, corn, beets, onions, parsnips, squash, pumpkins, tomatoes, cucumbers, berries, etc. There is also a little element in foods called vitamins which is destroyed by cooking and which is very important for the health and strength of the body. This being the case some foods should be eaten uncooked, such as fruits, nuts, lettuce, tomatoes, celery, etc. That is, those foods which can be eaten as well uncooked as cooked should be eaten that way. This element vitamin is also destroyed in eggs and milk by cooking, so they are more nourishing eaten raw. However, all vegetables eaten raw should be carefully disinfected as many dangerous disease germs are taken into the body on raw foods. This can be done by immersing them in a 5 percent solution of peroxide of hydrogen for about five minutes.

Take plenty of time to eat, in order that the food may be thoroughly chewed. There are a great many evils which follow the improper mastication of food. In the first place the teeth do not get the exercise which they need to make them healthy. The food is not thoroughly chewed and that causes it to remain in the stomach longer than necessary to digest. It is not well mixed with saliva causing imperfect digestion of starchy materials. It should be masticated up to the point of involuntary swallowing, but should not be held in the mouth so long that it becomes tasteless. Don't get into the habit of bolting your food, take time to eat, taste and enjoy what you eat as this will stimulate the flow of the digestive fluids of the stomach which acting on the thoroughly masticated foods will assure proper digestion. All foods in the fluid form should be sipped and not swallowed rapidly as in drinking water. Sugar in the concentrated form and candy should not be eaten between meals. The best time to eat candy is right after meals, and then it should be eaten sparingly by those who do not exercise much. Plenty of good pure water may be taken at meal time and it is well to drink plenty between meals also.

Do not eat when not hungry even if you miss a meal. Be guided by the natural taste and appetite as to when you eat and as to what and how much you eat. It is not well to eat more than enough to satisfy the natural appetite. When the appetite is in doubt it is better to eat less rather than too much.

Clothing.—It is also important to wear the right kind of clothing. The skin has been called the third lung, therefore good air concerns the skin nearly , as much as the lungs. The clothing should not be too tight, moderately warm and clean. Not only should the underclothing be loose and porous but the outer clothing should not be worn too tight nor composed of too closely woven fabrics. As a rule most garments are of such material as to prevent proper ventilation of the body. A person should not wear more clothing than is necessary to procure proper warmth. The clothing should be suited to the weather conditions and heavy furs only worn in the most severe cold weather. The body should be evenly clothed for if one part is bundled up and another part exposed, an uneven circulation of the blood will result which is detrimental to the system. Cotton or linen is far the best for underclothing as they not only take up moisture of the body quickly but also give it off rapidly. Woolens may be worn as outer garments but are not so good for underclothing. Although they are warm and take up the moisture quickly, they do not give it off rapidly enough and hence retain perspiration and moisture too long, which is detrimental to the skin. The feet should be well clothed, kept warm and dry as the condition of the feet has a great effect on the rest of the body. One who has learned to clothe himself properly will not be much affected by the changes in temperature.

DRUGS AND DRUGGING.

The harm done the system by the use of drugs cannot be overestimated. This is often begun early in life by the mother giving the babe soothing syrups, which, as a rule contain such drugs as opium and morphine. The practice is continued by the use of much advertised patent medicines which are claimed to be cures for most every disease the human body is heir to. No strong medicine or drug of any kind should be given to a child under any consideration if it can at all be avoided. They not only do irreparable damage to the delicate digestive organs, but also frequently destroy the teeth. Many of these medicines contain the habit forming drugs—cocaine, morphine, opium, caffeine, nicotine, alcohol, etc., and depend largely for their sale on the evil effects of these substances. Those who hope to have good health and to attain a high degree of physical and mental efficiency will do well to abstain wholly from the use of these. At least they should only be taken when given by a physician and discontinued as soon as possible. It has been proven by thorough experiments and on good authority that the long continued use of very minute doses of poison will ultimately do much harm. Some headache cures are two-thirds poison. What may stop the headache, may stop the heart too.

Alcohol.—Alcohol taken into the system in the form of beer, ale and all intoxicating beverages is not a food but a poison. Health authorities nowhere advocate it as a medicine, food or beverage. That its influence upon the human body is in no way beneficial, but extremely detrimental is shown by statistics taken from the records of forty-three of the largest life insurance companies, demonstrated by experiments performed by the world's leading scientists, and also proven by the experience of the most noted doctors and surgeons. Records of the insurance companies show that the death rate among men who might be classed as moderate drinkers, not taking more than a glass of whiskey or two glasses of beer per day, is 18 percent higher than the average. That the death rate among men who had drank to excess in the past, but who were accepted as standard risks was 50 percent higher than the average, and that the death rate among men who drank more than a glass of whiskey or two glasses of beer per day, but who were accepted as insurance risks, was over 80 percent higher than the average.

Reliable as are these statistics given above, they need not be accepted on their own strength. Laboratory experiments show that alcohol stimulates the heart, causing it to beat much more rapidly, but does not increase the blood pressure. It thus gives the user a sense of increased strength at the time of using, but leaves him weaker afterwards. It paralyzes the white corpuscles, and also reduces the resistance of the red corpuscles of the blood, thus leaving the body less able to resist disease. This last statement is proven by the fact that users of alcohol are more susceptible to colds, pneumonia, Bright's disease, typhoid fever, etc. It also seriously impairs the vision and produces a neuritis, which is sometimes called rheumatism. Every school child studying physiology is taught **the effects** of this poison on the stomach, kidneys, liver and other organs of the body. And yet, we have said nothing of the accidents, crimes, poverty and misery directly attributed to this great poison. It not only destroys the physical man, but lowers intellectual power, impairs memory, weakens judgment and reason, thus lowering man's efficiency in general. The evidence above given is unimpeachable, and the man who uses alcohol in any of its forms is bound to lose in life's battle physically, mentally and morally.

Tobacco.—Tobacco is also injurious to the body, although its effects are not as well understood as those of alcohol. That it lessens physical fitness is the experience of every athletic trainer. It has been found to have a depressing effect on the central nervous system, thus lessening the power of the voluntary muscles. It produces hardening of the large arteries, increases the action of the heart, causes heart palpitation, pain in the region of the heart, shortness of breath and many other serious effects. Few know that tobacco contains so much deadly poison. It is the drug nicotine that does the great harm. Two drops of this on the tongue of a dog will prove fatal. One drop on the skin of a rabbit will cause death. There is often enough nicotine in one ordinary cigar to kill two men if taken directly into the system. It has never been known to have a beneficial effect on the body.

HOME HYGIENE.

"Happy is the man who is the owner of a healthful house in healthful surroundings." The dwelling house should not be built on low lands, near swamps, marshes, stagnant ponds, or polluted creeks as these localities are very apt to be damp, chilly and breed malarious fevers. Good, high, dry ground is best for the

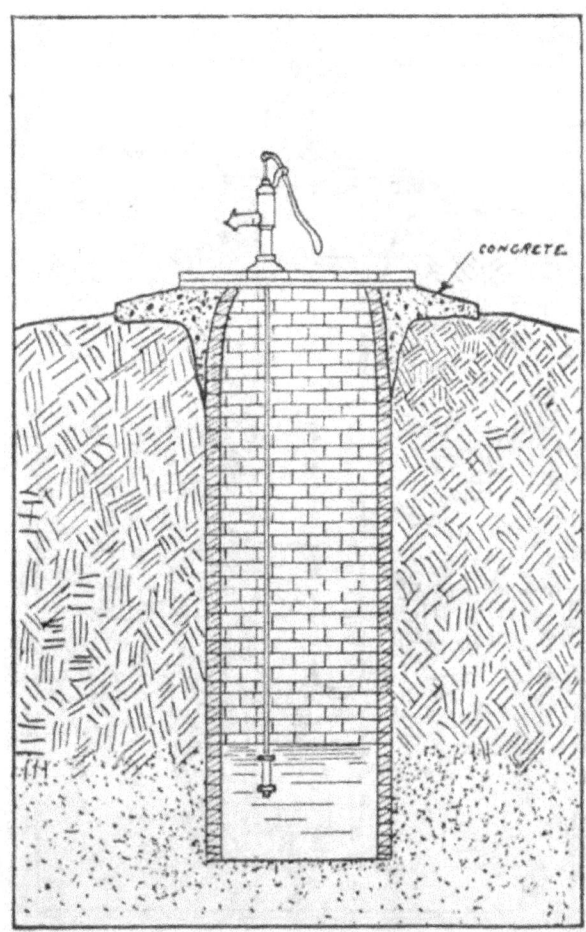

A Model Well, cased with brick laid in cement mortar, and properly graded, curbed, and protected.

building site. There should not be too much heavy shrubbery or too many trees about the house, as, although they are good for shade in hot weather and protection against severe winds, they prevent sufficient sunlight, deprive the house of proper currents of air, and promote dampness of the walls and cellar. The location should be so selected as to receive direct sunlight and pure outside air from all four sides. It should stand free and detached from other buildings. Do not build on "made" land as low ground is generally filled in with garbage, rubbish and decaying animal and vegetable debris, which are often the causes of impure air in the house. Good virgin soil is much preferred to such lots or to old torn down building sites. Lots which are honeycombed with broken drains, privy holes, or receive the soakage from barnyards, stables, or the surface drainage from adjoining lots are not desirable. Also the home cannot be sanitary which is located too near railroad yards, tannery, soap works, or such factories.

The Cellar.—The cellar of the dwelling house, in order to be sanitary, must

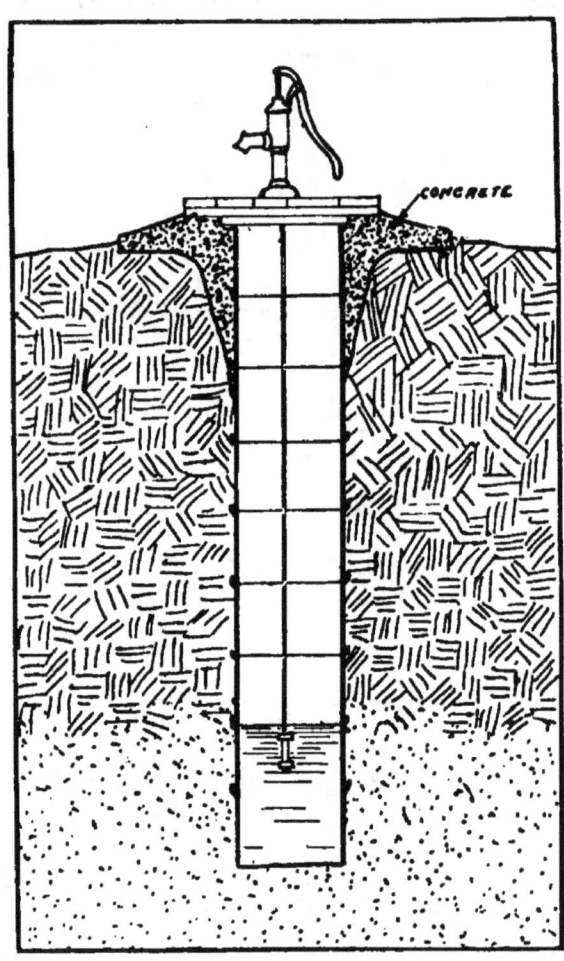

A Model Well, cased with terra-cotta pipe, curbed with concrete and provided with a water-tight platform and a pump. The water from such a well is unmixed with surface water or filth. Properly located such a well should furnish safe and healthful water.

be dry, airy and well lighted. A great aid in keeping the cellar floor dry is subsoil drainage. This can be effected by placing small porous tiles about two feet below the floor in parallel lines from ten to twenty feet apart. These all connecting with a main drain from the cellar. The danger of surface water creeping into the cellar and keeping the walls and floor damp and mouldy, can be prevented by proper grading around the house so as to drain off the water, also by the construction of proper foundation walls. A wall made of hollow tiles affords an air chamber which will greatly aid in keeping the cellar dry. When there is no cellar, the house should be set up on piers or posts in order to allow the free circulation of air underneath. If this is not done, unhealthful ground air will rise in the house. This can be prevented in houses with cellars by the cellar

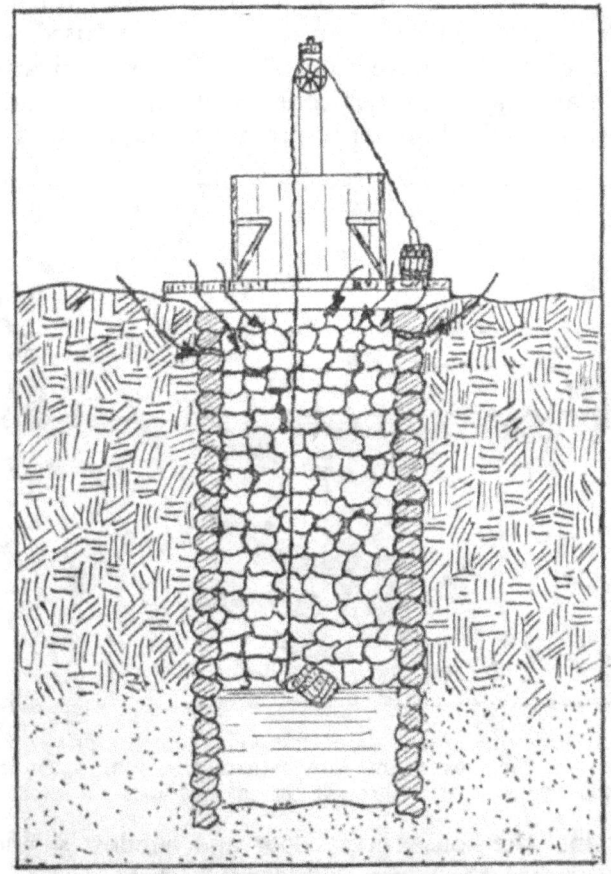

A Typical Insanitary Shallow Well. Filth enters such a well through cracks in the platform, is washed into it by surface water through holes under the platform, seeps into it through the loose casing, and is carried in by the bucket or the rope soiled by filthy hands.

floor being made of concrete, and thus being made practically air tight. Next to dryness, the cellar must be well lighted and perfectly ventilated. The necessity of this can be appreciated when we stop to think that most floors have crevices in them through which the cellar air rises and mingles with the atmosphere of the living and sleeping rooms.

The House.—Light and cleanliness go hand in hand. Each room in the house should have large outside windows. Bedrooms should be large, well lighted and airy. They should not be on the ground floor and never in the basement. The living room and especially the dining room should get plenty of sunlight, fresh air and be most cheerful. The most sanitary floor for the house is made of hardwood boards, tongued and grooved together which may be varnished or waxed and polished. This prevents the dust and dirt from collecting in the cracks and the floors can be easily cleaned by wiping them with an oiled cloth. Very little water should be used in cleansing these floors. With floors so constructed it is unnecessary to have carpets covering the entire surface, which at best are dirt and dust collectors and unsanitary. Small rugs can be used, which, not being tacked down, can be easily removed and cleaned often. Heavy draperies, upholstered furniture and the like, which collect and hold dust, and which are hard to clean, should not be used. In order to prevent the entrance of flies, mosquitoes

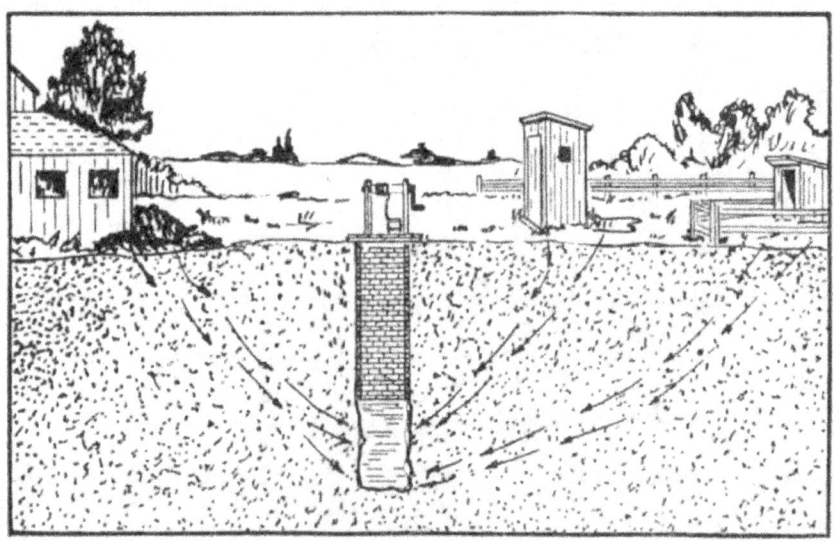

Heavy pollutions of the soil about the well from the privy, stable and hog pen will in time overcome the natural purifying agencies of the soil and will seep through the ground into the well.

and other insects into the house, every door and window should be thoroughly screened. The rooms of the house should not be kept closed up and dark for weeks. Both summer and winter they should be flooded daily with air and sunshine.

The mother or housekeeper, in order to safeguard the health of the family, will take special care that the kitchen, pantry, ice box and all places where food is stored and prepared, be kept scrupulously clean. Her house will be kept free from dust and dirt and all insects and vermin of any kind. Sinks, drains, water closets, bathtub, etc., should not only be cleaned daily, but scrubbed once or twice per week. Cellar should be kept clean and not made a gigantic pokehole for rags, cast-off clothing, old shoes, tin cans, rotten vegetables, garbage, swill or other offensive matters. The walls should be white washed once or twice a year. Cement floors may be washed each week and sprinkled with disinfectants. A shallow open vessel of lime or charcoal kept in the cellar purifies the air.

Surroundings.—The yard, outbuildings and premises surrounding the house should also be kept free from contamination and in a sanitary condition. Uncut grass, dense foliage, decaying weeds and wood will lower the sanitary condition. A well kept lawn immediately around the house is the most sanitary earth covering known. It prevents excess of moisture by evaporation and absorption and the purity of the soil is promoted by the action of the growing grass. Although the front yard in most places is well cared for, the back yard is often the dumping ground for all kinds of trash and rubbish. This should not be the case. All matter that is combustible should be burned. Tin cans and other debris which cannot be burned should be hauled away and buried. Also all gar-

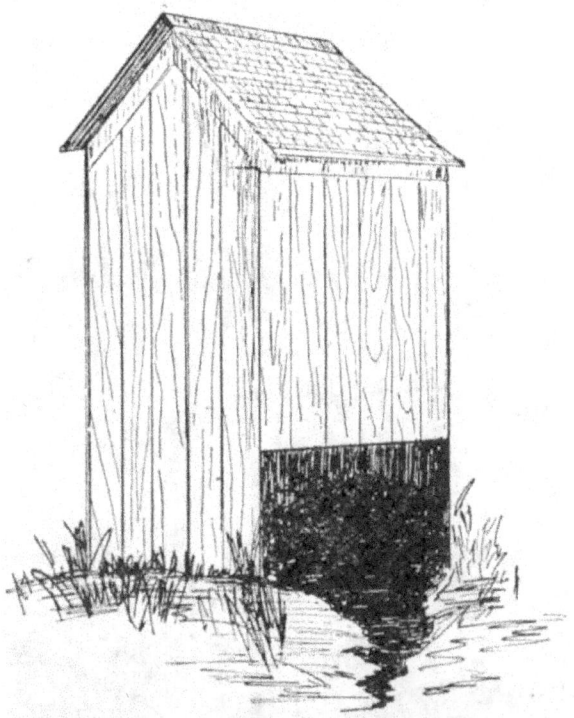

Figure 1.—Open, Insanitary Privy.

bage which cannot be fed to poultry or hogs. This should be taken care of often for if allowed to collect to any extent will draw flies, ants, vermin, and other insects. Proper disposal of sewage can be effected by some form of surface or subsurface irrigation, or if the dry closet is used, the sewage can be removed to distant fields and gardens. The open swill barrel should not be tolerated. If a barrel is used at all for this purpose, it should be kept tightly covered and some distance from the house. Manure should not be allowed to accumulate in barnyards, stables or poultry houses, as manure piles are the main breeding places of flies. It should be collected at least once a day, thrown into pits carefully screened or on piles which are well covered till it can be hauled out on the fields for fertilizer.

Water Supply.—The importance of an abundant supply of good pure water cannot be overestimated. The source should not be situated within several hundred yards of stables, barnyards, privy vaults, cesspools, or where they may receive the drainage from the same. Open wells are not safe sources of water supply. However, if used they should have tightly built walls so as to prevent the infiltration of impure water from the upper soil, also the surface around the well should be so graded as to drain the surface water away. The opening should be tightly covered to prevent dirt or vermin from falling into the well. Driven or tube wells are far better than those that are dug; also well filtered cistern water is often purer than the open well water. If the cistern is used, it is important in collecting water to allow the first washings from the roof to run off on the

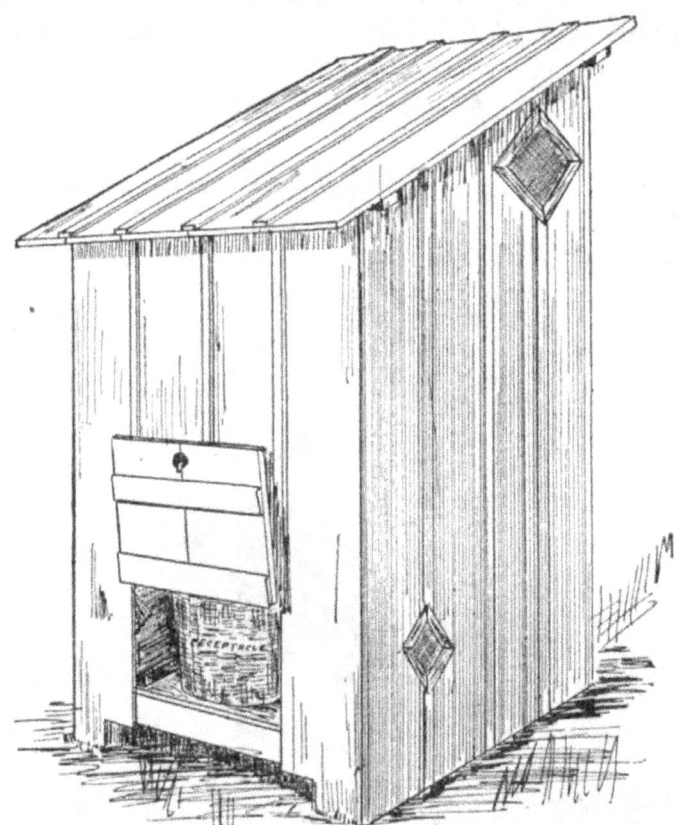

Figure 3.—Rear and Side View of Removable Receptacle Privy.

surface, as this always contains more or less organic filth in the shape of excrements of birds, leaves of trees, dust, etc. This water, in order to be pure, should be thoroughly filtered and the filter cleaned often. If there is reason to believe that the water is impure in the least, the best form of filtration cannot be depended upon to purify it. Often water containing the worst form of disease germs is clear as crystal, cold and good to taste. It should be examined by a chemist and if found to contain impurities, should be boiled or purified by chemicals. Any one can send a sample of water to the State Chemist for analysis, in case he is in doubt about its purity.

Disposal of Human Excreta.—The safe disposal of human excreta is of such vital importance to every community and home that it demands special mention. It is a well known fact that the germs of some of the most dangerous diseases are found in great abundance in human excreta (stools and urine). These germs come not only from persons suffering with the disease, but also from people apparently in good health who are known as "carriers" of infection.

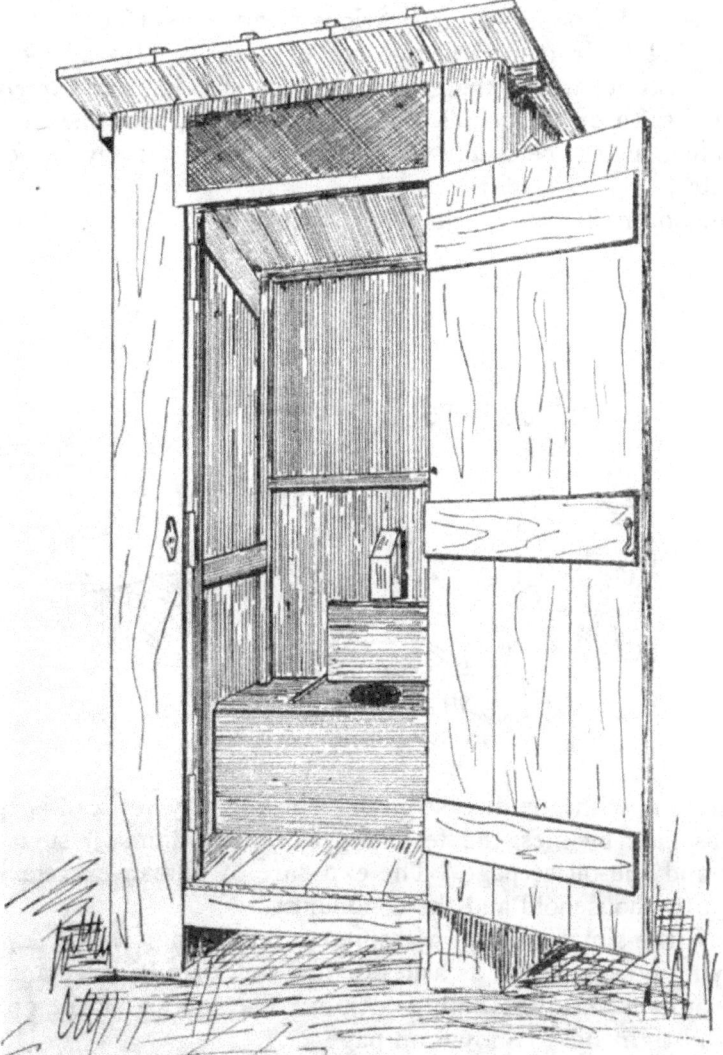

Figure 4.—Front View of Removable Receptacle Privy.

Although all forms of human excreta are considered very filthy and are instinctively shunned, yet through the improper disposal of the same we are often brought into the most intimate contact with them. Through the blind and unintelligent handling of this filth, it often gets into the water we drink, the food we eat, and on the skin of our bodies, thus conveying to our systems the germs which have come from the bodies of infected people. Such serious diseases as typhoid fever, tuberculosis, dysentary, and all kinds of worm diseases are contracted in this way. So we see that although the filthiness of human excreta is an important matter, the danger of this to the health and life is of still greater importance.

The highly perfected sewer systems of cities carry this matter a safe distance from the home at once. In the rural districts and at unsewered homes it is dangerously spread around by such various means as surface water or subsoil seepage, by the hands or feet of persons or by animals, also by flies and other insects. In all districts where there is no sewage system, we strongly urge for the sake of the health of the homes and the community, that one of the simpler methods explained below be installed for the safe and cleanly disposal of this poisonous matter.

The open, unsanitary privy shown in Figure 1 is often seen in the rural

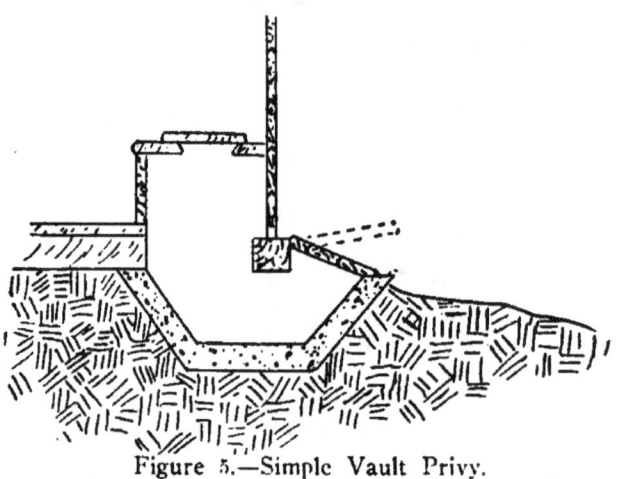

Figure 5.—Simple Vault Privy.

districts. The filth, with any disease germs which it may contain, is spread from a privy of this kind by flies, the feet of persons and animals, surface washing and drainage and subsoil seepage. The exposure of human excreta in this way is a menace to the household and the community.

Figure 2 is the simplest form of sanitary receptacle privy or dry closet. If used with drying powder, such as ashes or dry soil, or a disinfectant solution, it may be kept sanitary and practically odorless. The can should be provided with a good seat and tight lid. (Shown on page 27.)

Figure 3 and 4 show the front and rear views of the removable receptacle privy. These should have tight covers and be well screened in order to keep the flies and vermin away. The little windows at the sides and over the door should be well screened.

Figure 5 is a simple vault privy which is an improvement over those just described. The vault or receptacle is stationary and is made of concrete. The same principles of fly-proofing, ventilation, and use of drying powders and disinfectants used in those described above, apply to this. It should have a tight lid on the seat and also at the back where it is cleaned out. The main objection to this kind of privy is the difficulty of properly cleaning it.

Figure 6 and 7 show privies with septic tanks in which the human excreta undergoes fermentation. Through this process the solid matter becomes liquified and a great portion of the excreta is carried away in the form of gas and through evaporation. These are still a great improvement over those described above.

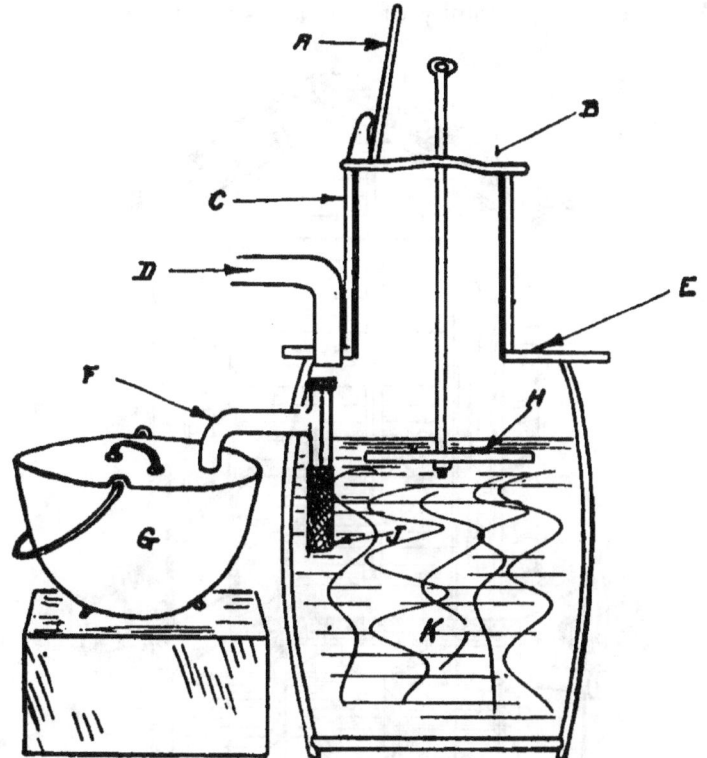

Figure 6.—"A" Automatically closing lid. "B" Seat. "C" Zinc lined box. "D" Ventilating pipe. "E" Floor. "F" Connecting pipe. "G" Effluent tank. "H" Anti-splasher. "J" Wire Screen. "K" Liquifying tank.
   The above illustration shows an ordinary vinegar barrel used as a liquifying tank and an iron pot for effluent tank.

The different parts of this privy are simple of construction and it can be made and operated by an intelligent person. (1) It consists of a water-tight tank to receive and liquify the excreta. This may be made of concrete, or it can be a tight barrel or iron vessel. (2) There is another tank connected with the first tank with a "T" pipe, both ends of which are covered with wire screens. This tank may also be made of concrete or it may be a water-tight can, barrel or iron pot. (3) A tight, zinc lined box fits tightly on the liquifying tank. This is provided with an opening on the top for a seat, which has a tight lid. (4) There may be an anti-splashing device used, as shown in the cut. (5) The ventilating pipe which connects the space under the seat with the open air. This may be made of a stove pipe or wooden flue.

In operating this form of privy, the receiving or liquifying tank should be filled with water to the point where it begins to trickle into the effluent tank. In order to start the fermentation, a little old manure should be added to the water. The surface of water in each container may be covered with a thin film of some form of petroleum in order to keep the insects away.

The size of the liquifying tank is governed by the number of persons to use the privy. For the average family of five, a 60-gallon tank should be used. In

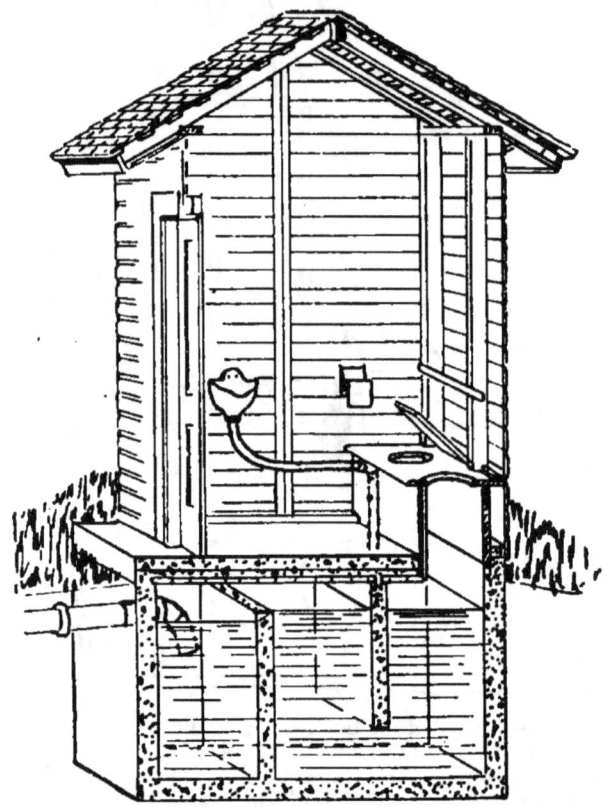

The Kentucky Sanitary Privy.

cold climates, the apparatus should be housed in a room where the temperature can be kept above the freezing point. Or the tanks should be sunk in the ground below the freezing point, or they may be imbedded in stable manure. In any case, they should be kept from freezing. The dry closet with removable receptacle may be used during the freezing weather and the septic vault the rest of the time.

In order to secure the best results with the use of this kind of privy, it is best to use the regular toilet paper. This will dissolve readily. Anything used which will not dissolve readily interferes with the successful working of the liquifying tank. If the apparatus is handled the way it should be, the tanks will seldom need cleaning—not more than once a year. However, the privy should be so constructed that it may be easily cleaned when it needs it.

It must be remembered at all times that the effluent from these privies are just as poisonous as the crude excreta and should be properly disposed of. It may be piped away on the top soil a safe distance from the buildings and the water supply. Also, since by means of these privies·the excreta is reduced to a small amount, it may be treated with a disinfectant. Whatever form of privy is used, the excreta or effluent matter should be removed a safe distance from the house and especially from the water supply.

Milk Supply.—As impure milk is the source of many serious disease germs, it should be strictly guarded against. The dairy cow should be in perfect health. No milk should be used from one suffering from any disease and special care

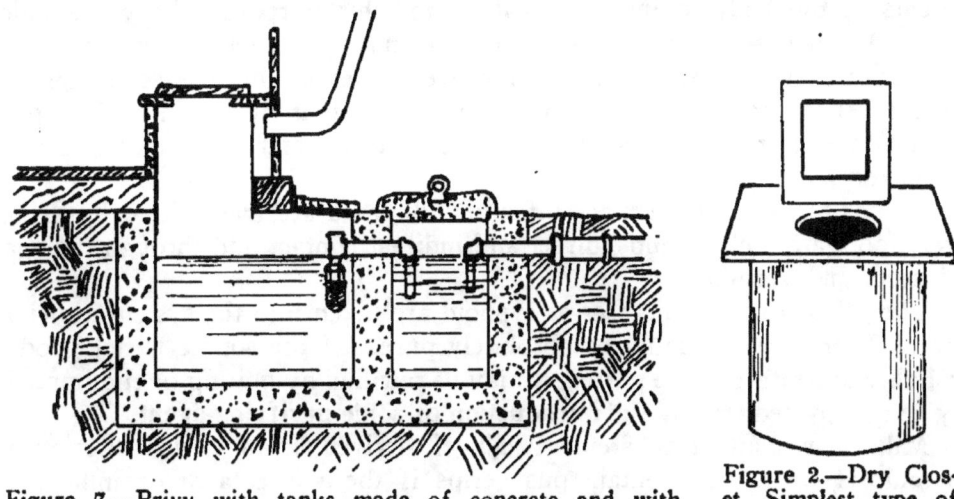

Figure 7.—Privy with tanks made of concrete and with direct distribution of effluent into top soil.

Figure 2.—Dry Closet. Simplest type of sanitary receptacle privy.

should be taken to detect cows suffering from tuberculosis. Neither should milk be used from any cow which has any disease of the teats or udder. All cattle used for dairy purposes should be examined by a competent veterinarian at stated intervals. They must be in the best of condition in order for their milk to be fit for use. The teats and udder of the cow should be thoroughly washed before milking, also the one who milks should have clean hands free from any local disease. The first stream of milk should always be discarded as it is very weak in food value and often contains many disease germs. Also all the milk which becomes contaminated in any way should be rejected. The narrow mouthed partly covered pail should be used and no loud talking, sneezing, coughing, tobacco spitting or general expectoration should be allowed during milking. The dairy barn and stables should be kept as clean as it is possible to make them. All milk should be carefully strained and cooled in strictly sanitary milk-houses, and all utensils used should be thoroughly washed and scalded out before using again. The importance of the above instructions can be realized when we stop to think that milk, butter and cheese are some of our most important articles of diet and that cow's milk is often the sole food of many delicate babies.

GERMS AND THEIR CARRIERS.

If the laws of nature are observed, if the rules of personal body hygiene and of home hygiene as set forth in the preceding pages, are strictly followed, there would be very little sickness and disease. The body that is kept in a clean, healthy condition is practically immune from disease. Many, in fact most diseases, enter the body in the form of germs, bacteria or microbes which are too small to be seen by the naked eye. These little organisms are like tiny little seeds which enter the system in the food we eat, the water we drink or the air we breathe. They may also enter the blood through wounds and cuts. However, these little germs or seeds, so to speak, cannot grow and multiply unless the soil is favorable. If the body is in a good healthy condition, these little organisms will be overcome by elements in the body intended by nature for this purpose. They are quickly destroyed and cast out as waste matter. Almost every one is exposed to the most serious disease germ at times, however, whether the disease is contracted or not depends largely on the condition the system is in at the time. One person may not take it at all, another in a very mild form, and still another in a very serious form.

As has already been stated, infectious diseases are transmitted by drinking water, food, air, soil, wounds, direct and indirect contact and through the agency of insects and vermin.

The germs of such diseases as typhoid are taken into the system in drinking water. Therefore, it should be absolutely pure. If the source is not good and it is liable to contain these germs, it may be purified by boiling or the impurities may be greatly reduced by the introduction of some purifying agent.

Milk may contain tubercule bacilli if derived from cows suffering with tuberculosis, or it may contain pus germs if there is catarrh or inflammation of the udder. It may also serve as the transmitter of the disease producing bacteria of diphtheria, typhoid fever, scarlet fever, dysentery or cholera. These germs may get into the milk on account of the unsanitary condition of the dairyman's home, dairy barn or from polluted water. It is wise, therefore, to have all milk pasteurized, which will destroy all germs, and which may be done by heating the milk to from 140 to 160 degrees F.

Such diseases as common colds, pneumonia, eruptive fevers, etc., are contracted by the breathing of foul, stuffy, impure air. As has been said before, there should be an abundance of fresh, pure air in every home. All debris and decaying matter which would pollute the air should be disposed of immediately.

One of the diseases most likely to be transmitted to the body from the soil is tetanus or lockjaw. Also puncture or incised wounds are infected by germs from the soil.

Diseases are contracted by direct or indirect contact with anything handled by a person suffering with the disease such as clothing, money, handkerchiefs, dishes, etc. These things should be thoroughly disinfected.

Flies.—Flies are great carriers of disease germs. On account of their filthy habits of swarming over decaying matter and filth, they become loaded with disease germs. The microscope has revealed thousands of germs on the legs of a fly, which are later deposited on dishes and food, and thus carried into the body. Not only should every window and door of the house be thoroughly screened to prevent their entrance and every device such as sticky fly-paper, fly-traps, etc., be used for catching and destroying those that get into the house, but every effort should be made to remove and destroy their breeding places. The premises should be kept clean by the prompt disposal of all filth and dirt. Manure from stables should be kept well screened or promptly removed to the fields. Privy vaults, cesspools and all such places should either be kept lightly covered or treated with kerosene or other oil. It is also well to sprinkle lime over such places. A ceaseless warfare should be waged against these germ-carrying pests.

Mosquitoes.—It has also been fully proven that mosquitoes are transmitters of such diseases as yellow fever, typhoid, malaria, etc., from one person to another. In fact some of these diseases can only be spread in that way. Mosquitoes breed in stagnant water, therefore, all pools should either be drained, filled in or treated with oil. The little larva can also be destroyed by the introduction of the little fish into such pools as they eat them up. Rain water should not be allowed to collect and become stagnant in barrels, tanks, cesspools, or old tin cans about the house. All cisterns should be tightly covered or well screened. In this way, the breeding places of these most dangerous germ-carrying insects can be done away with.

Vermin.—Rats, mice and other vermin are known to spread such serious diseases as the Plague. They should be carefully excluded not only from the house, but all other buildings as well, and if they gain access should be speedily exterminated. They are generally found in filthy locations, therefore, cleanliness is a safeguard against them as well as the diseases they carry.

DISINFECTANTS.

Not only can disease be prevented by the above named means of removing the agents for carrying and transmitting the same, but when it is in the family or community, the spreading of infectious and contagious diseases can be prevented by isolation and disinfection. The isolation should be as near absolute as possible. The person suffering with the disease should be placed in a room apart from the rest of the family from which all unnecessary drapery, furniture and rugs or carpets have been removed. He should be attended by one member of the family or trained nurse who should take every precaution not to carry it to other members of the family. All excretions, sputum, etc., coming from the sick room should be immediately burned.

Natural Disinfectants.—The proper and judicious use of disinfectants is also a great means of prevention and spreading of disease. Sunshine, dryness and cleanliness are important aids in this work. Extensive experiments have shown that very few disease germs can live long if exposed to the direct rays of the sun. The disadvantages of sunlight as a disinfectant are its superficial action, variability and uncertainty. It is a valuable adjunct to other methods and should be used extensively as possible. Dryness is also unfavorable to the development of disease germs.

Heat is the best, most available and cheapest disinfectant. It can be used in the way of burning, dry heat, boiling and steam. The germs in all materials which can be burned should be destroyed in that way. All disease germs, bacteria, etc., are destroyed when exposed to dry heat of 150 degrees F. for an hour. Most bacteria are destroyed at a lower temperature than this. Most objects which can stand the heat without injury should be disinfected in this way. Boiling is an absolutely safe sterilizer and disinfectant and is applicable to most materials and objects. Half an hour boiling will destroy all germs subjected to it. Steam kills all bacteria at once and all spores in a few minutes. It is very valuable for this reason, and because it can be applied to a great many materials and objects. All clothing, bedding, mattresses, carpets, draperies, etc., which cannot be disinfected by other means, should be sent to places where they can be steamed.

For the disinfection of materials and objects which cannot be subjected to the aforenamed means and for the disinfection of the sick-room, houses and places where the disease has been, chemicals are used in gaseous form or in solution.

Chemical Disinfectants.—Physical disinfectants, those previously described, cannot be used in many places and for many materials infected with disease germs. Therefore, such chemical disinfectants as Sulphur Dioxide and Formaldehyde are used. When sulphur is used the gas is best generated by placing the powdered sulphur in an iron pot and igniting it by the use of alcohol. In burning, it evolves the sulphur dioxide gas which is good as a surface disinfectant, very destructive to all animal life and one of the best insecticides known. However, it does not really kill germs or spores, it also weakens textile fabrics, bleaches vegetable coloring matter, tarnishes metals and is very dangerous to those doing the disinfecting. About five pounds of sulphur should be used to every 1,000 cubic feet of space.

Formaldehyde.—At the present time formaldehyde is used much more than sulphur. It is better for the reason that it is non-poisonous, a good germicide, has no injurious effects on fabrics and objects, does not change and can be used without danger to disinfect rooms with rich draperies, bric-a-brac, etc. It it not an insecticide but kills germs and bacteria in a very short time and spores in an hour or so. Paraform, from which the formaldehyde gas is generated when heated, can be bought in the form of pastiles or powder. It should not be burned as no gas is generated when it reaches the burning stage. The lamps used for disinfecting with paraform can be purchased anywhere and are very simple in construction. Two ounces of the paraform should be used for every 1,000 cubic feet space with an exposure of about 12 hours. Formaldehyde may also be used in the form of liquid formalin and either sprayed or sprinkled over the objects to be disinfected which are then placed in a tightly covered box and disinfected by the evolution of the gas.

In using either one of these gases, it is necessary to hermetically close up all cracks, apertures, openings where the gas might escape. This should be thoroughly done by placing over these gummed paper before the act of generating the gas has been begun.

The most common chemicals used in solutions as disinfectants are carbolic acid, lysol, lime and bichloride of mercury. In order for these to be effective they must be used freely for some time in the concentrated form and warm or hot if possible. They may be used by soaking the affected objects in the solution or by applying it as a wash or spray. The strength of the solution depends on the work to be done and the materials used. As a rule, **carbolic acid** is used for floors, walls, ceiling, wood work, instruments, all small objects, etc., by washing them with it.

Lime.—Lime is generally used in the form of whitewash and is produced by mixing the common lime with water. It is very often used to disinfect walls, ceilings, cellars, etc., by giving them a coat of whitewash. The milk of lime should be used freely to disinfect the excreta in privy vaults. It is good to use it wherever there is any decaying vegetable or animal matter.

Bichloride of Mercury.—(Corrosive Sublimate).—This is a very strong poison, however, a powerful germicide. If used in a strength of 1 : 500 it will quickly kill all germs, bacteria and even spores. It dissolves in 16 parts cold water or 3 parts boiling water, producing a colorless solution which should be carefully labeled or colored so as not to be accidentally used internally.

How to Use Disinfectants.—In order for the work of disinfection to be thorough and successful, it must be suited to the needs in each case and be performed conscientiously. It cannot be applied in the same manner to all objects and materials or used in the same way for all diseases.

Rooms are best disinfected by the use of formaldehyde as before mentioned. All cracks, apertures, holes and all openings from the room to the outer air should be carefully closed by means of gummed paper strips which can be obtained in rolls and need only be moistened and applied to the openings. Be careful not to overlook openings into chimneys, ventilators, transoms, etc. After all openings have been closed up and the disinfectant applied the disinfector should withdraw quickly and the room be left closed at least 12 hours. In cases of very infectious diseases and where the infection is liable to adhere to the walls, as in cases of tuberculosis, it is often well to remove all paper, kalsomine or paint and apply new. The walls may also be scrubbed with a disinfectant as a solution of carbolic acid or corrosive sublimate.

All iron beds or metal furniture may be scrubbed with soapsuds and then a solution of carbolic acid or some other disinfectant applied. Wooden furniture may be washed with the disinfectant solution and also subjected to the gaseous disinfectant. All sheets, table cloths, linen or cotton clothing or bedding may be soaked in a carbolic acid solution and then boiled. Mattresses, pillows, quilts, etc., should be moistened with a 5 percent solution of formalin and then taken to a place where they may be thoroughly steamed. Carpets may be subjected to the gaseous disinfectant and also steamed. As the steam sets or fixes all spots or stains they should be removed if possible before the material is sent away to be steamed. As steam injures woolen goods they should be subjected to the gaseous disinfectant or to the solutions. Books are very hard to disinfect and as they are dangerous as germ carriers, especially if handled by the patient, they should be burned. However, to disinfect them they should be well opened out and stood on end while being subjected to a gaseous disinfectant.

Those doing the disinfecting should understand their business, do it thoroughly and conscientiously, and be sure that their hands and clothing are thoroughly disinfected when they are through.

SPECIAL EXERCISE.

A strong healthy body is the most important asset a man can have. For this reason no part of it should be allowed to become weak and inefficient through neglect. The muscles and various organs of the body only become strong, able to accomplish their work and at the same time to throw off the waste material, through proper and regular exercise. Many fine bodies are weakened and made unfit for the work they are to perform just by lack of exercise or lack of proper exercise. Even in the bodies of those who say "We get plenty of exercise in our work," there are muscles which are left for long periods at a time without exercise. For this reason there are those whose bodies are very unevenly developed—parts strong and muscular—parts left to weaken and be a seat for disease because of lack of proper exercise. One must make every part of the body strong in order to get the most efficient service from it. We say, "A chain is just as strong as its weakest link," so the body is just as strong as its weakest part.

The best time for exercise is on rising in the morning. Exercise should not be taken within two hours after a meal nor just before going to bed, because with some people this causes nervousness and sleeplessness. Sometimes the muscles are rather stiff in the morning and the exercise makes them supple.

Exercising every part of the body makes it strong and healthy, the mind clear, and the disposition good.

Breathing.—Place the hands on the knees, keeping the knees stiff, raise the body with the hands extending horizontally in front of the body, and then throw them backwards as far as possible while inhaling, and return the hands to knees while exhaling.

Raise the hands to front of chest, inhaling deeply, thrust the arms forward forcefully while forcing the air from the lungs.

Keep the hands near together and rotate the arms and shoulders, first around the right shoulder then around the left, inhaling while raising the arms and exhaling while lowering them.

Inhale abdominally with the hands on the hips, press in with the fingers and bend the body to the front, then raise the body and fill the chest, exhale slowly.

Stand very erect with hands on hips, fingers pointing to the front, and pant like a dog. Do this till the diaphragm becomes very flexible.

Stand very straight with the chest thrown out, shoulders squared, hands clapsed behind the back, inhale deeply, by starting to breathe at the abdomen, raising the diaphragm and then filling the chest just as full as possible. Tuberculosis often starts in the part of the lungs which extends up under the shoulders and is scarcely ever used in just ordinary breathing, especially by one who does not carry the shoulders squarely.

Stationary Run.—Stand still and run on the toes, breathing deeply.

Chest Development.—Stand at arm's length from the wall and place the palms on the wall, then bend towards the wall till the chest touches the wall, return to the original position.

Kidneys.—Keep the knees stiff, bend the body at the hips and touch the floor with fingers, then raise the hands to the chest and repeat several times at the beginning. Keep this up till you can do it a dozen times.

Stand with the feet about two feet apart, extend the hands above the head and about two feet apart with the palms turned in; bend the body and touch the floor, keeping the knees stiff.

Liver.—Extend the arms to the side horizontal with the shoulders and bend the body to the right and left just as far as possible with the feet spread apart and knees stiff. The liver is like a sponge and is cleaned by expanding and contracting.

Bend the body far to the right and the left with the accompanying movement of the arms as if chopping wood. This is sometimes called the "Gladstonian Exercise."

Spine.—Keep the knees stiff, stretch up as far as possible with the hands raised above the head. Swing the arms in front of the body in a circle. Raise the arms again and stretch up as far as possible and repeat a half dozen times or more.

Constipation.—Lie on the back on a firm flat surface such as the floor or a firm couch, and place the hands under the hips, raise the knees to the chest and return to the floor. Repeat eight or ten times. Be very careful not to strain the muscles. Lie on a firm surface on the back with the hands under the hips, heels held together. Keep the knees stiff and raise the legs to a vertical position. Return to the floor and repeat eight or ten times. Do not strain.

Stand with the body erect, heels together, chest thrown out, abdomen drawn in, hands at the back of the neck. Draw the right knee as close up against the body as possible, as if taking a very high step. Do this about six times and repeat with the other knee. Breathe deeply.

Sit on a stool with shoulder squared, hands on hips, elbows thrown back and chest out, knees spread apart. Bend forward and back as far as possible. Repeat several times.

Back.—Lie on the back on a firm surface, place the hands on the legs, raise the chin to the chest, then raise the body to a sitting position, running the hands along the limbs, keeping the heels on the floor, and return to the floor. This is especially good for the muscles of the back. But great care should be taken not to strain the back. If necessary, place the toes under some object for support for a few times. Some people may not be able to do this exercise until they have practiced the others for a few weeks. It may help to throw the hands, clasped, in front of the body till the back is strong enough to throw the body to a sitting position without the aid of the hands.

Neck.—Bend the head forward as far as possible and rotate in a circle bending the head just as far each way as possible. Repeat six times, then reverse and rotate six times.

Legs.—Stand erect and rock on the toes and heels.

Hands.—Stretch arms out straight and open and close the hands forcefully.

A long brisk walk with shoulders back, chest expanded and arms swinging freely, is one of the best forms of exercise. The common slouchy gait is of little account. Put snap into the step, walk with the hips not knees. The feet should point straight ahead, not outward. Use the muscles of the back.

Swimming is said to be the very best form of exercise for all the muscles of the body.

The exercises should be followed by a cold bath. A cold plunge is excellent for persons who are strong, otherwise a shower or sponge bath is good. A brisk rub should follow the bath.

Each person should pick out one or two of each list and perform them conscientiously every day for at least two months, for their value cannot be tested in a week or so.

Of course if there is any sign of heart trouble, the exercises should be followed only under the advice of a physician. And should not be taken at times when good sense advises that all violent exercises should be avoided.

HOW TO PREVENT
COLDS—PNEUMONIA—TUBERCULOSIS—TYPHOID.

Aside from the instructions given in the foregoing pages on how to develop strong, healthy bodies, bodies immune to diseases, and the general means of preventing disease and ill health, we wish to take up the most important points in the prevention of some of the most serious diseases. These diseases are wholly preventive and yet cause an immense loss of life every year, not to speak of the countless thousands incapacitated by them. The nature and prevention of Common Colds, Pneumonia, Tuberculosis and Typhoid Fever, are taken up in particular. These diseases may all be prevented and yet tuberculosis alone claimed 98,194 victims in 1915 in the United States. Pneumonia was responsible for 89,326 deaths during the same year. However, the decline in the death rate of these dreadful maladies in recent years is very gratifying. For instance, the death rate of Typhoid Fever had dropped from 35.9 per 100,000 in 1900 to 12.4 per 100,000 in 1915. This is due to the great strides which have been made in sanitation and general prevention. These diseases may be practically eliminated by the proper means of prevention.

It is also extremely dangerous, in fact, criminal, for parents to unduly expose their children even to such infectious disease as whooping cough and measles. Statistics show that in 1913 measles caused a greater number of deaths than scarlet fever, and in 1914 and 1915 whooping-cough had that distinction. Jealously guard your own health and that of your children. **Prevention** is the word.

COMMON COLDS—THEIR NATURE AND PREVENTION.

It is definitely known that a cold is an acute infection of the air passage due to the presence of bacteria. There are several different kinds of these bacteria, any one of which may cause a cold. One of these is the dangerous pneumo-coccus, which causes pneumonia. These bacteria may lodge in the nose or some of the cavities opening into the nose. They may be in the throat, lungs, chest or even in the blood. They are as a rule present to a greater or less degree at all times. It is when the body is weak or in a rundown condition that these are able to do the greatest harm.

The common cold is much more serious than most people realize. The medical experts claim that a cold cannot be cured. It must run its course and in doing so it often so weakens the body that it is subject to any one of a number more directly fatal maladies. All that can be done in treating a cold is to aid nature in lessening the duration of the attack.

The greatest means to prevention of this common malady is the development of a strong, healthy body.

Harden the body against changes in temperation by the cold bath every morning.

Make the lungs, throat and air passages strong and healthy by breathing plenty of pure air.

Keep the system clean by keeping the bowels open, the kidneys active and the skin clean. This can be done by the external and internal use of plenty good water.

Keep the digestive organs working properly by not overeating, by regular meals, and by proper and sufficient exercise.

Keep your chest warm, but don't bundle up your neck with furs and thick collars. Leave the fur collar loose so the cold air can circulate freely.

Keep away from persons with colds. Sneezing and coughing spread the germs.

Keep the body warm and dry. Chilling makes it more susceptible to the germ attacks.

Keep the feet warm and dry.

Don't bundle up the throat and leave the ankle unprotected.

Dusty air causes colds. Avoid it.

Do not work, live or sleep in overheated, ill ventilated rooms.

Suit the clothing to the condition of your health and to the weather conditions.

Do not use tobacco or alcohol as these weaken your power of resistance.

Those who are peculiarly susceptible to colds should go to a good physician and have a thorough examination to learn the reason why, if possible. It may be due to unhealthy conditions of the mouth or throat, to obstruction of the nasal passages by adenoids or enlarged tonsils, or to faulty posture. In case the body is made susceptible to colds by any of these causes, they should be removed at once. Neglect or delay may cause serious results.

PNEUMONIA—ITS NATURE AND PREVENTION.

Pneumonia is a germ disease in which the germs affect the air passages. It is known as one of the "impure air" diseases. Germs from without invade the body.

Why is it that there is so much more pneumonia during the winter months than at any other time? Is it because there are so many more of the pneumo-cocci, the pneumonia disease germs, during cold weather than at any other time? All scientists tell us no. These germs are present everywhere, at all times and it is impossible to prevent their entrance into the body. However, we can prevent them from getting a foothold and growing. They cannot grow and multiply in healthy tissues of the body.

-If the body is kept in good healthy condition, all the tissues strong, it will be able to ward off the attacks of these germs. We must give our bodies a fair chance in the fight against disease. There is more pneumonia during the cold months of the year than at other times because our bodies are not in as good condition during the cold season. They are "run down" on account of insufficient fresh air, lack of outdoor exercise, insufficient good nourishment, etc. We shut ourselves up in ill ventilated stuffy, overcrowded houses, sleep with our bedroom windows closed tight, do not get enough outdoor exercise, do not bathe often enough, overeat, and dissipate in various ways. In these ways we weaken our bodies and make them more subject to disease.

Health is the strongest opponent of disease. Keep your body at its full "fighting strength" and you have little to fear from pneumonia or any other disease.

Follow fully the instructions given above for the prevention of colds and you will do much in the way of preventing pneumonia.

Especially give the body plenty of good, fresh air. Practice "deep breath-ing." Sleep with your bedroom window open **always.**

Stay out of stuffy, overheated, overcrowded, ill ventilated places.

Stay away from people who are sneezing or coughing, as disease germs are spread in this way.

Keep the body, especially the feet, warm and dry and prevent chilling.

Do not take alcohol into the system in any form as those who use it are particularly susceptible to the disease.

Avoid constipation, overeating and extreme fatigue.

Those at the extremes of life, the very young and the very old, need to be well taken care of as the disease is very fatal at those ages.

Pneumonia has been called, "Captain of the Men of Death," so the great-est care must be exercised during the pneumonia season.

If there is a generally achy feeling, severe headache, sore throat, pain in the chest and high fever, it is well to call the doctor at once. In the meantime, take a good hot foot bath, go to bed, cover up warm and then drink a pint of hot lemonade or flaxseed tea. This will cause free perspiration and relieve congestion.

TUBERCULOSIS—ITS NATURE AND PREVENTION.

Tuberculosis is preventable, but because it is so common and chronic, the health authorities cannot control it like the quarantinable diseases. Every person must be taught how to meet the dangers of this disease and protect himself against infection.

Tuberculosis is a contagious, probably never an inherited disease, as for years was supposed. It is contracted by breathing in or swallowing the germs which cause it. No one is so strong but that at some time he may contract tuberculosis, although robust health is a most valuable safeguard. Sometimes we can withstand the germs without becoming infected, but when we are weakened by fatigue, privation, intemperance or by other diseases, and tuberculosis germs enter the body, we become infected. Constant attention to details of prevention is necessary if we live or work with a consumptive.

The sputum or spit of the ordinary consumptive gives off daily, millions of tuberculosis germs. His saliva abounds in these germs and therefore they are left on his spoon, cup, glass and fork. If he touches his finger to his mouth in turning the pages of a book, he may leave the germs on the pages. If he covers his mouth with his bare hand while coughing, whatever he touches after that—food, baby's toys, another's hand, may become smeared with the germ or bacilli, which may then find their way to the mouth of another person. If sputum dries upon his handkerchief or bedding, any one handling them may inhale the infected dust. Flies carry sputum on their feet from the gutters to fruit, vegetables and any nearby food. It is not yet known which is the more dangerous—to inhale or swallow the germs—both may cause tuberculosis of the lungs.

We cannot get away from the consumptive for there are several millions of them now living in the United States, and the only way we can protect ourselves is to force those afflicted into proper habits of living. Public sentiment should encourage the enforcing of the anti-spitting laws in our cities.

Some early symptoms of the disease are: a slight fever in the afternoon is sometimes the only symptom for months, a loss of weight and strength, rapid heart beat, a sense of fatigue on slight exertion, indigestion or loss of appetite, slight pains in chest and hoarseness or cough. Any or all of these symptoms long continued, indicate need for consulting a physician. Never consult a doctor who advertises—you need honesty.

An early diagnosis of the disease is very important because proper treatment at this time will usually effect a cure and early cases are often dangerous carriers of infection. A sneeze may send many germs into the air to be breathed by those near by.

The germs are not destroyed by snow, rain or the lowest winter temperature; but sunlight kills them in a few hours, and good strong daylight in a clean room kills them in a few days. They live for months in dark rooms. Dirt protects them from light and thus preserves them. Dust carries them through the air A room should never be swept when dry nor a feather duster or dry cloth used to dust, as this just scatters germs. A moist cloth should be used and the floor should be scrubbed with soap and hot water. The consumptive's room should be without carpet. A boiling temperature kills germs almost immediately; therefore, boiling is the best method of disinfecting dishes, clothing, towels and bedding. Those things which would be spoiled by boiling may be rendered quite safe by hanging in the sun for a day or two. Antiseptics placed in basins in the sick room have no effect on the germs in the air, on the walls, etc. But antiseptics, such as strong lye or 5 percent solution of carbolic acid, should be put in spittoon and left there while it is being used.

The immediate destruction of all sputum from consumptives is the most important thing in the fight against tuberculosis, and promiscuous spitters should be reported to health officers and punished severely. Tuberculosis is curable, but is very serious even in the first slight stages.

HOW TO AVOID CONTRACTING TUBERCULOSIS.

Keep in good physical condition all the time. Cultivate a proper carriage of the body. Practice deep breathing, through the nose, in the open air several times daily. Bathe frequently—a cold sponge bath every morning will help ward off colds. Sleep with your windows open. Spend several hours outdoors every day and keep your room well aired where you live, work or study. Sleep nine hours every night, eat regularly and be temperate in all things. Avoid hot rooms. Do not move into a house vacated by a consumptive, unless it has been well cleaned and disinfected. Do not work in shop or office which is dusty or poorly ventilated. Never use a common drinking cup at a public fountain. Have your lungs examined once a year. Do not put into your mouth anything taken from the mouth of another person, such as a marble, whistle, candy, gum or partly eaten fruit. Do not allow any one to kiss you on the mouth. Do not allow children to play on the floor of a consumptive's room.

TYPHOID FEVER—ITS CAUSATION AND PREVENTION.

In the United States about 400,000 persons are incapacitated and about 30,000 are killed by typhoid fever each year. The rate of prevalence in recent years, for this country, has been from two to five times as high as in some European countries, although these countries formerly had higher typhoid fever rates than ours. Their reduced rates have followed improvements in sanitary conditions for typhoid fever is a preventable disease and practical measures for its prevention are known. Therefore, it is within the power of any community of intelligent persons to fix its own typhoid fever rate.

The improvement of sanitary conditions, especially in the rural districts, in respect to the disposal of human excreta, is one of the vitally important problems confronting us both as individuals and as a nation. And upon this problem does typhoid fever prevalence depend.

Typhoid fever results from the presence of certain little poisonous plants in the human body, which are called typhoid germs. These germs cannot be seen with the naked eye, but with the use of a powerful microscope, such bacteria become readily visible. Under favorable conditions, as in milk, meat, broth or nutrient jelly, each typhoid germ will divide into two, about every 45 minutes, and thus a few germs may, in a short time, give rise to thousands. Typhoid germs like wheat, corn and other plants, do not arise spontaneously, but come by natural descent from others of their kind. And, like other plants, must get into favorable soil in order to grow or multiply.

Typhoid germs reach the human body by being swallowed. Not every person who swallows typhoid germs has typhoid fever, nor does individual susceptibility to typhoid infection seem to be a matter of general health. In epidemics of typhoid, caused by heavily infected water supplies, it is unusual for more than one out of ten persons who drink the water to have typhoid fever. Some persons have two or more attacks of the disease. Therefore, one who has had an attack should not, for that reason, take any unnecessary risk of exposure to infection. When a susceptible person swallows typhoid germs, the germs multiply in the food canal, and from the intestine they invade the blood and are carried throughout the body. In the blood and tissues, the germs elaborate a poison, the effects of which, on the different tissues and organs of the body, give rise to the symptoms of the disease.

Typhoid germs come from persons. Myriads of living germs are discharged in the excreta from bodies of persons sick with typhoid fever. Every typhoid patient therefore should be regarded as a reservoir of infection and the excreta dealt with as a very dangerous poison. Also some persons in apparently good health harbor in their bodies and discharge in their excreta typhoid germs, just as do persons who suffer from the fever. Any person who, has ever been exposed to typhoid infection may be one of these so-called "carriers."

Typhoid carriers may be (1) persons in the "incubative" period of a few days or weeks immediately preceding the definite onset of the attack of fever; (2) persons who have mild or "walking" cases of typhoid fever; (3) persons recovered from a definite attack of the disease and (4) persons who have become infected but who have not recently had, and who may never have, definite manifestations of the disease. Man alone seems to be the source of typhoid infection. We have typhoid fever because we get something soiled or contaminated with human filth into our mouths and swallow it. Every person who has typhoid fever has recently swallowed some typhoid germs, which have come in some way from the excreta of some infected person. If human filth is prevented from reaching human mouths, typhoid fever will be prevented. This is the central fact in typhoid fever prevention. This can be accomplished only by the proper disposal of the excreta from all persons, both sick and well, at all times so that none of this dangerous matter will get

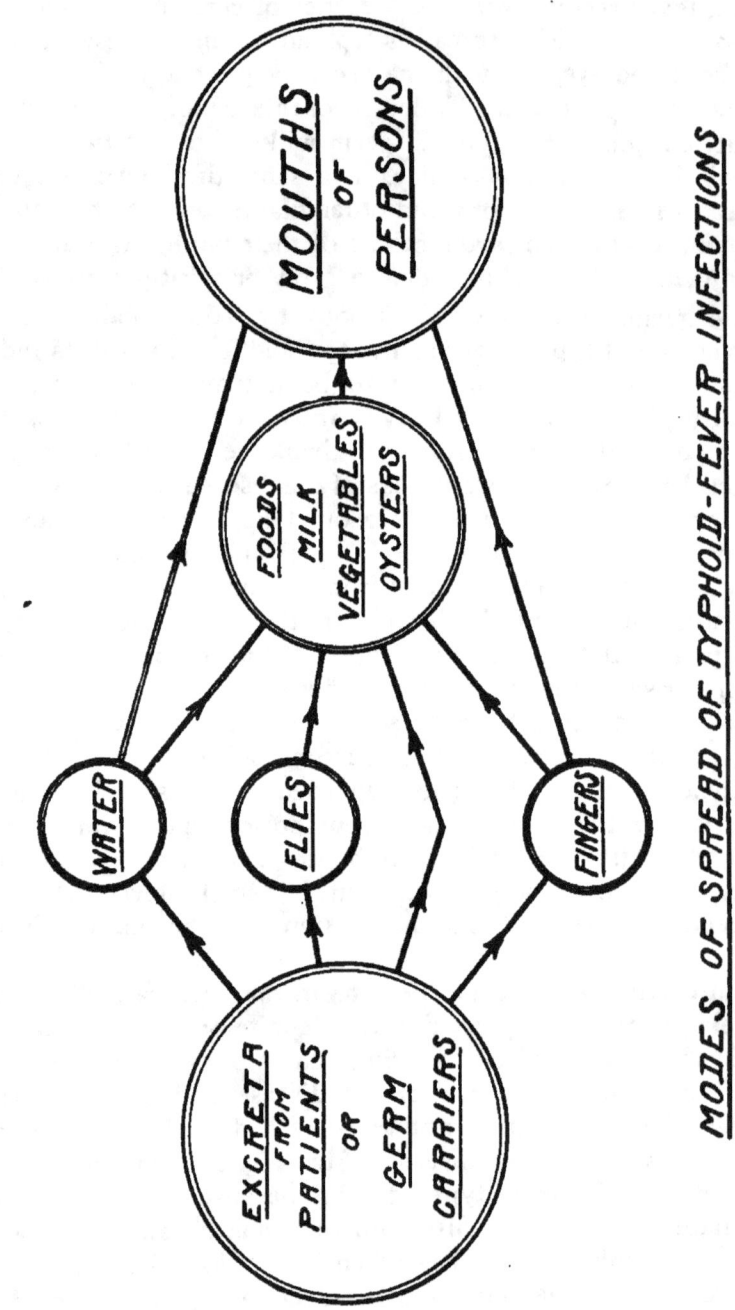

MODES OF SPREAD OF TYPHOID-FEVER INFECTIONS

into our mouths, our food or our drinking water. The sanitary disposal of this poison will also prevent dysenteries, hookworm, tapeworm and roundworm diseases, much of the diarrheas of infants and adults, and some of the tuberculosis. But sanitary disposal in rural districts is very exceptional.

Various Ways of Carrying Human Filth to Human Mouths.—It can be carried by washing rains or by surface drainage into water supplies, truck patches, fruit grounds, yards where the children play; it can be carried for a considerable distance by underground seepage into water supplies; it can be scattered by feet of poultry and persons, cats, rats, etc.; by flies directly to foods for persons, by hands to food or water; by contaminated water used for washing milk vessels or fruit, vegetables or water in which oysters or other shell fish are grown or stored.

Flies, the nastiest of all insects, feed on, crawl over and breed in human filth, from which they carry matter with all its germs, both within and on the surface of their bodies, and smear the filth from their feet and bodies on everything they touch.

Typhoid germs are very small. Twelve thousand of them placed end to end, or 36,000 of them placed side by side, measure only about one inch. They are colorless and cause no disagreeable odor or taste. Therefore, water which is clear, or milk which is sweet, if contaminated with even very small quantities of filth, conveyed on a fairly clean looking finger or fly, may be teeming with living germs of typhoid fever.

Milk is a favorable culture medium for the germs. Therefore, it is very important to exercise greatest precautions in handling milk. The typhoid germ is comparatively easy to kill. The boiling of water, the heating of milk to 140 degrees F. or 60 degrees C. for twenty minutes will kill germs.

Infected excreta may be made free from danger by the intelligent use of either heat or chemical disinfectants. A good and comparatively cheap disinfectant is compound cresol solution—one part of cresol solution to 50 parts of water; for use on the skin the strength should be one-half of this. A still cheaper disinfectant is chloride of lime solution, made by adding one pound of chloride of lime to four gallons of water. This solution should be kept in an air-tight vessel. Excreta may also be disinfected by pouring into the vessel containing the excreta about four times as much boiling water as excreta and cover vessel tightly for about one-half hour. All articles which may have come in contact with the infected excreta should be promptly and thoroughly disinfected.

Preventative Measures.—(1) Increase human resistance by anti-typhoid inoculation or "vaccination." This consists of three injections about ten days apart, given under the skin. The first injection contains about 500,000,000, the second and third about 1,000,000,000 killed typhoid germs. It is accompanied generally with only slight discomfort and is apparently free from serious danger. Persons who have been inoculated, it has been found by experiment, are about one-fourth as likely to develop typhoid fever as are those who have not been inoculated. But this treatment is not a substitute for sanitation. (2) Safeguard food and drink. Hands in any way soiled should be well washed before touching food or beverages. Prevention of fly-breeding is a preventive against typhoid fever. Water should be obtained whenever possible from sources safe from exposure to human excreta, but if this is not possible, water should be boiled or treated with "chloride of lime" solution. If milk is not rigidly safeguarded against contamination, the most healthful food becomes one of the most dangerous. If you are not sure that the milk has been rigidly safeguarded all the way from the cow to your table, it should be pasteurized (by heating to 145 degrees F. for twenty minutes). Garden truck and fruits, especially those eaten raw, should be protected against contamination. Excreta should not be used as a fertilizer in truck garden unless it has been thoroughly boiled. Oysters, clams, etc., taken from polluted water should be well cooked. (3) Proper disposal of human excreta is clearly the greatest single measure for the prevention of typhoid fever. Adequate sewerage systems should be installed in cities and towns, and less expensive machinery, but greater care by individuals, will safeguard rural districts from typhoid fever scourges.

HOW TO KEEP THE BABY WELL.

Baby's Rights.

1. Every baby has a right to be well-born, to have a father and a mother who are healthy in body, mind and morals.

2. Have your baby's birth properly reported and registered, thus insuring rights and privileges of citizenship.

3. Of the babies who die in the first year 30 to 40 out of 100 die in the first month. Give the baby a fair chance.

Food.

4. Nurse your baby. No other food is so good for the baby as the mother's milk.

5. Most mothers can nurse their babies if they are patient and persistent.

6. The act of nursing stimulates the production and flow of milk.

7. Do you know that 80 out of every 100 babies who die after the first month and before the end of the first year, are bottlefed?

8. The baby who is nursed by its mother is stronger to resist disease and danger.

9. Don't worry, fret, overwork, or lose sleep as this will reduce the milk supply.

10. Don't get angry or excited as this is liable to make your milk unwholesome and even dangerous to your child.

11. Wash the nipples carefully before and after each nursing.

12. Lead a simple life with regular and systematic outdoor exercise. Walking is best but must not be overdone.

13. Don't wean your baby much before it is a year old and then it should be done gradually.

14. Don't wean the baby during the hot summer months unless by physician's advice.

Bottle Feeding.

15. If you cannot nurse your baby, use cow's milk fresh and pure from healthy cows. This is the best substitute for mother's milk.

16. Consult your physician in preparing the cow's milk for the baby. The same preparation will not do for all babies.

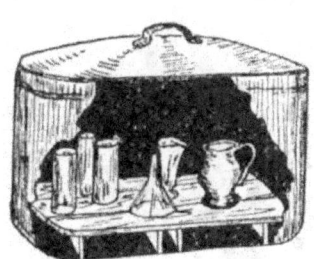

All Utensils for the Baby should be sterilized. The wash boiler with a loose-fitting false bottom makes an efficient steam sterilizer.

17. Keep scrupulously clean all milk vessels, bottles, towels, hands and whatever comes near or is used in preparation of baby's food.

18. Never use the feeding bottle with the tube attachment. It is a germ breeder.

19. Use the smooth, graduated feeding bottle, free from corners and angles.

20. After the first few weeks, never feed a well baby oftener than seven times in 24 hours. Six meals per day is better.

21. If your baby cries a great deal, it might be well to see your doctor. Crying is not a sign that he is hungry.

22. Don't use a "pacifier." It is unclean, unsafe and spoils the shape of baby's mouth.

23. Don't use "soothing syrups" or other "dopes." These are not kept in the home of the "Better Baby."

24. Keep the rubber nipples in a covered glass containing a solution of boric acid.

25. Turn the nipples inside out and wash them with soap and water at least once a day.

26. Keep a supply of nipples and bottles so that a clean boiled one may be used at each feeding.

27. Use nipples with small holes as it is best that baby feed slowly.

28. Each feeding time warm the bottle of milk by placing it in warm water deep enough to cover the milk, put the nipple on and shake the bottle well.

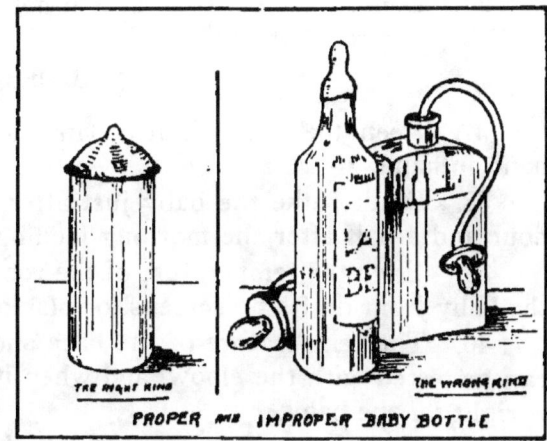

PROPER AND IMPROPER BABY BOTTLE

29. Never put the nipple in your mouth but test the temperature of the milk by sprinkling a few drops on the inner surface of the wrist.

30. Don't urge the baby to take more milk than it wants. Hold the bottle yourself while he feeds and then throw out what is left.

31. Immediately after feeding, rinse the bottle with cold water and fill it with cold water to which has been added a little baking soda.

32.   Before using again the bottle should be washed thoroughly with soap and water and boiled.

33.   Don't dry the bottles and necessary dishes with a towel. Invert and let dry by their own heat after boiling.

34.   Use the home-made sterilizer as shown in the illustration and sterilize all utensils for the baby.

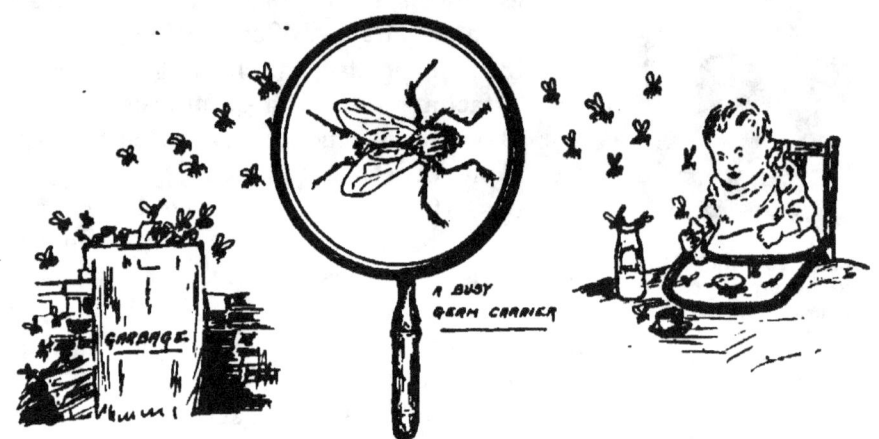

From the Garbage to Baby's Food. Result: Disease and Death.

35.   Keep the filthy germ-laden flies away from the baby and its food. They are the messengers of disease and death.

36.   Don't overfeed, especially in hot weather.

Bathing.

37.   Keep the baby clean. Bathe him every day. Dirt and disease go hand in hand.

38.   Don't bathe the baby just after feeding. The best time is about an hour and a half after the morning feeding, and after the bowels have moved.

39.   Have the temperature of the room about 70 or 72 degrees and protect the baby from drafts by screens, or blankets hung on chairs.

40.   The temperature of the bath should be about 98 or 100 degrees. It can be tested with the elbow, and when it feels neither too cold or too hot, it is right for the baby.

41.   Never add hot water to the bath with the baby in the tub and never leave the baby alone in the tub.

42.   Don't begin the bath until everything is ready at hand so there is no delay and danger of chilling the baby.

43.   The mother's or nurse's hands must be thoroughly clean, free from dirt and germs before the bath is begun.

44.   During very hot weather, sponge the baby off frequently with water a trifle cooler than the bath water.

Clothing.

45. Adapt the clothing to the climate and season. Dress the baby comfortably but not too warm. The garments should be simple, plain and loose, in no way hampering growth or freedom of movement.

46. Don't keep the abdominal band on longer than necessary. As a rule it is not needed after the first ten days. Don't pin it too tight as it is liable to

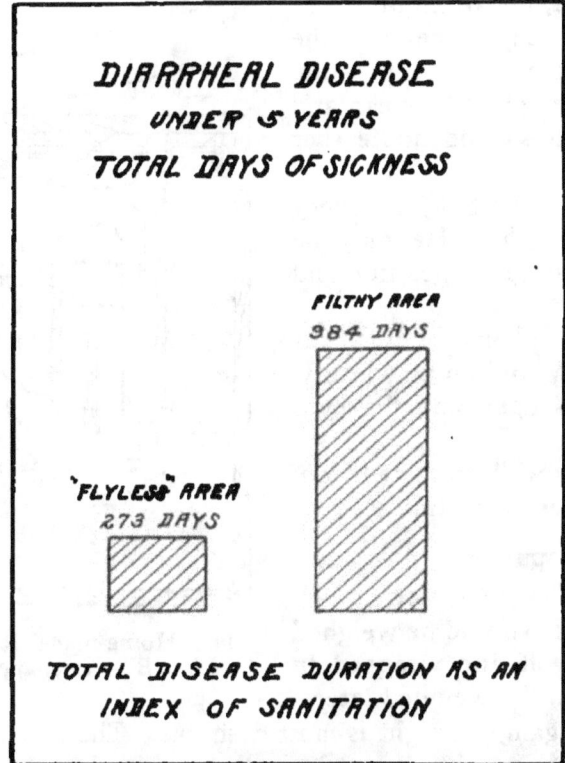

hinder the development of the abdominal muscles and favor a habit of constipation.

47. Change the diapers just as soon and as often as they are wet or soiled. Wash them with soap and water, rinse and hang in the open air to dry.

48. During cool weather the clothing should be of a mixture of fine wool and cotton. When three or four months old, the long skirts may be displaced by short skirts. Make the change on a mild day if possible.

49. In warm weather the baby should wear a light cotton-and-wool shirt and abdominal jacket (band), a light petticoat, a cotton dress and a diaper.

50. The night dress should be put on over a light knitted abdominal jacket and a diaper.

51. In cold weather the night dress may be closed at the bottom with a drawstring as long as the child will tolerate it.

Sleep.

52.   The new-born baby should sleep nearly all the time if healthy.   He often sleeps eighteen to twenty hours out of the twenty-four.   Until three years old a child should sleep twelve hours at night and have a nap in the forenoon and one in the afternoon.

53.   Train the baby to go to sleep at about the same time each day. He should "go to bed" and to sleep about 6:30 at night, for all night.

54.   Let him sleep alone after the first two or three weeks of his life. The bed and clothes must be clean and fresh, a firm mattress and no feather pillow.

55.   Don't take the baby up every time he cries at night.   He may be uncomfortable, change his position and let him sleep.

56.   Give him plenty of fresh air while he sleeps.   Wrap him up warmly, keep the windows open and his eyes well shaded.

57.   Keep him well protected from flies and mosquitoes at all times.

Development.

58.   Weigh the baby often the first few weeks.   He should be weighed with the clothing off and wrapped in a blanket which can be weighed later.

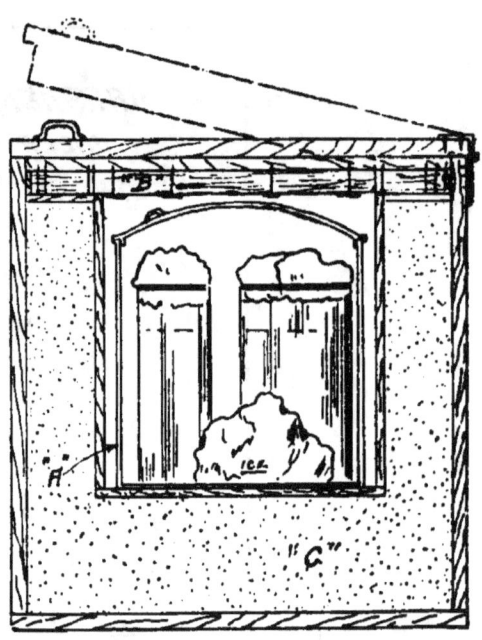

The Home-made Refrigerator. "A" Pail. "B" Newspapers. "C" Sawdust.

59.   A steady gain in weight is most desirable.   The first two or three days he will likely lose in weight; however, in five or six days he should attain his original weight.   If he does not make natural gain, is irritable, restless, dull, have the doctor take a look at him.

60.   At about four months he should hold up his head; at eight months, sit up; at nine months, stand; at one year, walk and probably form a few words.

61.   The teeth will begin to appear about the seventh or eighth month. From the very first the teeth should be looked after carefully and kept clean.

62.   Keep the baby off the floor and out of the draughts.

63.   Guard him against people who have colds or communicable diseases.

64.   Don't kiss the baby on the mouth or allow any one else to do so. Many infections can be communicated in that way.

65.   Don't rock the baby violently or trot him roughly on the knee.

66.   Don't allow him to play with dogs or cats as they are germ carriers.

67. Protect baby's eyes from the direct rays of the sun. Don't lay him on his back in the baby carriage with his eyes unprotected.

68. Don't have everything a glaring, staring white around the baby. Use some softer colors for his immediate surroundings and thus protect his eyes.

WHO AM I?

I am more powerful than the combined armies of the world.

I have destroyed more men than all wars of the nations.

I am more deadly than bullets, and I have wrecked more homes than the mightiest of siege guns.

I steal in the U. S. alone, over $300,000,000 each year.

I spare no one, and I find my victims among the rich and poor alike, the young and old, the strong and weak. Widows and orphans know me.

I loom up to such proportions that I cast my shadow over every field of labor, from the turning of the grindstone to the moving of every railroad train.

I massacre thousands upon thousands of wage earners in a year.

I live in unseen places, and do most of my work silently. You are warned against me, but you heed not.

I am relentless.

I am everywhere—in the house, on the streets, in the factory, at railroad crossings and on the sea.

I bring sickness, degradation and death, and yet few seek to avoid me.

I destroy, crush or maim.

I give nothing, but take all.

I am your worst enemy.

I am—CARELESSNESS.

SAFETY FIRST.

The Bank of Safety pays 100 percent and never fails.

Caution means Safety.

Cultivate personal caution.

The effectiveness of safety first is the big dividends it pays in human lives and limbs every day.

Everyone makes mistakes; some more than others. The efficient man never makes the same mistake twice.

Stop—Look—Listen. Think before you act. Keep your mind on your work and avoid accidents.

It often takes less time to prevent an accident than to report one.

Taking chances fills hospitals with men having mangled bodies and broken limbs.

The safe man or woman is and always will be the best man or woman.

Safety and duty mean about the same thing.

Get the good habit, the right habit, the safety habit.

Be first in the safety army, fighting to drive the careless from its ranks.

First aid to uninjured is safety first. First aid to injured is safety last.

A place for everything and everything in its place helps to reduce accidents.

Think of yourself and the doctor will not have to think of you—Safety first.

Keep off railroad tracks. Fifty-three percent of all railroad accidents occur to trespassers.

All accidents have causes. There are no accidents that were to be.

When you are reckless, you're wrong. Get right.

Stop and think—"Can I afford to get hurt?"

DON'TS.

Don't lose your head in case of accident.

Don't wash away blood clots, they are nature's protection.

Don't give alcoholic stimulants to bleeding patients.

Don't try to stop bleeding with cobwebs or tobacco.

Don't leave a wound uncovered after the bleeding has stopped.

Don't leave tight bandage on a wound too long.

Don't take the bandage off a wound that has been bandaged loosely, if blood soaks through the bandage put on more bandages.

Don't bring strong ammonia too close to the nostrils.

Don't touch explosives after dark.

Don't start a fire with kerosene.

Don't try to fill a lamp that is already lighted.

Don't try to fill a gasoline tank when there is any fire about.

Don't take a light into any place where gas has escaped.

Don't play with firearms.

Don't stand under a tree during electrical storms.

Don't use the telephone during electrical storms, the wire may have become charged.

Don't stand or sit near the stove or radiator during storm for any large metallic mass may become heavily charged with electricity.

Don't stand at the screen door, or near the chimney during an electrical storm.

Don't stand near a wire fence during an electrical storm.

Don't seek shelter in a small shed or building standing apart from larger buildings during a thunderstorm.

Don't cross the street without looking both ways. Keep eyes to the left until the middle of the street is reached, then to the right till the curb is reached.

Don't cross the street except at regular crossings.

Don't pass behind a car without looking to see whether another car, auto or wagon is coming in the opposite direction.

Don't run for street cars; the strain is too hard on the heart.

Don't jump on a moving car.

Don't try to get off a street car or train before it has stopped.

Don't get off a car backward, always face front.

Don't fail on leaving a car to look for passing wagons and automobiles.

Don't put your arms or head out of any vehicle when it is in motion.

Don't touch a wire in the street—the wire may be "alive."

Don't allow children to play on car tracks.

Don't allow children to "hitch on" or steal rides behind street cars, wagons and automobile trucks.

Don't allow children to play in the streets where cars, trucks and automobiles are passing.

Don't try to cross a railroad track before an approaching train.

Don't take chances.

Always "SAFETY FIRST."

Don't forget that health is the key to the garden of happiness.

Don't forget that life is not merely to live—but to be well.

Don't forget that a man may live forty days without food, five days without water, but less than five minutes without air.

Don't forget to ventilate the bedroom properly both in winter and in summer.

Don't forget to ventilate—better pay coal bills than doctor bills.

Don't forget that people are not so much overworked as they are victims of bad air, bad diet, poisons or worry.

Don't forget that daily exercise is nature's tonic.

Don't take violent exercise either immediately before or after meals.

Don't forget that there can be no health without exercise.

Don't eat just before you go to bed.

Don't forget—a simple diet is the best, for many dishes bring many diseases.

Don't forget that all can allow enough time to eat slowly.

Don't eat raw vegetables or fruits without washing them thoroughly. There may be germs of disease on them.

Don't allow flies in the house.

Don't forget to use the fly swatter.

Don't allow flies near the food, especially milk.

Don't buy foods where they are not carefully screened from the flies.

Don't allow the fruits or confections to be exposed to swarms of flies.

Don't allow flies on the baby's mouth or its nursing bottle.

Don't allow children to play with cats, they are germ carriers.

Don't go in a crowd when tired and not feeling well, especially when colds or grippe are about the town.

Don't cough or sneeze, without turning the face from others or covering it with a handkerchief.

Don't allow offensive odors about your person.

Don't neglect the daily bath, either a cold one on rising, or a tepid one before supper.

Don't go to meals with dirty hands.

Don't forget to wash the hands immediately before handling food stuffs.

Don't forget to wash the hands immediately after handling the sick or articles from the sick room.

Don't forget to wash the hands immediately after handling any dirty article.

Don't forget that a cook with dirty hands is liable to infect every person who eats food prepared by her.

Don't forget a nurse with infected hands can spread disease.

Don't forget that cleanliness and health go hand-in-hand.

Don't neglect to consult a dentist at least once a year.

Don't neglect to consult a good optician if the child's eyes trouble him.

Don't allow the child to breathe through his mouth or sleep in an ill-ventilated room.

Don't spit on the street or the walk for it dries and must be breathed by others passing.

Don't allow stagnant water or decayed material to remain about the house for such place are excellent breeding places for mosquitoes.

Don't use drinking cups or towels which have been used by others in public places, for they are carriers of disease germs.

Don't put anything into the mouth except water, food, a fork, spoon, toothbrush and dental thread.

Don't give a pacifier to the baby, it is unsanitary and disfigures the mouth.

Don't neglect to use the toothbrush night and morning.

Don't send the child to school or to play without first thoroughly cleansing the mouth.

Don't wear new stockings or socks without washing them first. The dye may cause blood poisoning.

Don't neglect to teach the child to properly turn the leaves of a book, affix postage stamps, and apply court plaster.

Don't allow the child to sit in a stooped position with head down and shoulders cramped.

Don't allow the child to work or play half heartedly—not breathing deeply.

Don't allow anything to become seated, keep the germ of disease moving by intelligent assistance.

Don't be irregular in the discharge of alimentary excreta.

Don't neglect the slight cough, for just such a cough often leads to pneumonia.

Don't forget to see that your feet are kept warm and dry.

Don't load the system with medicine when suffering with a cough, but learn the cause, then treat intelligently according to the seat of the trouble.

Don't cool off too quickly when very warm by taking ice cold drinks or ice cream; it is very injurious.

Don't take food or drink too hot or too cold.

Don't wash down unmasticated foods.

Don't eat in a hurry or when very tired or angry.

Don't abuse the appetite.

Don't live to eat, but eat to live.

Don't send the child to the store with a nickel when it craves sweets, but give it sugar bread or bake it some oatmeal cookies.

Don't save the milk from baby's bottle, throw it away.

Don't grasp a tumbler or cup around the rim, instead at the bottom.

Don't forget that alcohol has maimed more than battle.

Don't forget that the gymnasium has saved more than the hospital.

Don't be grouchy; it retards progress in anything.

Don't be ill-natured. It disfigures a woman's face far more than wrinkles.

Don't strain the eyes by reading in reclining position.

Don't be irregular.

Don't overwork.

Don't be worked to death but work like a man.

Don't carry the world's troubles on your shoulders.

Don't worry.

Trust the Eternal.

GET THE HABIT.

Get the habit—of early rising.

Get the habit—of retiring early.

Get the habit—of eating slowly.

Get the habit—of being grateful.

Get the habit—of being punctual.

Get the habit—of fearing nothing.

Get the habit—of speaking kindly.

Get the habit—of radiating sunshine.

Get the habit—of sleeping 10 minutes after the noon meal.

Get the habit—of getting away from home once in a while.

Get the habit—of seeking sunshine daily.

Get the habit—of promptness at meals.

Get the habit—of daily physical exercise.

Get the habit—of economy—not stinginess.

Get the habit—of eating but one **hearty** meal a day.

Get the habit—of healing a wound, rather than making one.

Get the habit—of keeping everlastingly at it—if it is right.

Get the habit—of always breathing through the nostrils.

Get the habit—of having a kind word for the stranger.

Get the habit—of hunting for good instead of evil.

Get the habit—of closing your mouth firmly—when angry.

Get the habit—of saying "thank you," no matter how trivial the favor.

Get the habit—of the bull dog tenacity—everlastingly holding on.

Get the habit—of laughing at misfortune—your own not others.

Get the habit—of looking for the good that is in your neighbor; you'll help the crop along.

Get the habit—of closing your mouth when passing from a warm to a less warm atmosphere.

Get the habit—of cleansing your teeth soon after you rise, after each meal, and just before retiring.

Get the habit—of masticating every mouthful of food until it near liquefies.

Get the habit—of stretching and tensing your entire body every morning before arising.

Get the habit—of gargling the throat with cold water after cleansing the teeth.

Get the habit—of being careful at meals; a sour countenance giveth a sour stomach.

Get the habit—of drinking one or more glasses of water (preferably cold), immediately after the morning gargle.

Get the habit—of always exercising before—not after—your morning bath.

Get the habit—of a daily bath, the temperature of the water being suited to the needs of the body rather than the whims of the mind.

Get the habit—of a vigorous rubdown while in the bath—not afterwards.

Get the habit—of a daily air bath, if only for a few minutes, after the cold water bath.

Get the habit—of a sun bath for the entire body whenever time and opportunity permit.

Get the habit—of allowing the sun to paint your face red rather than have your liver paint it yellow.

Get the habit—of not coddling yourself when winter comes; too much clothing is not desirable or hygienic.

Get the habit—of having fresh air in the bedroom the year round; better be carried off by a burglar than by an undertaker.

Get the habit—of relaxing mind and body when you retire; do not try to hold the bed up; let go.

Get the habit—of locking up your think-box when you wish to sleep; put the key under your pillow until morning.

Get the habit—of correct position at the table when eating; at the desk when writing. Do not crook your spine. Push back your chair.

Get the habit—of correct poise and carriage of your body. Do not let your breastbone get too near your backbone.

Get the habit—of the busy bee; while he does not stay long on one flower, he always keeps his mind on one job.

Get the habit—of daily thinking—the night time of the body is the daytime of the soul.

Get the habit—of going when you say "good-bye." When you get ready to go—go.

Get the habit—of the postage stamp. Its chief virtue is not in its size, but in the ability to stick to one thing until it gets there.

Get the habit—of realizing that your mental attitude today determines your success tomorrow.

Get the habit—of realizing that death holds no terror for those who have learned the lesson life.

Get the habit—of realizing that it is only your own grist that comes back to you in the mill of life.

Get the habit—of keeping your eye steadily ahead—and then move ahead. The headlight of an engine will light up a hundred miles of track—if the engine keeps her going.

GENERAL NURSING

Home Nursing.

With the increasing realization of the importance of systematic and intelligent care of the sick in the home, the general principles of ordinary rules of nursing should be made available to as many as possible.

In the great number of homes where the care of the sick must necessarily fall upon the mother or some other member of the family, it is most essential that they be able to accomplish this with little waste of time or energy.

The Home Nurse should culivate the habit of observation and not only be quick to note any change in the symptoms of her patient, but to observe every detail of surroundings with appreciation and understanding of their effect upon her patient's condition. Long practice in the habit of observation (for it is a habit which may be cultivated) will develop a quality very necessary to the nurse. Whatever observations are made, should be noted in a quiet unobtrusive manner, and as far as possible without the patient's knowledge.

The temperature, pulse, and respiration are the chief guides in noting or recording symptoms. Temperature above 98.6° or below 98° should be reported to a physician, if continuing for any period.

While taking the respiration, the nurse should observe whether the breathing is easy and natural, or short and labored.

Rate and quality of the pulse should be noted and recorded as it is very indicative of the patient's condition.

The condition of the tongue should be observed as many diseases have some action, direct or indirect, upon it. The nurse should note whether it is dry or moist, whether its color is normal, red, whitish, coated or otherwise, pale or flabby or swollen. The condition of the other organs or senses—eyes, ears, nose should be observed and abnormal conditions noted.

The nourishment of the patient is extremely important to convalescence. The following is quoted from Isabel Hampton Robb's Handbook of Nursing:

"Reliable information as to the condition of appetite and the amount of food taken by a patient can only be obtained from the nurse's observation; the exact amounts, whether of solid or liquid foods, which are taken should be noted, and also the hours at which they were given. It should be noticed whether the food is eaten with a relish or only with an effort, some patients are inclined to be ravenous, while in others the appetite is capricious, and can be tempted only by particular forms of food. Any inclination to nausea or vomiting should be recorded.

"When food is not retained, the fact should be recorded and reported, with the amount and character of the vomitus. In some instances, this may have peculiar characteristics; if so, it should be covered over and saved to show to the physician. The color and odor of the rejected material are of importance, especially where there is any suspicion of intestinal obstruction, for where this is at all serious the contents of the intestine, not being able to pass by it, are forced back into the stomach, producing vomiting of faecal matter. Small quantities of blood may be changed in the stomach from red to a dark brown color by the action of the gastric juice, so that the vomited matter has been described as 'coffee-ground' vomit. The position and nature of any pain associated with vomiting, and many other symptoms occurring with it should be inquired into."

Any unusual symptoms should be reported to the doctor.

The Home Nurse, whether mother, sister, wife or friend, should have such regard for her patient as to guard faithfully all confidences vouchsafed to her keeping, either by the patient himself, or by the physician.

Do not repeat family secrets or affairs to the first neighbor you meet.—Practice observation, and apply the Golden Rule.

The Nurse.

It is essential that the nurse give proper attention to the care of herself. This is especially true when everything falls upon the mother. She owes it to the entire family as well as to the sick person to guard herself from breakdown and, in caring for the patient suffering from contagious disease, to protect herself and the other members of the family from the disease. Neatness and simplicity should be the keynote of her apparel. Simple dresses of wash material are best and should have very little starch in them. The hair should be washed often enough to insure cleanliness, usually once in two or three weeks, being dressed simply and brushed well away from the face. A daily bath either tub or sponge, should be taken if possible. This is healthful as well as restful and refreshing. The teeth should be brushed and the throat gargled at least twice a day, to insure cleanliness. The hands require special care to prevent the spread of disease. They should be washed frequently and in case of contagion, a good disinfecting solution such as lysol, bichloride of mercury 1-10,000 or alcohol (75%) should be used freely. A solution of carbolic acid is often used but must be handled very carefully to avoid burns. Use of disinfectant should follow thorough scrubbing with soap and brush. The finger nails must be kept short and clean. When disinfectants are much used, a simple hand lotion such as rose water, or glycerine and water, half and half, is beneficial in helping to keep the hands in good condition. Try to keep the hands away from the face or mouth as much as possible.

All disinfectants must be kept from the reach of children. In contagious or infectious diseases, it is much safer for the nurse to isolate herself with the patient and avoid contact with the other members of the family, and other parts of the house, necessary supplies being specially provided for the sick-room. If a wet sheet wrung from bichloride 1-5000 is kept hanging over the outside of the door, the danger to the other members of the household is considerably lessened.

If the nursing and household responsibilities must be assumed by the same person, then a separate dress and cap, which completely covers the hair, must be worn when with the patient. The "all over" apron may be used to advantage here, being hung just inside the door of the sick-room. The dress worn outside is slipped off, before entering the room, and the apron put on before the nurse cares for the patient. If this may not be done, at least keep an "all over" apron inside the door and slip it on when going into the room. The door knobs are another source of infection and it is well to wrap them with a cloth which has been wet in an antiseptic solution. Here again, be sure that the hands are attended to before going to the other parts of the house. These precautions are very necessary to the protection of the other members of the household.

The importance of a certain amount of fresh air and exercise in the open together with a certain amount of sleep, cannot be over-estimated. To sleep with the windows open summer and winter and to take a brisk walk daily are essential to continued good health. To average less than six hours sleep in the twenty-four hours will soon break down the strongest resistance against disease. When there is not much assistance possible in the home, rest and exercise may have to be

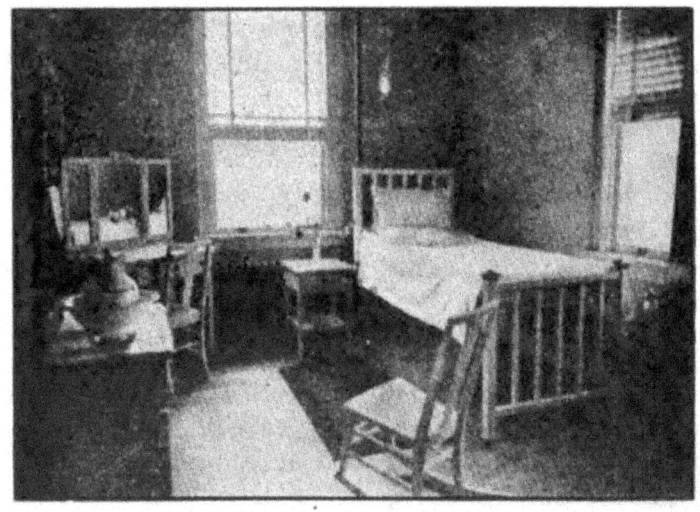

The Sick-room.

taken at various times, but no opportunity should be neglected. Regular habits, in regard to food, rest and exercise are necessary, as it is most difficult when not in good physical condition to give proper care to another.

Provision for the Care of the Sick.

Location of Sick-room.—In choosing the sick-room the chief considerations are means of obtaining proper ventilation, sunshine, and quiet. A room which may be entirely closed from the rest of the house is desirable in case of contagious diseases. For this reason it is often best to have the sick-room located on the second floor. Pure air, quiet and isolation are more easily obtained on the second floor as it is more removed from the household activities. At times this may be inconvenient, however, the room should be so located that it may be easily ventilated, kept quiet and where the disease, in case it is contagious, is least likely to spread to other members of the family. It is always best to have it lo-

- cated on the south side of the house, if possible, as plenty of sunshine is most desirable. The room should be sufficiently large to avoid the appearance of being overcrowded.

Furniture.—The furnishings of the sick-room should be of the simplest nature, in order that they may be properly and easily cleaned. Practically all unnecessary furniture should be removed from the room, such as heavy draperies, upholstered furniture, rugs and carpets which are not needed and are only dust and germ catchers. The simpler the furnishings of the room, the more restful it is to the patient and the easier it is to be cared for. Fresh, washable curtains for the windows, covers for the necessary stands and dressers and a few favorite pictures will redeem the room from too much plainness. A few fresh flowers are usually cheering. These, together with all **growing** plants should be removed from the room at night. A couch or cot for the nurse, an easy chair and one or two straight ones, a stand for the bedside and one or two more as needed, a dresser for bed linen, etc., is sufficient furniture. Above all things see that all openings are well screened with either screens or mosquito netting in order to keep out all insects which may annoy the patient and spread disease.

Lighting.—The amount of light in the room depends much on the condition of the patient and his illness. If the patient is suffering from disease of the brain or eye, the room must be darkened and curtains arranged so that there is no flapping of curtains or sudden flashes of light when the windows are open.

In such infectious diseases as scarlet fever and measles, in which the eyes are often affected, special care should be taken to protect them from the light. This may be done by placing the head of the bed toward the window or by placing a screen between the patient's bed and the window.

Ventilation.—Plenty of fresh air is very necessary. In warm weather this may be easily accomplished by opening two or more windows, one at the top and another at the bottom, or if there is only one window, open it at the top and bottom and open the door. See that the bed is placed well out of the air current so that the air does not blow directly upon the patient. In cold weather, proper ventilation is more difficult. Possibly the simplest way then is to open a window a few inches from the bottom and place a board across the opening or tack a stout piece of cotton cloth across it. If the board is used, a few holes bored through it allows the entrance of more air. This method allows the fresh air to enter between the sashes and be directed upwards. The window on the opposite side of the room may also be lowered a few inches from the top and the shade drawn down to cover the opening. A fireplace or a stove is a most valuable addition to a sick-room, as many impurities are drawn through the chimney. When it is too warm to use either fireplace or stove, lighted lamp, or candle placed in the grate of stove will accomplish the same results.

The air of the sick-room should be changed thoroughly several times each day. This may be safely done in cold weather by putting extra blankets over the patient, leaving only the face exposed, and opening the door and window wide for a few minutes, being careful always not to uncover the patient entirely until the room is warm again. If a very even temperature is required, as is often the case with the very sick or the aged, the room may be indirectly ventilated by opening the windows in an adjoining room and leaving the door open between the two. Don't be afraid of night air, it is often more pure than that breathed during the day.

Temperature.—A thermometer is indispensable in the sick-room and should be placed away from windows, heating apparatus or lights, and should be consulted frequently, regulating the temperature accordingly. This in most instances should range from 68 degrees in the daytime to 65 degrees at night. It should be remembered that the temperature of the patient decreases at night, especially between midnight and 4 a. m., during which time the vitality of the patient is at its lowest ebb. The heat of the room may be regulated by opening and closing the registers or by otherwise controlling the heat supply, by applying extra blankets, etc., avoid closing the windows, thus shutting off the supply of fresh air. If coal stoves are used, special care must be exercised to prevent air from becoming vitiated by escaping gases. In case the air is too dry and irritating, a kettle of boiling water may be kept in the room, or wet blankets or sheets may be hung around the stove or register. It is sometimes difficult to keep the sick-room cool in hot weather. However, this may be done by placing before an open window a tub of cold water to which has been added a pint of salt, allowing the air coming into the room to pass over the water, aids in reducing the temperature. Hanging wet towels or sheets in window or doorway, allowing the air to pass through often helps in cooling a room.

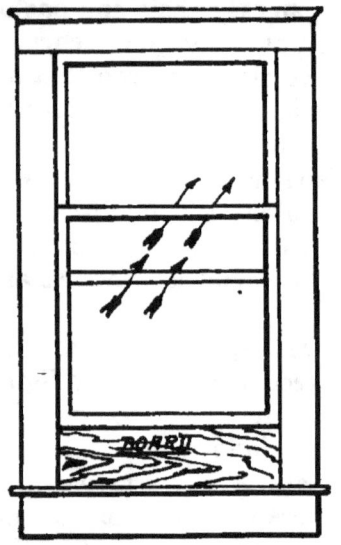

How to use the window-board in ventilating.

Quiet and Privacy.—The sick-room should be kept strictly private and protected from all unnecessary noises, should not be a congregating place for the members of the family or for visitors. All gossip, discussion of the home cares and troubles should be absolutely forbidden in or about the sick-room. Neither should there be any whispering or talking in an undertone as the patient may think his condition is being discussed. The rattling of windows, slamming of doors, squeaking of hinges, etc., should be prevented as these are often very annoying to the patient. Neither should there be allowed any hard rocking in rocking chairs, in fact, everything should be done to make the room quiet and restful.

Care and Cleanliness of Sick-room.—Dirt and disease go hand in hand, therefore it is of the utmost importance to keep the sick-room scrupulously clean. To aid in this, as stated above, it is best to remove all heavy carpets or rugs, draperies, etc., which will catch and hold dust and disease germs. Perhaps the best floor covering is two or three small rugs placed where they are most needed. These may be taken out and thoroughly brushed each day and the floor wiped up with a damp cloth. In contagious disease, the cloth should be wrung from water to which has been added a disinfectant solution. If the floor is covered with matting or carpet, it should be brushed with a broom which is dipped frequently in the solution, so that no dust is raised. The room should be thoroughly dusted each day, using a damp cloth, which lessens danger of contagion. Brooms, dust cloths, dust pans or other utensils used in the sick-room, should be thoroughly disinfected before used in other parts of the house.

Disposal of Excreta, Soiled Linen, etc.—It is of the utmost importance, especially in cases of contagious disease, that all bodily excreta, urine, stools, vomited matter, sputum, bodily discharges of all sorts, be promptly and thoroughly disinfected before being taken from the room and all waste material burned or deeply buried. All waste matter from the body is extremely infectious and unless so handled, liable to spread disease. It is also necessary to disinfect all bed linen, towels and other clothes used about the patient. This may be done by placing in a tub or wash boiler containing sufficient water to cover them completely. If clothes are boiled before being laundered this is a simple way of rendering them safe. Should boiling be impossible, then a disinfectant should be added to the water, and clothes allowed to remain in solution for a number of hours. For this purpose a solution of two ounces of powdered chloride of lime to one gallon of water may be used. Six tablespoonfuls of the 95 percent carbolic acid to one gallon of water is also excellent. Water which has been used for bathing the patient should be disinfected before being disposed of. This can easily be done by adding one teaspoonful of chloride of lime to each gallon of water, allowing it to stand for an hour. All spoons, dishes, glasses, etc., used by the patient, should be placed in a disinfectant solution and boiled before being washed for further use. Neither should these be allowed to come near the food of other members of the family even after being disinfected. All persons who have in any way handled the patient, bedding or utensils from the sick-room should disinfect their hands before performing other duties.

Management and Routine of Sick-room.—Where it is possible, it is always best for the one caring for the sick, whether nurse or mother, to isolate herself with the patient, this being especially desirable in cases of contagious disease. The same person should assume full responsibility for the management and care of the sick, receiving all instructions from the attending physician, thus avoiding mistakes or confusion regarding orders and treatment. It is well to do everything systematically, keeping a record for the physician. When the patient first awakens in the morning, take the temperature, pulse and respiration. After this wash the mouth and teeth, bathe the face and hands, brush the hair. In case an enema is needed this is generally given before the breakfast unless the patient is very weak, in which case it is given an hour or more after breakfast. After half an hour of rest the patient is given the treatment prescribed by the doctor. - The daily bath is usually given midway between breakfast and lunch or dinner. Following the bath, the clothes and bed linen are changed and the patient made comfortable. The sick-room is then cleaned and put in order. These essentials accomplished, the order for the rest of the day is left to the discretion of the nurse.

Care of Sick-room Supplies.

All dressing or surgical supplies, such as cotton and gauze, should remain in original packages until used. After opening the package the part not used should again be carefully wrapped.

All scissors, corks and bottles should be cleaned thoroughly by boiling before using.

Medicines or solutions should not be used when kept more than six months.

Always use fresh washcloths, towels, muslin, etc.

Never use cotton, gauze or dressing a second time. For each dressing, use sufficient of each article required. Burn old dressing, empty liquids and wash receptacles.

All appliances and utensils used during illness should be kept scrupuously clean by proper daily care.

It is well to wash and boil all dishes once each day, or in case of typhoid, pneumonia and other infectious diseases, after each using.

Hot water bags, douche bags, rubber rings, basins, etc., may be kept clean by scrubbing frequently and boiling when necessary. All rubber goods may be boiled if placed in sufficient cold water to more than cover articles. Put on stove and bring to a boil, remove from hot water and dry thoroughly.

Bedpans and urinals or douche pans should be thoroughly scrubbed with hot water, soap and brush each day, and washed with cold water after each using. A small brush may be used to reach the back part of bed- and douche-pan, and a handled brush for urinal. There is no odor about either bedpan or urinal if kept perfectly clean.

Dustcloths, dustpans, mops and brooms should be kept specially for the sick-room and should be carefully cared for after each day's use.

When there is no further need for medical or surgical supplies, or sick-room necessities, they should be thoroughly cleaned, carefully wrapped and labeled and placed in a convenient chest or closet where they may be ready for use if occasion arises.

Choice and Preparation of the Bed.

The Bed.—It is of the utmost importance, especially in the case of protracted illness, that the patient have the right kind of bed. If obtainable, a single or three-quarter-size iron or brass bedstead is best. These are usually light and can easily be moved about in the room. They are also easily cleaned and disinfected after the patient has recovered. The springs and mattress should be of the very best. If the springs are too weak, they will allow the patient to roll toward the center of the bed and in case a full-sized bed is used, this is not only very uncomfortable for the patient but very inconvenient for the nurse. The mattress should be firm and smooth as this will add greatly to the comfort and welfare of the patient, especially in protracted illness. Bed-sores are often due to an uneven mattress. The best mattresses are filled with good horse hair or Ostermoor felt. and covered with strong blue and white ticking, since these colors do not fade when disinfected. Although expensive, such a bed wears well and lends much to the comfort of the patient. In order to facilitate the handling of the patient it is best to have the bed high enough to bring the mattress on a level with the waist line of the nurse.

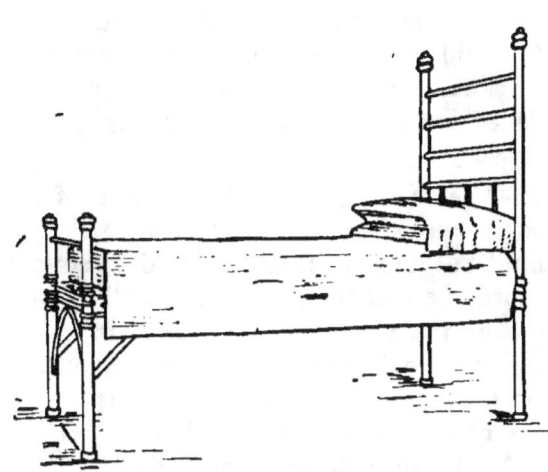

The proper kind of bed for the sick.

Bedding.—The sheets should be large enough to tuck in well at the head and foot and on both sides in order to protect the mattress and prevent wrinkling, keeping the bed smooth and comfortable. All the bedding should be of light weight but warm, and of a kind easily washed. Blankets being better than comforters. If comforters are used they should be made of wool filling and simple covering. This style of comforter is no less expensive than are good blankets and make less desirable covering. The pillows should not be too large or firm, should be made of feathers, the case should be large enough to protect the pillow well and be easily changed. In case of illness or when caring

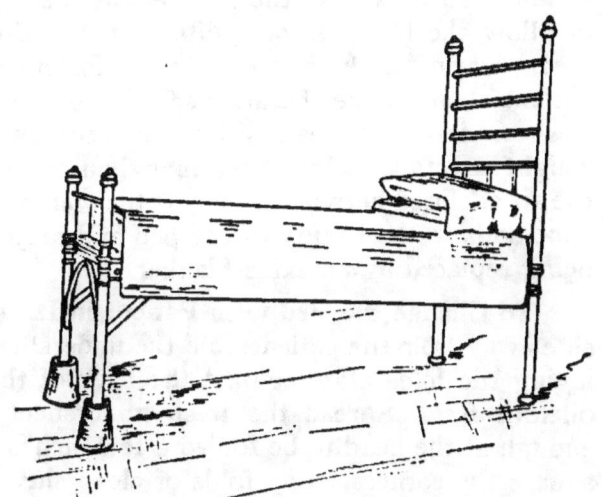

In cases of fracture or hemorrhage it is often necessary to raise the foot of the bed.

for an unconscious patient, or patient having head wounds, or one suffering from hemorrhage of the lungs, it is well to protect the pillow by encasing in soft rubber sheeting over which the usual pillow cover is placed. The bed should be covered with a light spread, or, if this is not possible, or the weight is uncomfortable, a sheet will do. All the bedding should be kept thoroughly clean and fresh, being frequently changed and aired.

How to Protect the Mattress.—To protect the mattress against accidents, which are very apt to occur when water is used for treatment or when the patient is too ill to be responsible, a piece of rubber sheeting or oil-cloth or even a pad of newspapers, in emergency, should be placed across the bed in the center, over the lower sheet, another sheet doubled and spread across the surface and tucked in well at either side. This is called the draw sheet and should be kept smooth and tight. When not necessary, the rubber or oil-cloth should be removed, and again placed under the patient when a treatment is being given or the bedpan is being used.

Making the Bed for the Patient.—The making of the bed is one of the most important duties of the mother or nurse who is caring for any sick person. Therefore, special attention should be given to this duty and directions carefully followed. In making a bed, turn the mattress, be sure that the lower sheet is spread smoothly and tightly over the mattress and tucked in on all sides. If the sheet is not large enough to reach well under the mattress, it can be pinned to the mattress top, bottom, or sides with safety pins. Care should be taken to put the sheets on straight for otherwise wrinkles will be formed or the sheet torn if pinned. Next, the rubber or oilcloth, if this is necessary, should be spread smoothly over the bed and covered with another and narrower sheet called the "draw sheet" which can be easily removed. These should both be well tucked in. Another sheet should be spread over these, and well tucked in at the foot and sides of the bed, but left long enough to fold well back over the blankets at the top, as it is irritating and unclean to allow the blankets or quilts to touch the neck and face of the patient. Clean, warm, blankets instead of comforters should be used as covering. The patient should never be allowed to sleep with the head under the covers, as fresh air is very necessary for the recovery from any illness. Several light weight covers are always warmer than one cover of equal weight because of the air enclosed between them. If the weight is not annoying, a white counter-pane adds to the beauty of the bed and may be removed and folded at night, being replaced by an extra blanket.

To Change the Bed with Patient in It.—First, loosen the bedding on the side away from the patient, fold the undersheet and the drawsheet fan fashion, laying the folds close against the back of the patient, leaving the rubber or oilcloth free. Spread the fresh undersheet smoothly and tuck in, leaving enough at the head to be folded a few inches under the mattress and mitre or square the corners. Lay folds of clean sheet also against back. If the sheet is short it can better be spared at the foot of the bed than the head. Now draw the rubber sheeting smooth and if not long enough to tuck in at both sides secure it to the mattress with two safety pins, laid flat. Then place a fresh clean sheet and tuck in and fold the same as the undersheet, laying all the folds as flat as possible against the patient's back. With one arm under the shoulder and one under the hip, well around the further thigh, turn the patient gently on the back. Put on the fresh gown. Turn patient to the other side and draw the folds of bedclothes slowly through, beginning with the soiled linen and bath blankets, which are quickly put out of the way. Then draw the undersheet tight and tuck in, then the rubber, and finally the draw-sheet, being sure that everything is smooth and tight. Spread a clean upper sheet over the bed, allowing enough at the top to fold over eight inches, draw

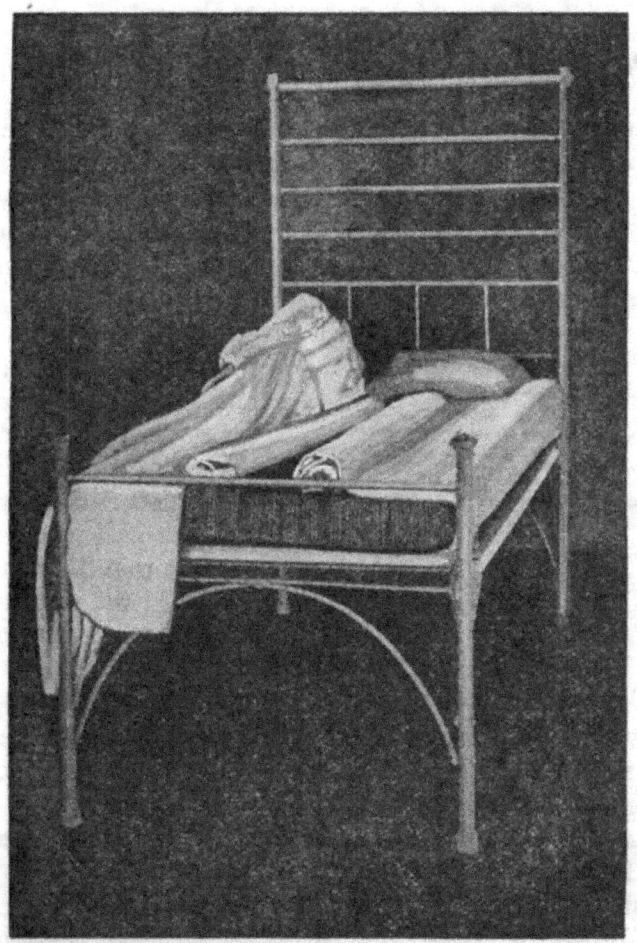

Changing the bed with the patient in it.

the upper bath blanket downward from beneath, without exposing patient. Tuck the sheet in well at the foot but be careful that it is not tight enough to draw across the feet. Put on the blankets or comforters and mitre the corners of these and the sheet in one. Then put on the spread which should be of light weight, if possible. This can be tucked in or not, as desired, but if tucked in, it is better to mitre covers separately. Allow the spread to come up high enough to fold in over the blankets a few inches and draw the fold of the sheet over this. Always put the top sheet on with the right side next to the patient, then when folded back the hem is right side out.

Where economy in laundry is necessary, sheets that are not badly soiled may be aired out-of-doors for several hours and used again. It is always well to air blankets, comforts and pillows frequently. Where a clean gown every day is not possible, one may be kept for the night and another for the day and thus be used for several days.

Care and Treatment of Patient.

Taking the Temperature.—Unless the patient is not responsible or in case of a small child, the temperature is usually taken by placing the clinical thermometer underneath the tongue to one side with the tongue pressed down upon it, the lips tightly closed for a period of two minutes. See that the patient has had nothing to drink for at least fifteen minutes previously. Temperature is also taken in the axilla or armpit, in the groin or by rectum. In an axillary temperature, the part must be wiped free from perspiration, the bulb of the thermometer pressed closely into the axilla and the arm held closely against the side for a period of five minutes. If taken in the groin the thermometer is laid lengthwise and the flesh held over it for the same period. In taking a rectal temperature, the thermometer is well oiled and inserted about one and one-half inches and allowed to remain in the rectum three minutes. In the first two methods 1 degree is added to the temperature registered, and in the last from ½ to 1 degree is subtracted.

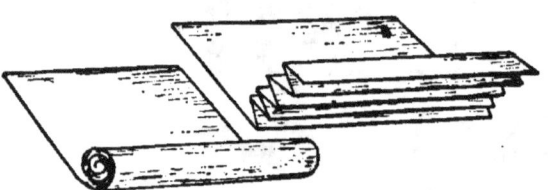

Different methods of folding the draw-sheet when changing the bedding.

However, the axillary and the rectal methods are only resorted to when caring for small children or irresponsible patients. After the temperature has been taken and recorded the thermometer should be shaken with quick jerks downward until the mercury registers below the normal point (98.6°), wiped thoroughly with cotton wet in alcohol and dried and returned to its case. Care is taken to "shake down" the thermometer after the temperature has been taken, also to look at it carefully before again using, thus avoiding all incorrect temperature registration. The doctor, nurse, and entire family have been very much disturbed at a mistaken rise indicated in the temperature, due to failure on the part of the nurse to "shake down" the thermometer. All such unnecessary shocks should be avoided.

The Pulse.—This is usually taken at the radial artery, the finger tips, not the thumb, being placed lightly along the inside of the wrist in direct line with the thumb of the patient. The pulsations are then counted with the eye on the second hand of the watch. They are counted for half a minute and then multiplied by two to obtain the number of heart beats per minute. In the normal adult this ranges from 60 to 80 beats, and in children from one to seven years of age, 80 to 120, and in babies 110 to 120 beats per minute. However, this varies much according to the condition of the patient. After a few trials the nurse will begin to detect the character of the pulse, whether it is full and bounding as in the early stages of fever, or thin and feeble where the vitality is low, due to age or hemorrhage or other causes, also whether it is regular or irregular or if there has been a decided change in any way. In case of noticeable change, the physician should be notified immediately.

Respiration.—This is the inhaling and exhaling of air, i. e., breathing. Therefore, the action of the two makes one respiration. The average rate for an adult in health is about eighteen (respirations) a minute. It is quicker in childhood than in later life and also varies much according to the physical condition. Respirations may be counted by listening closely to the breathing or by watching the rise and fall of the chest with the watch held sufficiently close for the nurse to see both motions and second hand at the time.

The Daily Bath.—This is very necessary to the comfort and well-being of the patient. Not only does it assist Nature by keeping the pores open and allowing the poisons of the body to escape, but the necessary rubbing stimulates the circulation and is very restful and refreshing. See first that the temperature of the room is not more than 72° and that the windows and doors are closed. Have everything that is needed at hand before beginning. For the ordinary bath this consists of a pair of soft blankets, a good sized bath towel, a face towel, wash cloth, soap and a bottle of 75% alcohol. Have a foot tub or large basin half full of warm water, a large pitcher of hotter water, a slop jar, and a table or chair which may be used as a washstand. Also have the clean bed linen ready on a chair close to the bed. In cold weather, it is better to place linen where it will be warm when needed, and it is a good plan to have a hot water bag or heated flat iron well wrapped at the patient's feet before beginning the bath.

When everything is ready, draw the patient to the most convenient side of the bed and replace the top covers with one of the bath blankets. To do this without exposure, spread the blanket over the patient first and then draw the bedding from underneath downward, folding the latter neatly over the foot of the bed. Turn the patient on her side, spread half the other blanket smoothly the length of the bed and fold in fan fashion the half nearest the patient and press it close against her back. Now turn her gently on her back and a little to the further side. Pull the folds of the blanket so that it is smooth beneath the body.

Then remove the nightgown. Use a mild soap such as castile or ivory and use it sparingly. Begin with the face and ears, then the arms, neck, chest, abdomen, thighs, legs and feet, washing each part separately and in the order given. . Dry each part thoroughly as soon as washed. Now turn on the side and wash the back and the rest of the body, using gentle but brisk friction. Rinse well after using the soap. Unless there is some reason for not doing so, place the foot tub carefully at the foot of the bed and place the patient's feet in the water for a few moments while the legs are being bathed. When the weather is cool or if the patient is sensitive to air, the bath is better given under the blanket. This is easily done by holding the blanket tent fashion with one hand a few inches away from the part being washed. In any case expose only the part being bathed, and when finished cover quickly. When about half the bath is finished, the water should be changed, being replaced by the heated water in the pitcher. After the bath and while the patient is still on her side, rub the back thoroughly with alcohol which has been kept standing in a pitcher of hot water for about ten minutes. If desired, the entire body may be rubbed with alcohol. Rubbing is not only restful, but stimulates the circulation, thus keeping the body in better condition.

When giving an alcohol rub, avoid the face. Begin with the neck and chest and then downward over the body as with the general bath. If it is difficult to move the patient, or there is reason for not doing so, then bathe and rub all but the back before the patient is turned on the side. While she is turned, change the first half of the bed so that one turning is all that is necessary.

Care of Teeth and Mouth.—The teeth and mouth of a sick person should receive special attention. In extreme cases where the tongue or lips are dry, or the accumulation of mucus or the brown excretion called "sordes" forms rapidly, attention may be needed every hour or so. However, in ordinary cases thorough cleansing morning and evening is sufficient. When the patient is able to use the brush herself this is made easier by having the head turned on one side at the doubled edge of the pillow and a small basin placed close to the mouth. Have a small pitcher of tepid water to which a good mouth-wash has been added (borax or listerine are very good), after using the brush thoroughly rinse the mouth freely. When the patient is too sick to do this, the nurse should use small squares of cotton wound around the index finger and wet with the mouthwash, gently go over the teeth and gums, roof of mouth and tongue, until they are clean. Several changes of compress may be necessary. The nurse should be most careful to have a piece of newspaper or paper in readiness to receive the soiled or discarded cloth. This should be burned immediately and the hands of the nurse scrubbed with soap, hot water, and a good brush before performing other duties. When the lips and mouth are dry and inclined to be sore as in fever, a solution of glycerine and water, half and half, is healing. Lemon juice added to the wash is both pleasant to the taste and cleansing. When a patient is on a liquid diet and especially when milk is given, it is well to rinse the mouth after each feeding. Next, the hands and face of the patient are washed in tepid or cool water, the hair brushed back from the face and she is ready for breakfast. If convalescent, she may be propped with pillows to a sitting posture or a straight-backed chair may be turned upside down with the front legs resting against the head of the bed and pillows placed at the back. (See illustration of back rest).

Care of the Hair.—Turn the patient's head to one side and tuck the end of the pillow in so as to leave the back of the head free. The hair should be evenly parted and braided in two braids—it is much more comfortable to lie on and easier to keep free from tangles. Place a towel to catch loose hairs and unbraid one side at a time and comb or brush gently. Beginning at the ends work upward. Hold the hair in one hand between the comb and the head so that there is no pulling. The braid should begin well below the ear. When the hair is very thick or has become matted it may be necessary to subdivide it and do only a little at a time. (Do not tire the patient). Now turn the head to the other side and proceed with the other braid, seeing that no loose hairs are left about. In doing up the patient, the time should be watched carefully so as not to have medicine, milk or nourishment overdue.

This method of procedure is practical when a patient is not critically ill or unable to be moved without danger and must be modified or changed to fit conditions. For instance, it may be necessary for two persons to give the treatments and bath and change the bed, or the patient may be too weak to have everything done at one time, and may need to rest at intervals; in any case great care should be taken not to tire or exert her more than is absolutely necessary. After the patient is resting comfortably, the room may be attended to.

Changing the Nightgown.—This is an easy matter if the gown is short and opens down the back as the hospital gowns do. Such gowns should be used for very sick persons or for those who should be moved very little. If an open gown is used, first remove one sleeve (always begin to remove clothing from the sound side first and clothe the injured side first) and put on the corresponding sleeve of the clean gown by reaching through the sleeve and grasping the patient's hand and drawing it through the sleeve. If the gown is a closed one, instruct the patient to bend the knees with the feet flat on the bed. Then pull gown up as far as possible. If the patient is helpless, pass the hand under the buttocks, raise the patient meanwhile pulling the gown up with the free hand. Place one arm under the head and shoulders of the patient (supporting the head by allowing the neck to rest in the bend of the arm) and draw the gown up around the neck. Then pass one hand through the upper armhole of the sleeve and grasp the patient's arm near the wrist, drawing off the sleeve with the other hand. Lift the gown over the head and remove. Put the clean gown on with the same movements reversed.

Making Patient Comfortable in Bed.—One of the most important duties in attending the sick is that of making the patient comfortable. In these days we know that the mind has much to do with the condition of the body. Therefore, many treatments and much medicine will not have the desired effect if the mind is not at ease and the body not comfortable. The mind of the patient should be made and kept happy. If there are household duties which are a source of worry to the patient, see that these (duties) are assumed by another and the patient's mind at rest, as this has much to do with her recovery. It is often well to explain the treatment which is being prepared for a patient, especially if she is at all anxious or alarmed.

The back should be rubbed with alcohol frequently. This hardens the skin and thus prevents bed sores as well as cooling the back and relieving the tired feeling. Rubbing the back with long strokes and using pressure on the upward strokes is sometimes very gratifying.

The position should be varied frequently and pressure on any part of the body carefully and frequently relieved.

Bedsores.

Bedsores are one of the most troublesome complications which may occur in any illness.

Bedsores result from continued pressure or friction on certain spots, and are provoked by wrinkles in the sheet, rubber or draw sheet, by dampness or uncleanliness of patient or bed. They are most apt to occur from pressure on the shoulders, hips, buttocks, elbows and heels from friction, between the knees and ankles, on the elbows, back of head or ears. The nurse should watch the patient's entire body. Keep the patient scrupulously clean, rub any reddened parts with seventy-five percent alcohol, powdered with cornstarch or bismuth and borax, equal parts.

Remove the pressure whenever possible by use of rubber ring, or the improvised cotton ring. Change the patient's position whenever possible.

Keep the bed very clean and dry, and the sheets free from wrinkles. The slightest wrinkle may cause a bedsore.

Of course, the condition of the circulation and the weight of the patient, as well as the length of the illness, effect the possibility of this most uncomfortable and deplorable occurrence, which it is sometimes impossible to prevent. However, bedsores are usually due to neglect, and are somewhat of a reflection on the care being given.

Great care in the foregoing details will usually keep the patient's body in good condition. Should a bedsore develop, the treatment is that required for any surgical case and is directed by the attending physician.

Helping the Patient Into Bed.—The simplest way to render the necessary assistance is to have the patient sit well over on the bed, resting both hands on the bed at either side. Then, the attendant places one arm around the patient's waist, the other under the knees. While the patient bears as much of her weight on her hands as she can, the nurse lifts the body and lower limbs, placing the patient comfortably in bed. With the combined effort of nurse and patient, this is easily accomplished.

Lifting Patient From Chair.—In lifting a patient from a chair, place one arm diagonally across the back, with hand in opposite armpit; place the arm under the thighs, just above the knees, and instruct patient to keep her body as stiff as possible and to place her arms across your back and chest clasping her hands on your farther shoulder. Be sure her arms do not rest on the back of the neck as the weight should be borne by the muscles of the back instead of the shoulder muscles.

If the patient is helpless, two persons should stand on the injured side or one on either side of the patient, and the first should pass one arm under the shoulders and the other under the small of the back. The second helper should pass one arm under the small of the back and one under the knees. Both should lift together and carrying the patient over the foot of the bed, place her on the bed. There are many other ways of lifting patients. The foregoing are among the simplest methods.

To Raise a Weak or Helpless Patient.—Have everything close at hand to slip into place and a second person to help. Place the hands well under the back, one from either side, and raise slowly. Do not let the weight of the body rest upon the end of the spine. A soft pillow tucked well down against the body, one under the knees and another, or a rolled up comforter, placed between the feet and the foot of the bed will help to keep her from slipping down uncomfortably. These things should be accomplished with as little exertion to the patient as possible. A patient sitting up in bed should be well protected about the shoulders. A bed table is easily made by sawing off the legs of an ordinary chair or sewing table about fifteen or twenty inches below the top. This is placed on the lap of the patient. (See illustration of bed table and breakfast tray). If a table cannot be obtained a firm pillow well flattened out, but not too heavy, will answer. Should it be necessary to use a pillow it is well to protect it against accidents, by covering with oilcloth or several thicknesses of paper.

Getting Patient Up in a Chair.—Usually the second step in convalescence is permission to sit in a chair from one-half to three-quarters of an hour. To do this, place a comfortable chair as near the bed as possible, in a position which will avoid draught, and where the patient can look out of the window, and so that as few steps as possible need be taken in reaching it. Place a soft pillow in the seat and one at the back. Over these spread a blanket cornerwise, leaving it long enough to cover the feet well. Put kimona on the patient by turning her on her side, placing the kimona so she will lie on the back width, turn her on her back and then the sleeves can be readily slipped over the arms. Fasten the kimona. Turn the stockings so that a part of the foot is turned into the leg so that the foot can be put in first and then they can be drawn on more easily. Bedroom slippers may then be put on. Draw patient to one side of the bed and lift as before described. She should be given as much support as possible while walking. When in the chair, she should be wrapped loosely in the blanket. Special attention should be paid to adjusting the head comfortably, placing extra pillows if needed. A small footstool or hassock under the feet not only gives needed support, but keeps the feet off the floor, thus helping to avoid a draught. Sometimes just the right angle of the chair can best be obtained by placing a book under the rocker at the front of the chair. Care should be taken not to allow the patient to sit up too long the first day. Unless the physician has stated the exact length of time, a half to three-quarters of an hour will probably not be too long. However, if the patient shows signs of fatigue it is better to help her into bed, and allow her to sit up again later in the day. In case of protracted illness, it is very restful to the patient to sit up for an hour or so at bedtime. Thus entirely changing the position and allowing the bed to be freshened and cooled, before completing preparations for the night.

Carrying the Patient in a Sitting Position.—(Four-handed seat).—If the patient is not too sick or helpless to sit up she may be carried on a four-handed seat made in the following way: The nurse should stand on one side of the patient and assistant on the other and together raise her to a sitting position. Then each one should clasp her own left wrist with her own right hand, then grasp each other's right wrist with the left hand. Place the seat thus formed in a position so that the patient can easily seat herself on it. She should support herself by putting her hands over the shoulder of each attendant, and be carried where desired.

Use of the Knee Rest.—Sometimes it is necessary to keep the patient's knees flexed and for this purpose a support is easily made consisting of two boards fastened at the top to form an angle. The center of the lower edge of the board next the patient is cut out so as to permit the giving of the bedpan without removing the support. It is well to secure the support by strapping to either side of the bed; the angle or part of support coming in contact with the patient should be carefully padded with a pillow or comforter. The patient may be kept from slipping down in bed by placing a box of desired size, which

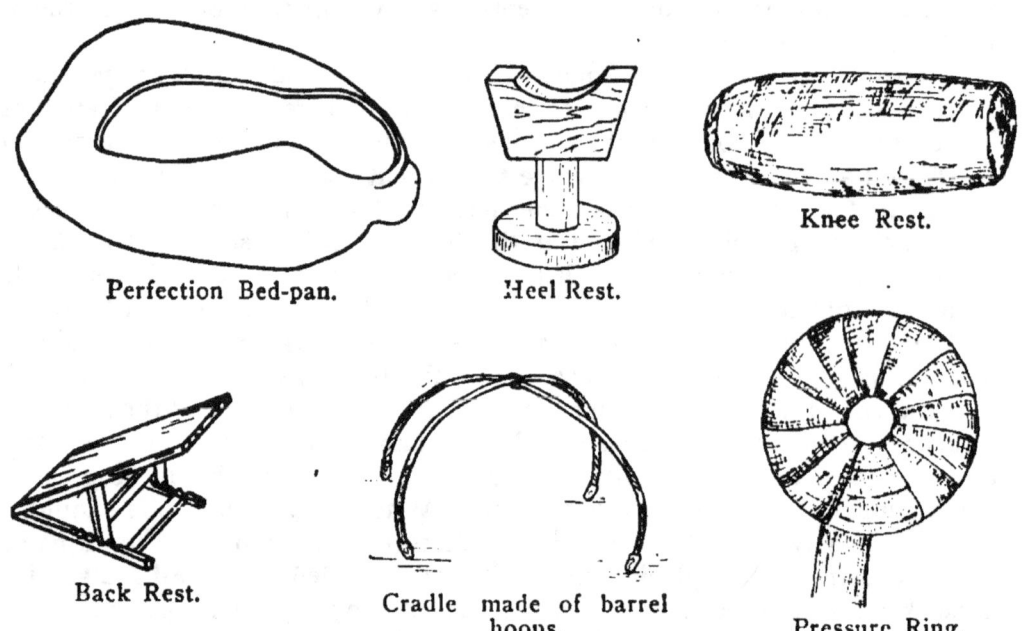

Perfection Bed-pan.   Heel Rest.   Knee Rest.

Back Rest.   Cradle made of barrel   Pressure Ring.
                    hoops.

is covered by a pillow, between the feet of the patient and the foot of the bed. A very simple means of giving support to patients is accomplished by placing a pillow under the knees, and likewise, if desired, at the feet.

Use of Back Rest.—When a patient is convalescing from a long illness, the physician usually permits her to sit up in bed for fifteen or twenty minutes several times a day, until she has gained sufficient strength to sit in a chair. For this a support to the back is necessary. This is usually accomplished by an improvised back rest. (See figure above). A canvas back is probably the best, however, a straight-backed chair may be used by turning upside-down, thus placing the top of the back of the chair at the base of the patient's spine—the seat against the head of the bed. The space between the patient and the chair should then be filled with a pillow or folded blankets. This makes a very comfortable and easily improvised rest. If the patient needs support while the rest is being adjusted, have everything in readiness, then draw the patient toward the head of the bed, lift her to a sitting position and support her by passing your arm, which is nearest the foot of the bed, across her chest, allowing her to lean on it while the rest is being placed.

Use of Cradle.—If the weight of the bed clothing causes discomfort, which is frequently the case, supports called bed cradles should be used. A cradle may be made by sawing a barrel hoop in halves. After securely fastening the hoops together in the center (X) of the semi-circle, they should be padded with sheet wadding or cotton batting and wrapped with bandage either torn from an old sheet, or a surgical bandage may be used if more convenient. This support should then be placed over the part of the body from which you wish to remove the weight of the bed clothing. The regular surgical cradle is usually made of cane, being of light weight and made in various sizes, is therefore more satisfactory. This cradle may be purchased at any surgical supply house for a reasonable amount.

If protection is required for the foot and leg, pillows may be so arranged in the bed as to remove the pressure. Air rings, or rubber rings, and improvised heel cushions are all devices used to relieve pressure on various parts of the body. A ring such as the one pictured may be made in varying sizes, and is usually made by taking several sheets of sheet wadding and folding in thirds, cutting across in the center and bandaging from the center, covering the outer parts and shaping the ring with bandage pressure to make it round. This may be used under the ear, which often becomes tired and sore, at the elbow, at the heel and between the knees. If the patient lies on the side the knees frequently becoming sore from pressure. Relieve pressure, as evidenced, by frequent rubbing with alcohol is the treatment indicated.

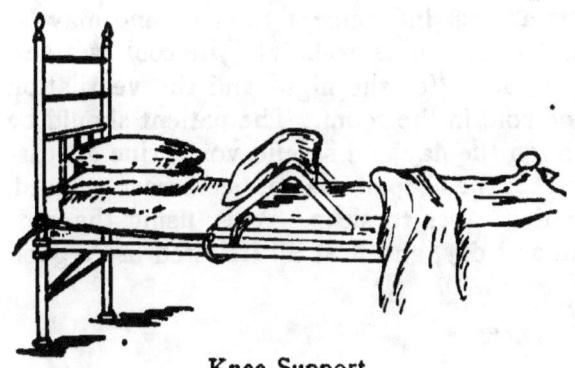

Knee Support.

Clothing of the Patient.— The patient's comfort and recovery are aided very materially by the use of proper clothing. Plenty of loose durable nightgowns, a loose kimona, stockings and bedroom slippers should be near at hand during the period of convalescence. All clothes used by the sick should be well aired and warmed before wearing. As soon as any article of clothing or the bed of the patient becomes damp or soiled, it should be changed immediately as such condition is not only uncomfortable but also endangers the patient's welfare.

Care of Patient at Night.—As night approaches, care should be taken to get the patient into a quiet, restful state of mind. If the patient is at home do not try to quiet every sound because it is too hard to maintain absolute quiet, but do not allow sharp noises. If the patient is restless and is not soothed by some treatment, he becomes very nervous and miserable. The watchful, careful attendant will find many things to do which are very soothing. A few suggestions may be helpful along this line.

It is a good plan to wait one hour after supper before beginning preparations for the night. The mouth and teeth are first attended to and, if it has been a trying day it will be most refreshing if the patient has a second bath. This time it should be of tepid water with a little alcohol or baking soda added and very little or no soap used. If this is not possible, wash the face and hands, then give a thorough alcohol rub, proceeding in the same way as the one given after the morning bath. It is only necessary to use an upper blanket for this. In rubbing, use long, even, up-and-down strokes, with firmer pressure on the upward strokes and very little on the downward. Short, choppy rubbing is often very irritating and should be avoided. Give special attention to all parts that are under pressure, such as the hips, buttocks, lower part of back, shoulder blades, elbows and heels. These very easily become irritated and sore. It is at these points that bedsores are found. For this reason no patient should be allowed to lie in one position too long at a time. And here the plan of having one gown for the day and another at night is advantageous, for it is another addition to the comfort of the patient to put on a cool, aired garment. If the same gown must remain on, be sure that there are no crumbs under the patient and if any have collected there or in the bed, brush them out with the hand or small clean whiskbroom, kept for the purpose. Loosen the drawsheet, rubber protector and undersheet and, beginning with the latter, draw them tight and smooth and tuck them well under the mattress. Then brush and braid the hair and take the temperature. If she feels so inclined and the supper has been light, give a glass of warm milk, malted milk or something of the sort. A warm drink is a great inducement to sleep and may be resorted to during the night when the patient is wakeful. In cool weather, be sure that there is extra covering put on for the night and the ventilation so arranged that it will not grow too cold in the room. The patient should be urged to take water frequently through the day and should void urine at least three times in the twenty-four hours. If the bedpan has not been recently used, give it the last thing before the patient goes to sleep. After using the bedpan be sure that the parts are clean and dry, and if at all irritated use a good powder freely.

Diet.

The matter of diet is of such prime importance in caring for the sick, that it should receive special attention. There is, however, only time to give it brief consideration and to make a few general suggestions regarding points in serving, outlining a possible menu for various illnesses, and adding a few recipes for making certain dishes.

The recipes have been taken from various books on invalid cookery. The patient's menu should be carefully planned in conjunction with the physician and with consideration given the individual's taste, if possible. Meals should be served with regularity and promptness.

The materials used should be of the very best, well cooked, carefully seasoned and daintily served.

All **hot** foods should be very hot, and all **cold** foods should be very cold. Hot dishes should cover all hot foods in order to keep them so; the cover also adds to the joy of the meal by awakening the patient's curiosity as to the covered contents.

The odors from food while being prepared should never be allowed to reach the sick-room.

The tray should be sufficiently large and well covered with a fresh tray

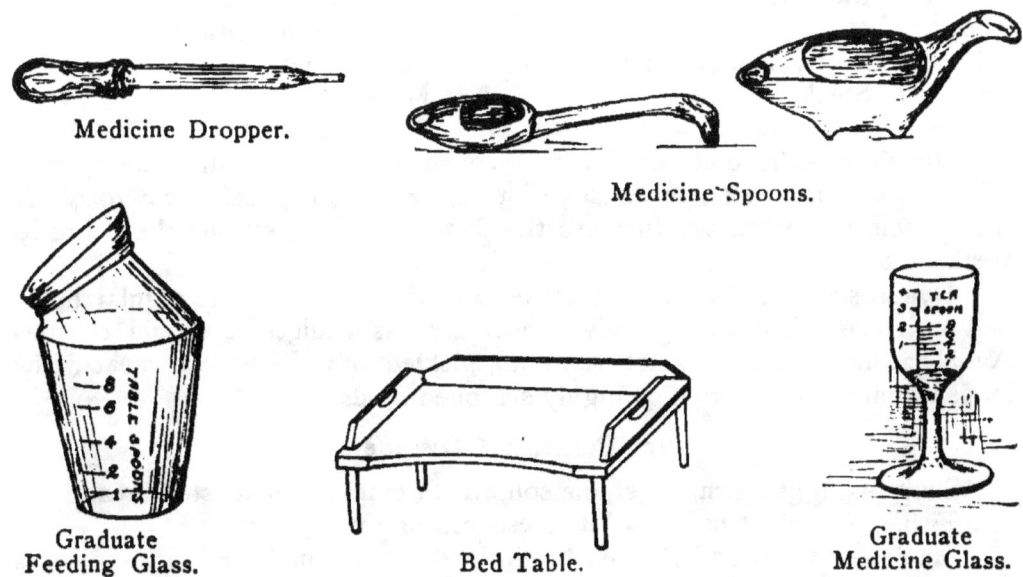

Medicine Dropper.

Medicine Spoons.

Graduate
Feeding Glass.

Bed Table.

Graduate
Medicine Glass.

cloth, the napkin spotless, the dishes the prettiest in the house and the silverware shining. A cut flower, a spray of autumn leaves, or rose petals in the fingerbowl all add to the attractiveness of the tray and to the joy of the meal. A real good joke or apt quotation clipped from some magazine or paper, and laid on the tray will often divert the patient's thought.

The face and hands should be washed just prior to serving the tray.

In long continued illness the nurse often finds it difficult to vary the menu, therefore, the following suggestions have been made in the hope of assisting her:

Diets for Special Diseases.

Anemia.—Anemia or other blood disorders require easily digested foods, and those rich in salts, such as milk, eggs, rare beef, sweet fruit and green vegetables.

Cardiac Diseases.—When the kidneys are also affected, the quantity of protein foods should be limited. Only carbohydrates and fats which are easily digested should be used. During an acute attack the patient should be kept on a milk diet.

Chronic Constipation.

Morning.
Two hours before breakfast—orange juice.

8 A. M.—
Milk with coffee,
Graham bread and butter,
Two soft-boiled eggs.

10 A. M.—
Glass of cider.

Noon.
Broth with one egg,
Steak,

Carrots,
Beans,
Graham bread,
Stewed apples.

4 P. M.—
Buttermilk.

7 P. M.—
Scraped beef,
Graham bread,
Stewed prunes,
Cider.

9 P. M.—
Figs or buttermilk.

Diarrhea.—The diet for diarrhea consists of foods with just opposite effects from those used in constipation—milk, soups, gruel, arrowroot. As the trouble abates slowly increase the diet, by adding scraped beef, broiled steaks, etc.

Dyspepsia.—Foods should be taken in small quantities, at regular hours, and well masticated. Only those which are easily digested should be used. Avoid fat meats, sausages, lobster, crab, pickled or warmed-over meats, fried foods, candies, and all rich or highly seasoned foods.

Liver Functional Disorders.

Soups.—Light broth, vegetable soup, with crackers or toasted bread.

Fish.—Broiled or boiled, white fresh fish or raw oysters.

Meats.—Mutton and chicken broth, beef tea, in small quantities, oysters,

Farinaceous.—Whole wheat bread, graham bread, dry toast or crackers, cereals, tapioca, arrowroot.

Vegetables.—Mashed potatoes, fresh vegetables, plain salads, watercress, lettuce, dandelions.

Desserts.—Plain milk pudding of tapioca or cornstarch, junket, stewed or fresh fruits, without sugar.

Liquid.—Weak tea and coffee or hot water without sugar or cream.

Avoid.—Highly seasoned foods as pies, pastries, foods rich in fats, fishes of oily nature, cheese, sweet wines.

Rheumatism.—Do not give much red meat, berries, sugar or tomatoes, but drink a great amount of water, milk and thin gruels.

Meats.—Mutton and chicken broth, beef tea, in small quantities, oysters, chicken, boiled fresh fish, raw clams, sweetbread.

Bread.—Whole wheat bread, corn or brown bread toast.

Vegetable.—Rice, green vegetables and fruits except strawberries and bananas. All sweetening should be done with saccharine.

Tuberculosis.—Treatment in tuberculosis is very usually that of building up the system by a plentiful supply of nourishing food, fresh air and rest.

In addition to the regular meals, lunches are usually served during morning and afternoon and at bedtime. However, this should not be done to the point of making the patient unhappy by feeling overfed.

Fresh eggs, milk and red meat are especially valuable foods in treating tuberculosis. All food should be served regularly and according to a definite schedule. The following may prove helpful:

A. M.—
      5:30.—A glass of hot water while still in bed.
      7:30.—Breakfast fruit, cereals, eggs and toast, a little meat, if desired, milk or water.
    10:30.—Eggnog with crackers.
P. M.—
    12:30.—Dinner should be the largest meal. It may consist of most any series of well-prepared nourishing foods, desired by the patient. A rest of an hour should follow the dinner.
      3:30.—Eggnog and crackers, hot gruel or soup.
      6:30.—This meal should consist of light and easily digested foods, eggs and milk, whole wheat bread, vegetables, etc.
      9:30.—Glass of hot milk with crackers.

Fever.—Fever patient should be served easily digested foods, such as milk, junket, baked potato and egg albumen, custard, ice cream, but not immediately after a meal. It should be remembered that the digestive juices are diminished in amount, and that peristaltic action of the stomach and intestines is weak. During convalescence the diet is most important and the diet list under anemia could be used. The following schedule may be taken as a sample menu for fevers in general:

First Day.—
    Breakfast.—Poached egg on toast.
    Lunch.—10:30, milk punch.
    Dinner.—12:30, raw oysters, cream crackers, light wine, if desired.
         4:00, one cup hot meat broth.
    Supper.—6:30, milk toast, wine, jelly and tea.

Second Day.—
    Breakfast.—Soft cooked egg, milk punch, coffee with sugar and cream.
    Lunch.—10:30, cup of soft custard.
    Dinner.—12:30, cream of celery soup, sippetes of toast, barley pudding with cream, sherry wine.
    Lunch.—4:00, milk punch.
    Supper.—6:30, water toast, buttered, wine jelly, tea.

Typhoid Fever.—Probably the most difficult patient for the home nurse to care for is the typhoid fever patient. A more liberal and varied diet is being allowed in this disease than years ago. Many varieties of broths may be given, Gelatine, white of egg and fruit juices furnish a range in methods of preparations of foods. The following menu may be suggested for the typhoid patient. The "standing order diet" of Lakeside Hospital, Cleveland:

High Calorie Typhoid Diet.

This is used the same as the old Shattuck Diet. As the name implies, it gives as great a number of calories of food as possible to typhoid patients, and takes away the undesirable feature of a solid diet which would enhance perforation and irritation to an ulcerated and inflamed bowel.

Milk, hot or cold;
Koumiss,
Whey,
Buttermilk,
Peptonized milk,
Junket,
Modified, with lime water, soda water,
  apollinaris or vichy,
Tea,
Coffee.

Soups.—Cream soups or pure with all vegetables strained, clear soups, broth, oyster stew, with oysters removed.

Gruels.—Of any cereal not containing very high percent cellulose and always strained through fine strain.

Albumen Drinks.—Water, plain or flavored with fruit juices; milk, plain or flavored with fruit juices.

Ice cream or ices without solid particles of fruit or nuts.

Eggs.—Soft cooked or raw, or eggnog or custard.

Meats.—Finely minced chicken or beef or scraped beef.

Crackers soaked in milk or broth.

Soft puddings, gelatine, apple sauce, strained.

Recipes.

Cocoa and Chocolate.—These have some nutritious value but are quite hard to digest.

Tea and Coffee.—Tea and coffee are stimulants but not nutritious.

Beef Juice.—Beef juice given either hot or cold is very good for the sick. To extract juice from meat, put the meat on the fire in cold water and gradually heat. Allow it to simmer but not to boil. Allow to cool, remove fat and heat to serve.

Beef juice may also be prepared by placing 1 pound of lean beef in a buttered skillet, heat to a steaming heat over a slow fire, but do not cook, squeeze with a hinged pot, masher or fruit press, leaving the juice fall into a hot cup and serve the juice with salt and pepper.

Beef Tea.—Chop fine 1 pound of lean beef, put in bowl and cover with cold water. Let stand until water is red, then press juice out of the meat with a pot masher. Make hot, season and serve.

Junket.—Slightly warm 1 pint of new milk, stir into it 1 large dessertspoonful of liquid rennet or 2 tablespoonfuls of powdered rennet and stand in a cool place till set. Serve with cream and sugar.

Potato Soup.—Boil 3 large potatoes, 1 stalk of celery, ½ small onion till tender. Mash smooth, then add 1 cup of cream, 1 pint of milk and 2 table-spoonfuls of butter. Season and serve hot. Strain before serving.

Creamed Celery.—Mash the outer stalk of a bunch of celery and cut in ½ inch pieces and boil in salted water till tender. Make a white sauce by melting 1 tablespoonful of butter, thickening with flour and when smooth adding 1 cup of hot milk. Stir till smooth and add to cooked celery. Serve hot with nicely browned toast.

Creamed Egg.—Warm a small dish or baking cup and butter. Break into it 1 or 2 eggs, season with salt and pepper, and cover with cream. Cook in hot oven until set and serve hot.

Eggs in Milk.—Heat 2 tablespoonfuls of milk and ½ teaspoonful of butter in a small pan. When warm, stir in 2 eggs and add a little salt. The egg should be beaten till yolks and whites are well blended. Stir until thick and serve hot with thin slices of toast.

Apple Cup Custard.—Pare and core three large cooking apples. Steam until tender, then press through a colander. While hot add 3 large tablespoonfuls of sugar, 1 tablespoonful of butter, beaten yolks of 3 eggs, ¾ cup of milk. Bake in small custard cups, when done spread meringue made of the sweetened whites; brown slightly and set to cool. Serve cold.

Orange Jelly.—Soak ½ box of gelatine in ½ cup of cold water. Dissolve 1 cup sugar in 2 cups of boiling water. Add this to the gelatine with 2/3 cup of orange juice and juice of 1 lemon. Strain into molds and set away to cool. Serve cold.

Shirred Eggs.—Butter an individual custard cup and drop an egg in it whole, dust lightly with salt and white pepper. Place in a moderate oven till set and serve at once.

Broiled White Fish.—Wash and dry a white fish and free it from bones. Place on an oiled baking sheet with the flesh sides up and broil under the flame. When a nice brown, season with butter, and serve plain or add a white sauce.

Baked Oyster.—Dry large oysters on a soft towel, dip into melted butter and roll in fine cracker crumbs which have been seasoned with salt and pepper. Place in rows in a dripping pan and bake in a very hot oven. When nicely browned pile on a hot platter garnished with parsley and serve at once.

Sippets.—Mince cold roasted meat or fowl, put into a pan and cover with cream, add butter and when hot stir in the meat, seasoned with salt. Let boil until it thickens enough to spread on hot, buttered toast.

Invalid's Beef Steak.—Take a piece of beef from the round steak, scrape carefully on both sides. Add salt and pepper to the part that scrapes off, make into pats and broil as other steak.

Cream of Tomato Soup.—Heat 2 tablespoonfuls of tomato juice, add ⅛ teaspoonful of soda. Heat ½ cup of milk, add 1 tablespoonful of butter, 1 tablespoonful of flour or bread crumbs, ¼ teaspoonful of salt and pepper. When ready, serve hot with crackers.

Oatmeal Gruel.—Soak 1 pint of rolled oats in 1 quart of water over night. In morning press through a gravy strainer till all the milky substance is pressed through. Add 1 quart of boiling hot milk and cook in a double boiler for an hour and a half or more, then add salt and 1 cup of cream. Strain and serve hot.

Omelet.—Separate the white and yolk of 1 egg, beat the white till stiff; cream yolk; add 1 tablespoonful bread crumbs and 1 tablespoonful milk. Mix and add ¼ teaspoonful salt and pepper, fold in the stiffly beaten whites. Place 1 tablespoonful butter in an omelet pan, heat, add mixture, cook on top of stove slowly till well risen; place on rack in oven till firm. Remove carefully to a hot plate, garnish with parsley. Serve hot. May use minced chicken or meat of any kind in place of bread crumbs.

Prune Whip.—Cook 1 cup of prunes, strain through a coarse sieve, removing stones. Add 1 tablespoonful of lemon juice, fold in the white of 1 egg beaten stiff, and add 1 teaspoonful sugar. Pile on a buttered plate, stand in the oven for about one minute or until set. Serve cold with whipped cream or thin boiled custard.

Egg Lemonade.—Beat 1 egg with 1 tablespoonful of sugar until very light; add 3 tablespoonfuls of cold water and juice of a small lemon. Fill glass with pounded ice; see that ice is pure. Drink through a glass tube or clean straw.

Milk of Albumen.—Put into a clean quart bottle 1 pint of milk, whites of 2 eggs, pinch of salt. Cork and shake for 5 minutes.

Methods of Giving Baths and Treatments for Therapeutic or Curative Effects.

Hot Water Baths.—These are usually given to induce perspiration or to relieve muscular tension, as in convulsion.

Bath to Induce Perspiration.—If the patient is able to get into a bathtub, fill the latter half full of water at 100 degrees F. This temperature is maintained from ten to fifteen minutes after which put the patient quickly into a bed which has been well supplied with hot blankets. The blankets should then be tucked around the patient so that no air is allowed to enter. Plenty of water should be given to drink during the bath as this induces profuse perspiration, thus aiding in carrying off the impurities of the body. After the patient has been closely covered for about an hour, the blanket should be gradually removed, the body quickly sponged under a bath blanket with alcohol and water, and dried with brisk friction. Then turn the patient onto a dry blanket, using the same method as when changing the bed after a daily bath, being careful not to expose the body, as the pores of the skin are so opened as to make undue exposure dangerous.

Hot Bath for Convulsions.—This method is used for children. Fill the tub about two-thirds full of water 108 to 110 degrees F. Strip the body and lay the child full length in the tub, immersing the feet first, and gradually the whole body, supporting the head on your arm. Keep an ice cap or ice compress on the head. This bath usually controls the convulsions within ten or fifteen minutes and the child is removed. If the rigidity still continues after this length of time the temperature of the water should be reduced to about 95 degrees F. It may be heated again if necessary. If the temperature of the bath is reduced, it is well to add a paste of mustard for a counter irritant, but in a hot bath this effect is negligible. The usual proportion is one tablespoonful of mustard powder to a gallon of water. The powder should always be mixed to a smooth thin paste before being added to the bath.

Sponge Bath for Reducing Temperature, Etc.—Place beneath the entire body of the patient, a rubber sheet or oilcloth covered with a cotton sheet or thin blanket; remove the top covers and cover the body with an extra sheet. Place a hot water bag to the feet and a cold application to the head; an ice cap, a hot water bag filled with ice water and small bits of ice or a cold compress across the forehead. Have a foot tub or large basin filled half full of water between 70 and 80 degrees F. (or as designated by physicians), a basin holding a few small pieces of ice, with which to lower the temperature as the water is made warmer by the body, a large soft wash cloth, two bath towels and a warm blanket. In giving a bath to reduce a patient's temperature, the more the body is exposed, the quicker will be the evaporation, which causes the reduction. A towel may be laid across the loins, but otherwise the patient may be uncovered. Remove the upper sheet and give light friction for two or three minutes before beginning to sponge. Friction consists in rubbing the skin quickly but lightly with the bare hand, making the strokes rapidly but without pressure. Dampen the wash cloth and wash with a long downward stroke with one hand, while keeping up a light friction with the other. Follow the same plan as in the daily bath beginning with the face, and proceeding with the neck, chest and arms, abdomen, thigh, legs, feet, back and buttocks. Use plenty of water and as it becomes warm, add a small piece of ice, noting the temperature of the water frequently. It is much better to have two people to give this bath as the friction can then be kept up continuously, but if this is not possible, stop the sponging at short intervals and give friction with both hands for a minute. Friction is an important feature of all cold baths. Sponge under the arms and in the axilla or armpits frequently. Having used water freely the under sheet is very wet, therefore, care must be taken in removing it, not to wet the bed. Turn the patient on one side and fold the sheet. Roll the wet sheet and the rubber or oilcloth together in folds close to the back of the patient as in changing the bed (see page 63). Let the fold of the dry sheet drop down over the back, allowing enough to be pulled through to the other side to cover the bed and tuck in. Place a blanket over the sheet and turn the patient on his back and slightly to the other side, while the rubber and wet sheet, followed by the folds of the dry sheet and blanket, are pulled through and removed. In this way the patient is enveloped in a dry sheet and blanket. Dry the body by making friction over the sheet, cover with the blanket and give a warm drink frequently. Broth and milk are harder to digest and should not be given after a cool bath. Leave the hot water bag near the feet and let the patient remain wrapped in this way until warm again, then remove blanket and put on nightgown. If the patient continues to feel cold, make friction over the blanket until this passes. The patient's pulse should be watched during the bath, and the temperature taken in about twenty or thirty minutes. If the patient reacts well, this treatment may be repeated every four or six minutes, if necessary.

Partial Temperature Bath.—When a patient is too sick to be turned, a cold, wet sheet may be applied to the exposed parts of the body only. The bed may be protected by putting the strips of rubber or oilcloth, or even several thicknesses of newspaper covered with towels, close under the sides and arms and under the legs. The wet sheet may be kept wet by sprinkling with a whiskbroom. In the partial bath, be sure that the arms are well away from the body and the legs separate, so that as much evaporation as possible can take place. The back and buttocks are then attended to by wetting the hands with alcohol (75%) and rubbing gently. The usual after care is given (see page 65).

Alcohol Bath.—When a patient is very sick, or there is danger of hemorrhage, or any other reason why there should be very little moving, it is not wise to attempt to put the rubber sheet, etc., beneath the body. In such a case, an alcohol bath is the best substitute for the temperature bath. For this, about a pint of alcohol (25%), will be sufficient. Take one part of alcohol and three parts of tepid water, place a bath towel on either side of the patient and one beneath the legs, to protect the bed, and keeping the wash cloth only ordinarily wet in the alcohol solution, sponge with long downward strokes, as in giving a plain bath. Treat the back by wetting the hands in alcohol and working under the body, rubbing as well as you can without moving the patient. Practice will enable you to do this easily. In case where the physician prefers the tepid bath, with the large amount of water necessary to accomplish good results, and the patient is too sick to be moved with safety, rubber strips or pieces of oilcloth covered with towels and placed close under the sides and under the legs will protect the bed, if sufficient care is used. The back may then be cooled as in the alcohol bath.

Sitz Bath.—This bath is usually given for pain or congestion in the lower abdomen or rectum. There is a special tub for this but if such is not obtainable, a good substitute is an ordinary washtub with a blanket folded over the edge and an old pillow or another folded blanket placed in the bottom for the patient to sit on. The tub is filled about a third full of water at 110 degrees F. If the patient is too sensitive for this, it may be begun at 100 degrees F. and gradually raised to the desired point, but it must be hot to do any good. If hot water is added while the patient is in the bath, the hand of the nurse must be kept between the hot stream and the body of the patient. The tub is placed in an armchair, tilted to an angle comfortable for the patient, and with the edges of the tub well padded, and the feet placed in another chair, she may sit this way for some minutes. An undershirt and stockings keep the patient from exposure. While the patient is sitting in the tub a blanket is also pinned about the shoulders and allowed to cover her. The bath usually lasts from twenty to thirty minutes, but in some cases must be shorter.

Foot Bath.—Various kinds of foot baths are given for relief in other parts of the body. These are helpful in case of a cold, headache, abdominal disturbances, etc., and are often great aids in inducing sleep, drawing the blood from the afflicted part. It is very easy to give a foot bath to a patient while sitting up, but when in bed it is more difficult. For either case, have a foot tub or large basin half full of water 108 degrees F. and when sitting up, place the feet in this and cover the tub and knees with a thick blanket, allowing the feet to remain in the bath for eight or ten minutes, then add more hot water until it reaches 112 degrees F., being careful not to expose the limbs too much. Move the water constantly with the hand to guard against burning the patient, while putting in additional hot water. Cover the feet quickly and let remain for another fifteen minutes or so. After thirty minutes, dry quickly with brisk friction and keep the patient warm.

To Give Foot Bath in Bed.—Fold back the bedding from the foot of the bed to about the middle of the thighs, and flex the knees. Cover the legs with a small blanket, place a bath towel doubled near the feet and put a folded towel or soft cloth over the edge of the tub which will come next to the patient. Put the tub close to the feet, and lifting the latter by holding the further foot in one hand and letting the nearest one rest on the forearm, lift them gently into the tub which may be pushed into the place where the feet have been. Let the blanket down well over the sides and if one blanket is not thick enough, add another. Add hot water as when giving the bath sitting up. When the time required has elapsed lift the feet, blanket and all, in the same way that you lowered them into the water. Pull the tub out of the way with the free hand and draw the folded bath towel into place for the feet to rest upon. Remove the tub from the bed and dry the legs and feet quickly, still under cover of the blanket. Place a second hot water bag at the feet, remove the extra blanket and draw up the covers, being sure that the bed is perfectly dry. Mustard is the medication perhaps the most commonly used in foot baths, but when the temperature of the water is high enough there is little gained from its use.

Soothing Baths.—There are several kinds of medicated baths used in various skin diseases, the most common of which are the sodium bicarbonate or baking soda, the starch, the sulphur and the bran baths, and are usually given in a bath tub. In giving any of these there should be enough water to cover the body while the head is supported by means of a cushion on an ordinary bath seat, or piece of starched canvas let well down into the tub and firmly attached on either side. To do this the canvas must be comfortable. Never leave a patient alone in a bath of any sort.

Soda Bath.—For the soda bath dissolve six or eight ounces of soda in each gallon of water used. This is very helpful in case of prickly heat, or any itching of the skin. It is very cooling in hot weather, whether there is irritation or not.

Starch Bath.—For the starch bath, mix half a pound of starch in a small amount of cold water and add slowly enough hot water to make a mixture about as thick as cream which is then poured into the average size bath and mixed thoroughly.

Sulphur Bath.—Sulphur baths are very soothing to the nerves of the skin. For this purpose, sulphurated potash is used in the proportion of one to two ounces for the average bath. The temperature of this bath is usually about 90 degrees F. In giving any of these baths, the patient is kept in them for fifteen or twenty minutes and is then put into a warm sheet and **patted gently** until dry. Never use any friction after a bath of this sort.

Mustard Bath.—In direct opposition to the above mentioned **is the mus**-tard bath, which is used as a counter irritant and when given for this purpose the temperature of the bath should not be above 75 or 80 degrees F., as the virtue in the mustard is destroyed by too much heat. The proportion is one level table-spoonful of mustard to each gallon of water. Then general procedure is as for any of the above baths.

Salt Bath.—The salt bath is another counter irritant and is made by dis-solving ten or twelve pounds of sea salt in a tub half full of hot water. Let this stand until it is down to about 75 de-grees F. Rub the patient quite vigorously with the hand. This should, of course, be done while the patient is in the tub. Place her in a warm sheet after ten or fifteen minutes and dry by **rubbing briskly** over the sheet.

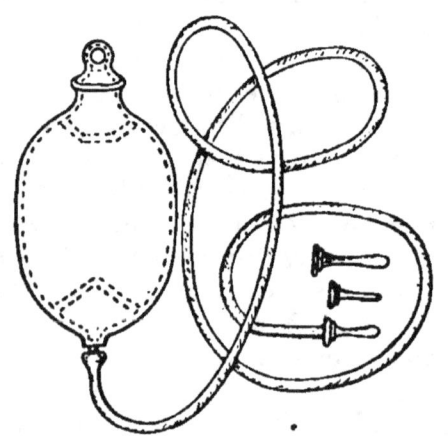

Fountain Syringe.

Salt Rub.—To give a salt rub, rub the patient with warm salt for about ten min-utes or until the skin is red, rinse thor-oughly, remove from bath, wrap in dry sheet and pat until dry. If sea salt is not to be had, coarse ordinary salt will do, but it is not so beneficial.

Giving an Enema.—After breakfast the patient should rest for about half an hour while things are being made ready for the treatments ordered by the physi-cian. If the daily movement of the bowels is dependent upon an enema or injec-tion, this is given first. Sometimes this is given before breakfast. However, it takes some time and if the patient is weak, it is better not to give it before nour-ishment has been taken. Unless otherwise ordered, it is usually of soapsuds made with castile or ivory soap and just warm enough to be comfortable when poured over the back of the hand. From a quart to three pints of soapsuds is prepared. A rubber bag with a hose attachment commonly called a "fountain syringe" with a small rectal tip is the best thing with which to give it. Turn the patient on her left side with her limbs drawn up against the abdomen. Place a slopjar close at hand. A small cotton pad or soft cloth should be placed upon the bedpan where the body rests and in cold weather everything that comes in contact with the patient should be warmed. Let the water run through the tube into the slopjar until it is warm, then insert the rectal tip, which has been covered with vaseline, and let the water flow. Draw the tip back a quarter of an inch to let it start freely and hold the bag about two feet above the level of the patient. If she complains of pain and the inability to take more than a little water, close the tube for a moment or two and then begin again. Do this until enough has been taken to insure a good result. (If given this way, the water works well up to the bowels and softens the stool).

Now turn the patient onto her back, slip the bedpan quickly into place and put a towel or newspaper up against the knees to protect the bedding. An extra pillow under the shoulders is a help in expelling the water. When a patient is too weak or irresponsible to hold much water, the injection may have to be taken lying on the back with the bedpan already in place. After removing the bedpan, see that the patient is thoroughly cleansed, then remove the extra protection from the bed. (A patient should always be given an opportunity to wash her hands after using the bedpan).

Giving a Douche.—In case of a female patient the douche if ordered, is given after the enema and is usually medicated according to the physician's directions. If there is no regular douche pan, it can easily be given on the bedpan, care being taken not to let it overflow. It is best to remove and empty when half the water has been used. Then the rest may be given in safety. The covered oilcloth or rubber sheet is placed well up under the hips before beginning and two quarts of water, which has been boiled and cooled to a temperature that is comfortable when poured over the back of the hand, is the usual amount. This may be used considerably warmer than that used for the enema. Here again, the cold water is allowed to pass through the rubber tube before the tip is inserted. The latter should be boiled five minutes before being used and should not be allowed to touch anything before it reaches the patient. Allow the water to flow freely, all being given in about twenty minutes, thus insuring full benefit of the heat as well as irrigation.

Absolute cleanliness is very necessary in giving a douche. The water, while cooling, should be well covered, and never tested with the finger, as this contaminates it. The douche bag should be put into tepid water and brought to a boil before using, this should be filled and placed two feet above the body of the patient. Any other daily treatments ordered by the physician usually follow this and should be given before the bath.

Counter Irritants.—Counter irritants may be hot or cold applications of any sort used to reduce inflammation, to relieve pain, or to localize infection of any sort. Unless there is definite knowledge of the trouble, and the necessary remedy, these applications should be made only under the direction of the physician. Otherwise, heat might be used when cold is the proper thing, etc., and in some cases great harm done to the patient.

Heat is a favorite counter irritant and may be applied simply by the use of a well covered hot water bag, from which the air has been carefully excluded by squeezing the bag tight above the water and screwing the stopper in before releasing the bag. The bag should not be more than one-fourth filled with water. Great care should be taken not to have it hot enough to burn the body. Usually anything that is really hot when pressed to the cheek is sufficiently hot to produce the desired effect.

Patients who are in an unconscious state, or whose circulation is sub-normal, are very easily burned. Therefore, the greatest care must be taken to protect the body from contact with hot water bottle, bricks or other applications of heat.

Poultices and Plasters.—A poultice is a soft composition as of bread, bran, or a mucilaginous substance, to be applied to sores, inflamed parts of the body, etc.

Flax and Linseed Meal Poultice.—Make a flannel protector to fit the part to be covered. If for the chest, cut to fit about the neck and arms properly, the same as when making one for the compress to the chest (see figure below).

Linseed meal is better than flaxseed as it contains more oil. Sometimes a poultice for both back and chest is required and in this case it is best to make two separate poultices. Cut four pieces of cheese-cloth or old muslin to fit the chest as does the flannel protector, allowing a two-inch margin at all edges, spread a towel flat, placing on it the flannel protector, covered by one thickness of the muslin. For an adult prepare the poultice as follows: to three pints of boiling water slowly add enough flax or linseed meal to make

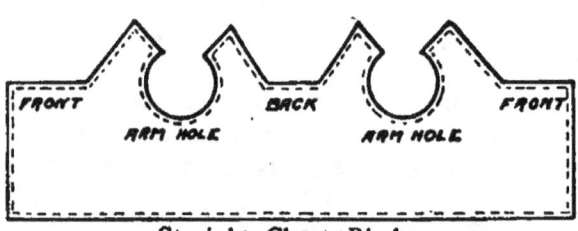
Straight Chest Binder.

it stiff enough to drop, but not run from the spoon. Keep the water boiling constantly while adding the meal, then add two teaspoonfuls of bicarbonate of soda (baking soda) and beat thoroughly until the poultice is light. Pour one-half of this on the muslin and spread quickly about one-third of an inch thick. Fold over the edges two inches and place the second piece of muslin over the top. Cover this for a minute or two with a towel while you prepare the other half of the poultice in the same way. Slip towel and all under the patient's back, being sure that it is in position. Place the other half over the chest and cover with oiled muslin or soft rubber sheeting and a piece of cotton batting. Draw up the edges of the binder and pin fairly tight down the front and over the shoulders. It is a good plan to rub a little vaseline into the skin before applying the poultice as this prevents blistering. Be sure that the poultice is not too hot. Cool it by lifting slightly from the skin a time or two, or until it is comfortable. Poultices are usually changed hourly, as they are usually not warm enough to be effective if allowed to remain on longer. Where economy is necessary the discarded poultice may be put into a steamer, on a plate or pan and steamed until thoroughly heated again and applied; this is not desirable, however, if new ones can be made each time.

Mustard Poultice.—Mustard is added to flax or linseed to make this poultice. It is usually proportioned one to eight parts mustard for an adult, and one to sixteen parts mustard for a child. Dissolve the mustard in warm water, and add to the poultice after the latter is of the right consistency, beat the while until it is light.

Mustard Paste or Plaster.—This is a favorite home remedy. It is made by mixing one part mustard to eight or ten parts of flour. Mix the mustard and flour with tepid water until you have a smooth paste, then spread between two pieces of muslin. Rub the part well with vaseline to prevent blistering. The plaster should remain on the patient until the skin is well reddened.

Complete Hot Pack.—Be sure that the room is warm (at least 76° F.) The first thing to do in a bath of this kind is to tie an ice cap or a rubber bag filled with ice water on the patient's head. If neither of these are available, wring a cloth from ice water and apply across forehead. Cover the patient with a bath blanket, then draw the covers from beneath downward as in giving a regular bath. Place a rubber sheet or piece of oilcloth between the blankets and pass it beneath the patient. This should be large enough to cover a single bed at least. Remove the nightgown and place a folded towel between the blanket and the patient's chin.

Soak two old blankets in a tub of water about 150° F., leaving about six inches at each end out of the water so that they may be wrung without burning the hands. Have someone to assist, and each person take one end and wring in opposite directions. Wring very dry. Have a pail with a hot soapstone or hot bricks in the bottom close at hand and drop the blanket in, still folded as when wrung, cover quickly with a piece of carpet, paper, or any clean covering which will keep in the heat. Now, in the same manner wring the second blanket quickly and very dry. Unfold it and see that it is not too hot to touch the body. Shake it gently for a second if too hot and then apply to the back of the patient, making sure that it comes up high enough to be folded over the shoulders. Turn the patient on her back, pull the ends of the blanket out and place over the sides and, lifting the dry blanket tent fashion, away from the chest, etc., quickly spread the second hot blanket from the pail, over the body and tuck well in at the shoulders, sides, and feet, so that no air is allowed to enter. Now allow the dry blanket to drop into place. Place hot water bag, heated flat irons, or bricks at the feet and along the sides, being careful not to have them too hot. Tuck in tightly and cover with the usual bed clothes. While the patient is in the pack, take the pulse at the temporal artery, which is just in front of the ear, and keep the head application cold by changing frequently. Give as much water to drink as possible, or, if there is objection to this, give warm broth, hot lemonade, etc. Patients are usually kept in the pack for twenty minutes if there is no reason for shortening the time. At the end of this time, fold the bedding back over the foot of the bed again, and under cover of the dry blanket which covered the patient, remove the wet blankets and rubber sheet, turning the patient on the side, as in changing the bed after a bath. Be careful not to expose the body. Dry the body by giving brisk friction with the hands over the dry blanket. Wrap the blanket which was under the rubber and which you have left on the bed, up over the sides and tuck well in, now remove the blanket over which you have been rubbing, draw up the bed clothes, leaving the hot water bag at the feet and the cold application at the head, and let the patient rest. At the end of an hour, unless the patient is asleep, dry by rubbing over blanket thoroughly and under cover of the same, rub the body with alcohol (50 or 75%), again being careful to avoid exposure.

Partial Hot Pack.—Sometimes only a partial hot pack may be called for, as in treatment for a rheumatic arm or leg. In this case the member may be elevated on a pillow and the rubber and blankets placed beneath, as previously stated. A piece of flannel of the right size to cover the part well is placed in a large towel, the ends of the towel are gathered into the hand hammock fashion with the flannel in the middle, the towel is dipped into water from 170 to 180° F. until the flannel has become saturated. The towel is then wrung in opposite directions until very dry and the hot flannel shaken out and applied quickly to the affected part. The blanket is then folded over it and it is kept well covered for ten minutes or perhaps fifteen if it remains hot. This treatment is usually kept up for an hour or more, or as directed by the physician, and then repeated at stated intervals. After the pack is removed, rub the part with alcohol and wrap in flannel, cotton batting or rose cotton so that it will keep warm. If any liniment or ointment is to be applied it should be done immediately after giving the pack. In all such treatment, the things to avoid are burning, undue exposure, and too sudden changing of temperature, either by ventilation or by hasty removal of extra covering. Watch carefully that the patient does not become exhausted.

Complete Cold Pack.—Place the patient on a rubber or oilcloth with a blanket over it as before stated (see page 79), then remove the nightgown and cover with a sheet, folding all other bedding neatly across the foot of the bed. Fill a foot tub half full of water between 60 and 65 degrees Fahrenheit. Unfold two small sheets and gather them up loosely, lengthwise, and put them in the water. Place the hot water bag at the feet and the cold application, such as ice cap, rubber bag filled with ice water, or cold wet cloth, as the case may be, at the head. Place a dry towel across the loins. Wring the sheets only moderately dry, turn the patient to one side and spread one of the wet sheets smoothly, folding enough against the back, fan fashion, to be drawn through. Now turn the patient on her back, pull folds through and bring up all around the sides, between the legs and arms and body and over the shoulders. Remove the top sheet and place the second sheet over the patient, also putting folds between the legs and arms and over the shoulders. Keep the legs apart and the arms well away from the body. As soon as the sheets are in place begin giving friction and continue to give at intervals of three or four minutes during the pack. Keep the sheet wet by sprinkling generously with water shaken from a whisk broom. This pack usually lasts fifteen or twenty minutes. The after care is the same as that of a sponge or of a temperature bath. (See page 79).

Cold Pack for the Chest Only.—This pack is used in cases of congestion of the pulmonary organs, frequently in cases of pneumonia and bronchitis, but is often beneficial when there is a heavy cold and cough, and especially if there is rise in temperature. Make a binder of two thicknesses of flannel cut after the fashion shown in the illustration on page 84. It should be sufficiently large to go around the body and extend well down under the chest. Cut three or four thicknesses of cotton cloth or old outing flannel as you would cut a waist for an old fashioned Mother Hubbard dress, so that it fits under the arms and about the neck. Make this in two pieces, one for the back and one for the front. Put these into water between 60 degrees and 65 degrees Fahrenheit. Remove the nightgown and cover the patient with a small blanket or something of the kind. Wring the cotton compress quite dry. Place the flannel binder out smooth on a table and spread the compress for the back on the corresponding part of the binder, raise the shoulders slightly and slip both under together (the moist part, of course, next to the body). When this is under smoothly with the flannel extending a few inches below the wet cloth, apply the other to the chest, making it smooth over the shoulder; bring the binder to the front and pin loosely up the front and over the shoulders, being sure that it is not too tight under the arms to allow free circulation. This may be left on one-half to three-quarters of an hour and then changed or removed as symptoms indicate. The after care should be the same as that following cold pack—the chest rubbed lightly with alcohol and the patient placed in dry clothing. Sudden exposure should be avoided.

Hot Compress for the Eye.—The least irritating material for this purpose is absorbent cotton, or folds of soft old muslin cut in squares about an inch thick and large enough to cover the eye. Be sure that everything, including the basin for the hot water, is very clean. Place the compress in a small towel, in the same manner as when applying hot stupes as before described, apply to the eye and cover with a soft piece of dry flannel. These applications are usually changed every three or four minutes for thirty minutes, or as physician specifies. If both eyes are affected, keep the compress separate, never allow the compresses to be transferred from one eye to the other, as this may prove very serious, even causing second infection. Separate basins for each eye should be used instead of one, and if there is any discharge, do not use the compress a second time. Much harm has been done by causing double infection through lack of care in this matter.

Cold Compress for the Eye.—Make the compress as for hot applications. Fill a basin about one-third full of cold water, place in the center a cup turned upside down and on this place a piece of ice about the size of the cup or larger. Wring the compress from the water and lay upon the ice for two minutes and apply to the eye placing another compress on the ice to get cold in the meantime. These applications are usually changed every three or four minutes for a certain period and the same care is observed in keeping them separate as in the hot applications.

The Hot Compress.—The hot compress or stupe of flannel wrung from very hot water and applied directly to the skin is another easily applied counter irritant. These are often medicated according to the physician's directions.

To apply to the abdomen, pass a straight piece of muslin wide enough to extend from the pit of the stomach down to the hips and of sufficient length to go around the body and lap over several inches. Have sewn into a pad, large enough to cover the abdomen, three thicknesses of flannel. Place this in the center of a stiff towel or piece of cloth as in the partial hot pack, keeping both towel ends out of the hot water. Place in a basin and pour boiling water over it freely and let it stay there while you turn the bed clothes down to the thighs and cover the upper part of the body with a blanket. Wring the stupe very dry by twisting the dry ends of the towel in opposite directions. Have a hand piece of oiled muslin an inch larger all around than the flannel. A piece of cotton batting or heavy flannel laid between two pieces of muslin as large as the oiled muslin may be used as a substitute. Remove the flannel stupe from the wringer, shake it an instant, then lifting the blanket place it slowly and smoothly over the abdomen. Place over this the oiled muslin or dry flannel and the batting pad, then pin the binder down the medium line, being careful not to pin it too tightly. The stupe should be changed in one or two hours as ordered. In changing, have the second compress ready to apply before removing the first and see that it is changed under the blanket, thus avoiding exposure. A hot water bag, filled according to directions mentioned before, will help to keep the compress warm. The bag should be applied over the binder. In some cases the stupes are applied every three or four minutes, for ten or fifteen minutes and then discontinued for two or three hours. When discontinuing them in either case, wipe the abdomen dry and apply a cotton batting pad. In applying a compress to an arm or leg, the same general rules may be followed. The compress is then usually wrapped around the member. The same care is taken about exposure. Always remember to wring the compress until you can squeeze no more water from it.

Turpentine Stupes.—Turpentine stupes sometimes are made by adding a teaspoonful of spirits of turpentine to a quart of water and allowing this to boil for several minutes. However, the turpentine does not blend well with water and sometimes causes a burn, therefore, it is better to mix the turpentine with oil or lard, (one part turpentine and two parts oil, for adults and one part turpentine to six parts oil for children). After the abdomen has been well oiled with this mixture, apply the hot wet flannel as in the plain hot stupe.

GENERAL TREATMENTS.

Cramps.—May be due to a diversity of causes.

Where not due to some serious inflammation of one of the internal organs (gall bladder, appendix, etc.) the following may be of use:

Syrup of Ginger—½ tablespoonful in a little hot water.

Spirits of Peppermint.—10 drops in a little hot water.

When due to gastric fermentation, a little baking soda may be tried.

A hot water bag may be applied with benefit in some cases.

Where cramps are severe, do not trust to remedies, but consult a physician.

Headache.—Is only a symptom—it is Nature's way of saying that you have "trouble somewhere." It may be due to the eyes, nose, stomach, bowels, kidneys, etc. If possible, ascertain which organ is causing the headache, especially when of frequent occurrence.

To temporarily allay the pain, heat or cold may be applied to the head, and a hot mustard foot bath may be given (one tablespoonful of ground mustard to a gallon of water), or a mustard plaster may be applied over upper part of spine.

The following may prove useful:

One-half teaspoonful of Effervescent Sodium Phosphate (laxative), dissolved in one-half glass of cold water.

In so-called "nervous headache"—due to fatigue—fifteen to twenty drops of Aromatic Spirits of Ammonia, may be dissolved in two tablespoonfuls of hot water and slowly sipped.

For applications for headache: Use a handkerchief or folded gauze or other cold cloths placed to the head, the cloths should be dipped in a bowl of water containing a small piece of ice, and a hot water bottle to the feet, or a hot foot bath may be given.

See that the light is carefully shaded. Rubbing the back and limbs with alcohol and fanning till dry will greatly relieve one suffering from heat. Position of the patient should be changed often, and the pillows shaken out and aired well, then rearranged. It is well to divert the patient's mind from herself by reading something interesting to her or telling her stories, talking with her, etc.

If the patient is suffering from sleeplessness, give a hot bath and rub with alcohol, or if a hot bath cannot be given, relieve with a hot foot bath. Many times a cup of hot milk and a cracker, or a light lunch will have a quieting effect by drawing the blood from the head to the stomach. Keep the feet warm. Place a hot water bottle at the nape of the neck. Use a gentle head massage.

Never wake a sleeping patient unless by special orders, for healthy sleep is a better restorative than any you can administer.

Head Lice.—Moisten the hair with vinegar, so that the nits can be easily removed with a fine-tooth comb. Then, before retiring, tie a towel saturated in kerosene around the hair, and leave it on till morning.

Nasal Wash.—Made by dissolving one-half teaspoonful of salt in one-half cup of water.

Nose may be douched, using Birmingham Nasal Douche, or by snuffing the solution. Care must be taken in douching the nose. Throw head back and let water run into nose, then throw head forward, and let it run out again. Under no circumstances blow it out, as this may lead to middle ear disease. Douche to be thoroughly boiled after each use.

Sore Throat.—Every sore throat should be examined, using handle of spoon to hold the tongue down so that the tonsils may be seen. If the throat only seems inflamed, use a good gargle, if there are white spots consult a physician at once.

Treatment.—A good gargle for sore throat is made by dissolving a pinch of salt or two teaspoonfuls of alcohol in four tablespoonfuls of hot water (as hot as throat will stand without burning), and gargling throat with same every half hour. The cup should be boiled after use.

"Summer Diarrhea."—"Summer Diarrhea" is usually caused by indiscretions in diet. The offending particle of food by its presence in the alimentary tract irritates the bowels and keeps up the diarrhea. The logical sequence is to remove the irritating food as quickly as possible, and this can be best accomplished by giving one or two tablespoonfuls of castor oil.

Do not attempt to check the diarrhea until offending material has been removed.

Toothache.—Take a small piece of cotton, saturated with oil of cloves or creosote, and pack carefully into cavity of the aching tooth.

Swelling of gums or face usually means an abscess. Do not attempt to treat this yourself, but go to a dentist at once.

Have your teeth inspected at least twice a year by your dentist.

Brush them after each meal—it prevents decay.

Good teeth properly used (i. e., thorough mastication) **prevent indigestion.**

Antiseptics.

Bichloride of Mercury (Corrosive Sublimate).—Dissolve a 7½-grain tablet in a pint of water to make 1:1,000 solution. As a dressing for ordinary wounds, it is usually diluted from five to ten times, making a 1:5,000 or 1:10,000 solution, as the case may be. It corrodes instruments.

Tincture of Iodine is a fairly good antiseptic solution to apply to small wounds.

Carbolic Acid.—Not very generally used in treatment of wounds. Is more useful in sterilizing instruments in the strength of 1:20. Made by adding 1½ tablespoonfuls of pure carbolic acid to a pint of water.

Alcohol.—Very good antiseptic.

Boracic Acid (Boric).—A weak but soothing antiseptic. Very useful in inflammation of the eye. Five teaspoonfuls to a pint of water makes a saturated solution.

Another solution is one tablespoonful of boric acid powder to one pint of boiled water.

Normal Salt Solution.—A normal salt solution is one level teaspoonful of common salt to one pint of boiled water.

Soda Bicarbonate Solution.—This is usually in the proportion of one tablespoonful of baking soda to one pint of cold water.

Mouth Washes.

Salt.—Normal salt solution.

Borax.—One teaspoonful of borax in a half tumblerful of water.

Borin.—One tablespoonful of borin to one-half tumblerful of water.

Tincture of Myrrh.—A few drops of tincture of myrrh to one-half tumblerful of water.

Listerine.—One tablespoonful of listerine to one-half tumblerful of water.

Lemon Juice.—One teaspoonful of lemon juice and two tablespoonfuls of glycerine to one-half tumblerful of water.

Alcohol.—Equal parts of alcohol and water.

Gargles.

Alcohol.—Two tablespoonfuls of alcohol to one-half tumblerful of hot water.

Peroxide of Hydrogen.—Two tablespoonfuls of peroxide of hydrogen to six tablespoonfuls of cold water.

Salt.—Hot normal salt solution.

Borax.—One teaspoonful of borax to one-half tumblerful of hot water.

Alcohol and Listerine.—Two tablespoonfuls of alcohol, two tablespoonfuls of listerine to six tablespoonfuls of water.

Dobell's Solution.—Two tablespoonfuls of Dobell's solution to six tablespoonfuls of hot water.

Common Laxatives and Doses.

Epsom Salts.—One teaspoonful to two tablespoonfuls dissolved in a small quantity of hot water and cooled.

Rochelle Salts.—One teaspoonful to two tablespoonfuls dissolved in a small quantity of water.

Seidlitz Powder.—One powder (2 papers) dissolve each in one-third of a glass of water and mix.

Compound Licorice Powder.—One teaspoonful to one tablespoonful dissolved in a glass of water, or take dry.

Castor Oil.—One teaspoonful to two tablespoonfuls.

Aromatic Cascara.—One teaspoonful to one tablespoonful in an equal quantity of water.

Rhubarb.—Five to ten grains.

Calomel.—One to two grains in divided doses. This should be followed in the morning by a dose of salts.

Puberty.

The care of the child during the age of puberty should be given special consideration. Dr. Walter Reeve Ramsey gives the following most helpful suggestions on this subject in his Text Book for Trained Nurses, "Care and Feeding of Infants and Children."

"Puberty is the transition period between childhood and adolescence. The age of puberty begins earlier in girls than in boys, the average for girls being 13 years and for boys 15 years.

As this time approaches the child shows evidence of change, both physically and mentally. Instead of the tom-boy girl, who romped with boys and girls alike, we begin to notice a reticence and discrimination of sex. In girls, the breasts begin to develop and a growth of hair appears under the arms and about the genitals. Menstruation begins usually from the 13-14th year, occasionally as early as the 12th.

The first evidence of the approach of adolescence in boys is often a change in the quality of the voice, and at the same time there is a growth of hair under the arms and about the genitals.

During this time there is liable to be a marked instability of the nervous system. Children are prone to be irritable and there is a greater tendency during this time to nervous affections. Girls frequently suffer from anaemia.

The age of puberty should be considered one of the critical periods in the life of the individual.

During this period children should not be crowded with their studies, and if the general health is below par the child should be taken out of school for a time and sent to the country, and sometimes away from the other members of the family.

Only plain, nutritious food should be permitted.

Many children are prone to sit about and read sentimental novels, or frequent morbid picture shows, when they should be playing out of doors. This, of course, should be discouraged, and the child should be kept interested in out-of-door pursuits, which will tend to develop both the physical and moral side of his or her nature.

A proper amount of intelligent supervision during this period of a child's life will be repaid many fold.

Painful and irregular menstruation in girls should always be brought to the attention of the physician, as it is frequently due to a simply secondary anaemia, which can usually be readily corrected. Under no circumstances should local examinations or treatment be permitted except for urgent medical indications.

Menstruation.—Menstruation is a periodic flow of blood or bloody fluid from the uterus or female generative organs. The usual length of time elapsing between periods is twenty-eight days. However, this varies in different cases. Irregularity in the growing girl need cause no uneasiness as Nature usually adjusts herself within a year or so. Do not give hot teas, drugs or liquors to bring on the flow as this is probably Nature's plan to economize the blood for the growth of the body.

Painful Menstruation.—This may be due to various causes such as, anaemic condition, misplacement of the generative organs, exposure to cold and dampness, over exertion, excitement, or it may be due to tight lacing.

Nursing.—Give a hot mustard footbath, using 1½ teaspoonsful of mustard to one gallon of water. If this does not give relief, a sitz bath may be helpful. To do this fill a foot tub or other vessel half full of water and allow the patient to sit in this with thighs and hips immersed. Cover the patient's shoulders well. Give hot teas such as pennyroyal, tansy, hops, peppermint, or ginger. These should be given during the bath. After taking the footbath or sitz bath, and drinking the tea, the patient should be put to bed with a hot water bottle at the feet, back or abdomen, and covered with warm comforters and allowed to rest for several hours. This treatment should relieve the patient.

Hot flaxseed poultice, turpentine or mustard fomentations applied to the lower part of the abdomen, and a hot water bottle to the back and feet after which hot ginger tea should be given, will promote the circulation and often give relief. Do not give drugs unless advised by a physician.

Excessive Menstruation.—This may be due to inflammation of the ovaries, uterus, or tubes, or may be caused by tumors in these organs or some diseased condition of the uterus. It may also be caused by getting up too soon after confinement.

Nursing.—Put the patient to bed and keep as quiet as possible. If the flow is alarming, elevate the foot of the bed by means of bricks or blocks so that the patient's head and shoulders will be lower than the feet. While waiting for the physician, dressings should be changed frequently. The bed should be protected by rubber and draw sheet. Hot applications of vinegar may be applied to the abdomen and pelvis. This may be done by using the method as described in applying stupes or fomentations. (See General Nursing, page 87).

Suppression of Menstruation.—Suppression of the menses may be due to a number of causes such as anaemic condition, pregnancy, nursing, non-development of the generative organs, or the removal of the ovaries. The flow is very often suppressed during severe illness, or by over exertion or exposure to cold and dampness. Any condition tending to lower the vital forces such as insufficient nutriment, overwork, worry, unfavorable environment in general, may cause suppressed menstruation.

Nursing.—Build up the general condition by placing the patient in healthful surroundings. Give plenty of good, wholesome food. The patient should take plenty of outdoor exercise, but not become too tired. Use the hot sitz bath and hot mustard bath before going to bed. Also hot drinks, such as ginger tea, pennyroyal tea, etc., are beneficial. Tonics containing iron are sometimes good to build up the system, but should be prescribed by the attending physician.

Leucorrhea (The Whites).—This is a troublesome condition very general among women and commonly called "the whites." It is a discharge of mucus from the uterus and vagina, and resembles very closely a catarrhal condition of the head. It is not a disease itself, but is a symptom of inflammation of the uterus or vagina.

Nursing.—Improvement of the general health is the first thing to be considered. Take plenty of out-door exercise, eat nutritious food and build up the body. Cleanliness is very important and much relief may be obtained by douches or vaginal injections which may be given with a syringe, a fountain syringe being preferable. First cleanse the parts thoroughly with warm water to which has been added white castile or ivory soap. After this, a douche of one of the following may be used:

Witch Hazel.—Use a tablespoonful to a quart of warm water.

Slippery Elm.—Make an infusion of slippery elm bark and use for injection. This is very soothing.

Lysol.—Use warm water to which has been added a few drops of lysol.

Boric Acid.—Use one-half ounce of boric acid solution to a gallon of water.

Menopause. (Change of Life).

This is the cessation of the menses which usually takes place between the age of forty and fifty, and extends over a period of three or four years. It generally appears earlier in unmarried women than in married women who have borne children, and is a somewhat critical period in which the weak points of the constitution show up. The menses may stop suddenly, due to sudden shock or illness and cause the woman great discomfort. However, a healthy woman may pass through this period without much trouble and only a reasonable amount of discomfort.

The symptoms are irregularities in the flow, both in quantity and duration, there may be more pain than usual at the time of menstruation. The time between menstrual periods may be longer, extending from five to eight weeks, or it may be shorter. Often the menstrual periods are prolonged, lasting seven or eight days. A general discomfort common to all women are the so-called "hot flashes." A sudden wave of heat passes over the body, making it feel intensely warm. This lasts for two or three minutes and may be followed by a chilly feeling or profuse perspiration. This condition may occur several times a day or more frequently. There is usually a feeling of depression and there may be congestion causing headache, dizziness, sleeplessness, and the sleep is frequently disturbed. The generative organs diminish in size during this period.

Plenty of sleep and exercise in the fresh air are necessary during this period. Choose cheerful company and be free from worry. Keep the bowels open. For congestion of the head use a hot foot bath to which mustard may be added. Bathe the eyes, using an eye cup, several times a day. Take warm baths frequently. Avoid exposure to cold and dampness, especially wet feet, as it may cause sudden depression. Do not take a cold bath at the time of menstruation. If bleeding is profuse, call a physician. At this time the family should be considerate and patient, relieving the mother of responsibilities and heavy work as much as possible. A change of environment is often helpful.

Pregnancy and Emergency Care.

Signs of Pregnancy.—The first signs of pregnancy are: cessation of menstruation, changes in the breasts, morning sickness, disturbances in urination.

Cessation of Menstruation.—This is the most common indication even though there may be other causes for the suppression of the menses. Especially is this true if two successive periods are missed when the flow heretofore has been regular.

Changes in the Breasts.—At the time of cessation of the menses there is an unusual stinging and prickling sensation in the breasts which also feel tender to the touch.

Morning Sickness.—This is a feeling of nausea with or without vomiting, and usually occurs upon rising in the morning. This is one of the most common indications of pregnancy, and may be especially severe during the first pregnancy.

Disturbances in Urination.—In the beginning of pregnancy, urination may be troublesome, there being the desire to empty the bladder frequently. There may also be other annoying symptoms all of which are the result of irritation caused by the pressure of the growing uterus against the bladder. The acute irritation generally subsides after the first few weeks of pregnancy.

The Quickening.—The movement of the child in the uterus, commonly called the "quickening," is one of the surest signs. This is usually felt by the mother between the fourth and fifth month. When these symptoms are present there is little doubt as to the patient's condition and a physician should be consulted at once.

Duration of Pregnancy.—Pregnancy usually lasts about thirty-nine weeks, or 273 days. One method which physicians commonly use to reckon the date at which a given birth will occur is to count forward 280 days from the beginning of the last menstrual period, thus allowing seven days for the menstrual period.

The easiest method is to count back three months and add seven days. This will probably not give the exact date, it may occur a few days sooner or later. For instance, if menstruation began on October 30, count back three months to July 30 and add seven days. This will give August 6 the approximate date.

Abortion.—One of our best medical authorities describes abortion in the following manner:

"Abortion, miscarriage, and premature labor are all terms which indicate the premature discharge of the foetus from the cavity of the uterus. When the embryo is expelled before the end of the third month of gestation, the word 'abortion' is, technically, the correct term to employ; while from the end of the third month up to the earliest date at which the child can, by any possibility, live (about six and a half months) the term 'miscarriage' is used. If the woman is delivered at any time after the middle of the sixth month and within about two weeks of the proper end of her pregnancy, the birth is described as 'premature labor.'

The first symptom of either abortion or miscarriage is usually pain of an intermittent character, followed soon by bleeding due to the separation of the placenta from its uterine attachment. In some cases the bleeding appears first, and the pain, which is of a "bearing down" type resembling that of labor, comes later.

Premature emptying of the uterus at any time may be caused by fright, grief, or other form of severe nervous shock; it may result from disease of the mother or of the foetus, or from external injury, such as a fall, or a blow or kick over the abdomen. In the latter class of cases the element of fright must also be considered.

Abortion and miscarriage are by no means the trivial matters that they are so commonly supposed to be by women in general. The process is distinctly an abnormal and unnatural one, and as the uterus is not prepared to cast off the placenta as it would at the normal end of pregnancy, some part of it is almost certain to be retained in the cavity of the uterus. These retained fragments of placental tissue cause chronic inflammation of the membrane lining the uterus, even if they do not decompose and result in "blood poisoning," with the possible death of the patient. In any event the outcome is bound to be serious unless the case is most carefully and intelligently treated, and even in those cases in which the entire ovisac has apparently come away a thorough curettage under general anaesthesia is usually indicated as the safest procedure to follow. The nurse should use all her influence to impress upon patients the serious nature of abortion and miscarriage when proper treatment is neglected or refused; and it is safe to say that the dangers to the woman are considerably greater than are those which follow in the train of a normal labor at term.

An abortion is spoken of as complete when the entire uterine contents are expelled. It is called an incomplete abortion when some part of the membranes or placenta is retained. Here there is often much hemorrhage and discharge. A threatened abortion indicates a possible loss of contents of uterus but with proper care pregnancy may not be terminated.

Miscarriage.—Miscarriage is most likely to occur before the sixteenth week of pregnancy as it is not until this time that the union of the placenta and the uterus becomes firm. Frequently the cause cannot be determined. However, it may be due to the imperfect development of the embryo or to some constitutional disease of the mother in which case it cannot be avoided. It is very frequently the result of heavy work such as lifting or moving heavy objects, running a sewing machine, washing, sweeping, reaching high over the head, etc., or it may be brought on by violent exercise such as skating, dancing, golf, tennis, climbing or riding over rough roads.

Prevention.—Carefully guard against over-exertion of any kind during the early weeks of pregnancy. This is necessary in the prevention of miscarriage. If miscarriage has taken place a number of times, it is well for the patient to remain in bed for a few days at the regular period of menstruation until pregnancy is well established.

Nursing.—At the first sign of miscarriage which is bleeding and abdominal pain, the patient should go to bed at once and keep perfectly quiet until the condition again becomes normal. If miscarriage takes place before the sixth week, it may appear as a profuse menstrual flow. If quietness does not relieve the patient, a doctor should be summoned immediately, especially if this occurs after the first six weeks.

It is unfortunate and absurd that a miscarriage should be looked upon as something to be kept secret or to be ashamed of. It should be regarded as any other illness. The patient should have proper care and should be very careful during the regular menstrual periods following, as over-exertion may cause excessive loss of blood.

Labor.—The progress of labor is divided into three stages. The first stage is occupied with the dilatation of the mouth of the uterus; the second stage with the expulsion of the child; the third, with the expulsion of the placenta or "afterbirth." The first stage is the longest. The mouth of the uterus which is small in diameter must increase to three and one-half or four inches in order to allow the child's body to pass. This may take a number of hours and is very trying to the patient as she often feels she is not making progress. The pains recur with increasing severity and at shorter intervals during the period of labor. When pains begin, the patient should call the nurse if she is not already at hand, and notify the doctor, who will watch the case and be within easy call.

During the first stage, unless contrary to the advice of the doctor, the patient should take a warm bath, and an enema of soapsuds should be given previous to the delivery. The bed should be prepared, a rubber sheet or oilcloth, or a pad made of several thicknesses of newspaper covered with a clean cloth should be placed over the mattress to protect it.

The second stage is shorter than the first and the patient feels she is making progress. The pain may be lessened by the use of an anaesthetic if the doctor decides to do so. During this stage, the "bag of water," as the fluid surrounding the child is called, is ruptured. When this bag of water is broken earlier, the birth is spoken of as "dry" and proceeds more slowly.

After the baby is born, the third stage, which is the expulsion of the placenta or afterbirth, proceeds. When the uterus is empty it contracts, causing "after pains." These after pains are not usually felt in the first pregnancy.

Emergency.—In case the baby should be born before the arrival of the doctor or the nurse, it is necessary for the prospective mother and her family to know what to do.

The bed should be prepared by covering the mattress with a large piece of rubber sheeting or oilcloth. If the oilcloth is not at hand, a pad made of several thicknesses of newspaper covered with a clean cloth and fastened with safety pins to the mattress, will protect the bed. Also have a large covered kettle of boiled water and the sterilized dressing, not opened, and scissors at hand. Sterilize "by boiling" a piece of cord or tape for the baby's cord.

The patient should have a soapsuds enema and a warm bath during the first stage. When the "water has broken" and the pains occur every five minutes, the patient may be up and about, later when they occur every few minutes (two or three minutes) she should be put to bed. Someone should be present to render assistance and be with the patient constantly.

The attendant should scrub her hands with soap and water, using the brush for her finger nails, then soak them in an antiseptic solution of either bichloride of mercury or alcohol. The attendant should then prepare the patient by bathing the genital organs first with soap and water, always washing downward, then cleanse with bichloride of mercury or lysol solution. With each pain the patient should bear down but not strain unless necessary.

While the head is being born, the perineum should be supported by the hand, while at the same time the baby's head is pushed upward, thus relieving the strain and lessening the danger of a "tear."

As soon as the head is born the attendant should feel about the neck for the umbilical cord, and if it is found it should be drawn gently to one side or the other until it can be slipped over the head. No force should be used in loosening the cord, for fear of injuring it and causing bleeding.

The mouth, eyes, nose and throat of the infant are now to be carefully cleansed from blood and mucus with cotton or gauze dipped in boric acid solution and the face must be held up so that it does not lie in the pool of blood. There is no occasion whatever for haste in the delivery of the body, even if the face of the infant becomes distinctly blue. In another moment the uterus will again contract and the body of the child will be expelled.

If the child does not cry vigorously, it may be spanked energetically, but without too much force, or held up by its heels and slapped sharply on the back four or five times. In holding the baby up by its heels, care must be taken that no traction is allowed to come on the umbilical cord. The cord should not be tied until pulsation has stopped. The attendant should then tie the cord twice, once two inches from the child's navel, and once two inches nearer the mother. Sterilized or boiled string should be used, then the cord may be cut with the sterilized scissors between the two places where it is tied. There will be very little bleeding if the cord is tied tightly. If the bleeding should continue, the cord should be tied again a little closer to the navel without disturbing the first tying. The baby should then be placed in a soft, clean warm blanket and removed to a safe place while the attendant takes care of the mother.

In most cases from ten to thirty minutes after the baby is born, the placenta or afterbirth is expelled. The placenta and the soiled pads and dressings should be removed and kept for the doctor's inspection. This is important as the attending physician always wishes to examine the placenta. The attendant should then carefully wash the area about the vagina with an antiseptic solution, using sterilized gauze or absorbent cotton. The abdominal binder and sanitary pads should be applied. If the patient feels chilly, place a hot water bottle at the feet, give hot milk to drink and cover with a warm blanket. Usually she will fall asleep.

As a rule, there is a considerable amount of blood discharge at first, however, if there should be excessive bleeding before the doctor arrives, the attendant should attempt to stop the flow. Raise the foot of the bed so that the feet are higher than the head. An ice bag may be applied over the uterus to help in contraction. Cold compresses also help. In case of laceration, the doctor will attend to this when he arrives.

It is of the utmost importance that the physician be summoned early enough to be present at the time of delivery. However, the above instructions should be followed carefully if the baby is born before his arrival.

BABY DEPARTMENT

The object of the Instructions to Expectant Mothers and the detailed "Care of the Baby" is to increase the efficiency of our nation through the Promotion of Public Health.

The greater part of the material regarding the "Care of the Baby" is taken from Mrs. Max West's book on "The Care of the Infant," a monograph prepared by Mrs. West, and issued by the Federal Children's Bureau. The work is so complete and helpful we feel every mother should study and profit by it.

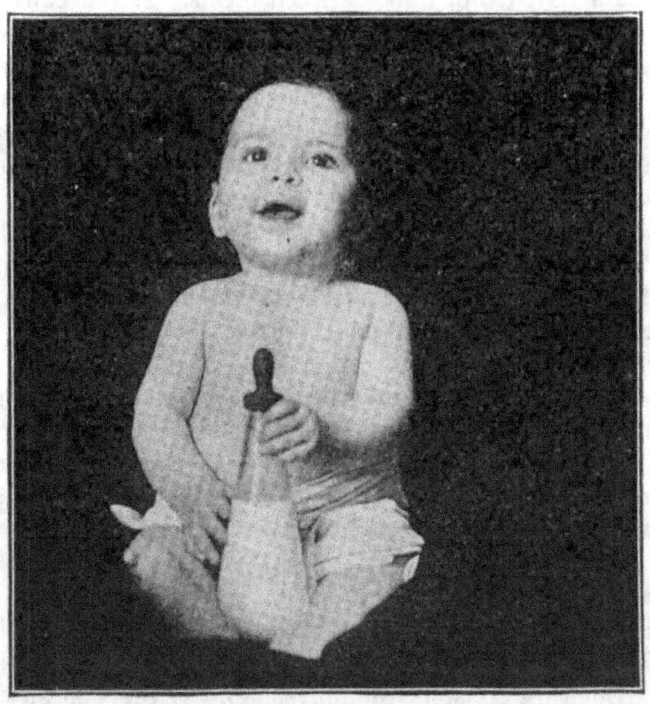

The Baby.

INSTRUCTIONS TO MOTHERS.

The average woman has a keen sense of duty toward her children. It is her lack of knowledge that causes her to fail in doing the very best for her child. But in these days of artificial living, it requires a great deal of thought and study; constant watchfulness; hard work and devotion, to care for the child properly from birth up through childhood, in order that he may reach adult life sound in body and in mind. The more normal the child the better chance he has to succeed in later life. The vast majority of abnormalities start in the early years. Lack of success in life is due, in many cases, to physical defects that might have been avoided by intelligent care in youth. "Every child has the right to be well born."

Birth is not the commencement of the life of the child, therefore it is necessary to consider the welfare of the mother and its effects upon the child.

Healthy motherhood is natural, and with proper health, knowledge and care, child-birth should cause no fear of trouble.

The expectant mother should put herself under the care of a doctor early. A good physician wishes her to consult him for advice. Every expectant mother should have a simple examination in order to remove all the difficulties possible before confinement. Should labor threaten before the expected time, she should go to bed at once, and send for the doctor.

Food and Drink.—Eat a good quantity of simple nourishing food regularly three times a day, drink milk between meals. If the baby is to be strong, the mother must have proper nourishment (food) during pregnancy. It is desirable to have meat, fish or chicken once a day. Bread, thoroughly cooked cereals, fresh fruits, fresh vegetables, plenty of milk and eggs, simple soups, broths and cocoa. Drink water freely—eight to sixteen glasses a day. Do not eat highly seasoned or spiced foods. Do not drink tea or coffee more than once a day. Drink no beer, whiskey, or any alcoholic stimulants.

Exercise, Rest and Sleep.—Daily walks in the open air should be taken during the entire course of pregnancy. Moderate housework with the windows open is a good tonic. Avoid heavy lifting or violent exercise. An extra amount of sleep is needed. Rest for an hour or two during the day. The windows should be kept open during sleep.

Clothing.—The clothing should be loose and warm but not too heavy. It should be supported largely from the shoulders. Do not wear round garters. Avoid getting the feet and clothing wet. This is for the comfort of the mother and the welfare of the baby. At the time of confinement use only clean clothing for the baby and bed. Have the bed prepared according to the nurse's instructions. Be sure that your clothing and the baby's are clean, complete and kept in separate places.

Bowels, Skin and Kidneys.—Keep the bowels, skin and kidneys active. At least one free movement of the bowels should take place daily. If there is any difficulty about this, consult your physician. If there is any swelling of the hands, feet or face, continued headache, nausea, blurred sight or spots before the eyes, backache, pain or bleeding or if passing only small quantities of urine, send at once for a doctor. Do not send, but take to the doctor each month or oftener, a sample of urine. Report to him if you have a discharge.

In some cases a laxative diet of either fresh or cooked fruits will accomplish the desired effect.

Medicine.—Take medicines only when they are prescribed by a doctor. Patent medicines are apt to be poisonous both to mother and child.

Bathing and Cleanliness.—Bathing is necessary for your health. Daily sponge or shower baths with soap and moderately warm water will keep the pores of the skin open. Give particular care to cleanliness of the nipples. Keep them free from undue pressure by the clothing, and if necessary draw them out gently a few minutes each day with clean fingers. It is important for both you and your baby that everything be clean about the home.

Care of the Teeth.—The teeth should be thoroughly brushed after each meal and before going to bed, and the mouth well rinsed, after an attack of vomiting. An excellent wash for the teeth and mouth is a half teaspoonful of common baking soda or table salt dissolved in a glass of warm water (this to be used once each day).

Articles Needed for the Expectant Mother.—

Sufficient bedding.

Six nightgowns.

Piece of white oilcloth, 1½ yards square.

Plenty of old newspapers.

Plenty of old muslin.

One pound of absorbent cotton.

Two pounds of sterile gauze or equivalent in old muslin which has been sterilized.

Useful bed pads can be made by enclosing several newspapers in old muslin. If these are to be used, at least twelve of them should be prepared.

Necessary Articles for Confinement.—

Cord dressings of old muslin.

Sterilized tape for tying cord.

Castile soap.

Blanket (old and soft) to wrap the baby in.

Clothes-basket for baby's bed.

Two abdominal binders (roller towels may be used).

Sufficient quantity of perineal pads which may be made either of absorbent and sterilized gauze or of old sterilized muslin.

Two breast binders from 8 to 10 inches wide.

Boric acid powder (5 cents worth).

Small bottle of alcohol.

Two dozen safety pins, large and small.

Oil or lard for greasing baby.

Scissors.

Before the nurse or attendant is dismissed the mother has had her first lessons in the school of motherhood.

Birth Registration.

One of the most important services to render the new-born baby is to have his birth promptly and properly registered.

In most States the attending physician or midwife is required by law to report the birth to the proper authority, who will see that the child's name, the date of his birth, and other particulars are made a matter of public record. Birth registration may be of the greatest importance when the child is older, and parents should make sure that this duty is not neglected.

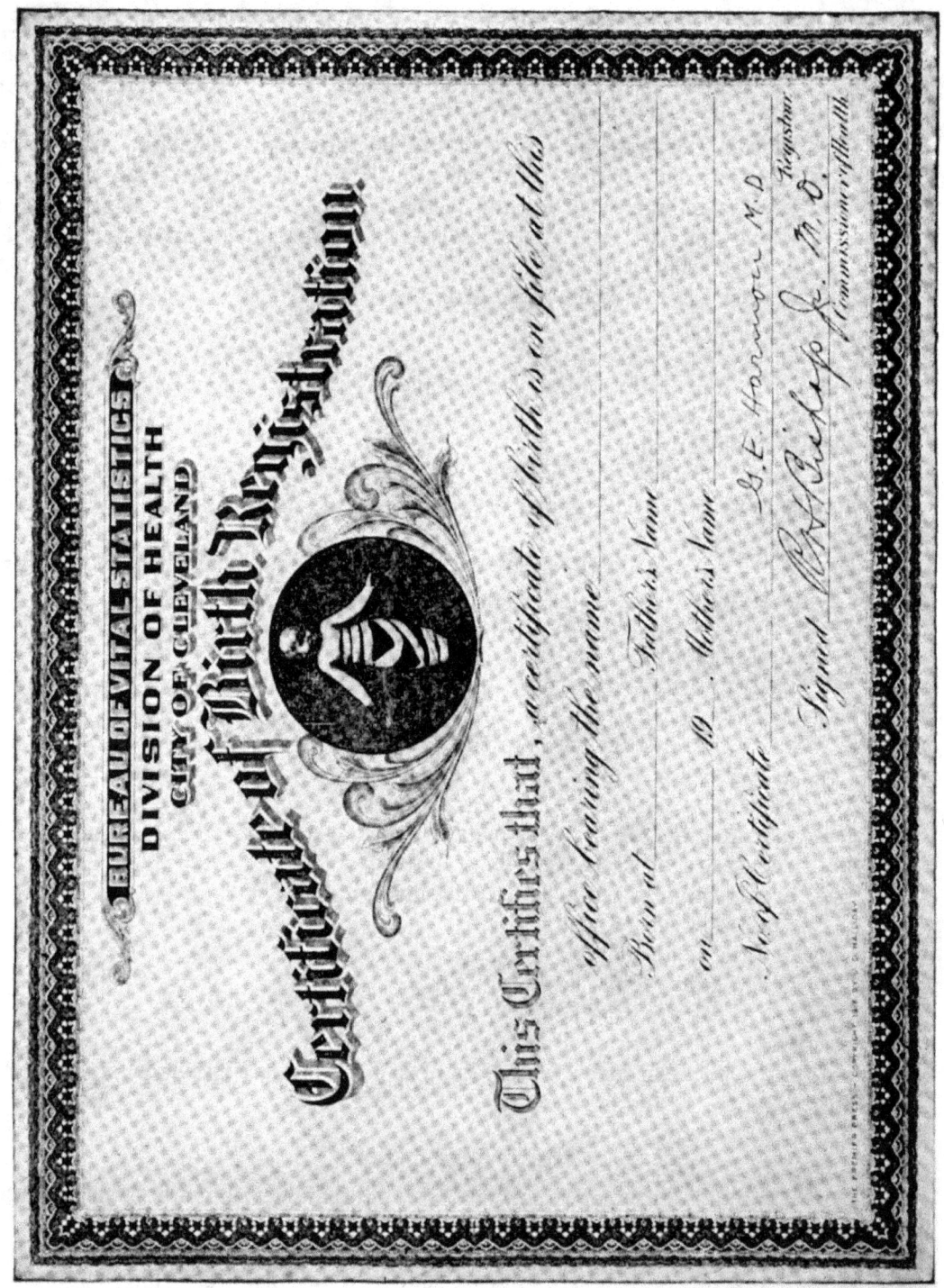

Baby's Room.

Light and Ventilation.—Sunshine is as necessary for the baby as for the plant, and a baby deprived of it will pine and droop just as a plant does; there fore the room in which the sun shines for the longest period of the day should be chosen for the nursery.

The room should have a constant supply of fresh air, as the baby will be much less liable to illness than when he is deprived of it. To "air" a room at intervals by opening the windows is well, but a far better plan is to have a continual stream of fresh air flowing through. To do this the windows must be opened on opposite sides of the room in order to secure a cross draft, which is always necessary to real ventilation. The bed should be as far away from the windows as possible and in a corner out of the direct draft. If this is impossible a blanket may be pinned around the crib so that the wind will not blow directly upon the baby.

The temperature of the room should be 65 to 70 degrees. A thermometer should be hung in the room above the bed.

Overheating is the commonest error in the city. In the country perhaps the most usual mistake is draughty rooms, floors, cold halls and unventilated rooms.

The room being cold the night clothing should be warm, varying with the temperature.

Weak or sickly infants and babies under six weeks should be kept in a warmer room.

Heating.—It is desirable to have a heating system which is readily controlled, so that the temperature of the room may be raised or lowered when necessary. Hot-air furnaces are considered more healthful than steam or hot water, because they provide for the circulation of fresh, moistened air. Gas and oil heaters should be avoided if any other method can be had, as such heaters exhaust the air of even a large room in a short time. An open grate in the room is an advantage, both because extra heat may be had when needed and because it helps to keep the air in the room in circulation.

Cleaning.—The floor should be bare, so that it can be kept clean by wiping it with a damp cloth or dust mop. There should be no heavy draperies nor upholstered furniture to catch dust. Painted walls which can be washed are sanitary and easily renewed.

Bed.

The first bed may be made from an ordinary clothes basket or from a light box, such as an orange crate. Later, a metal crib with a firm spring is desirable. Table padding or "silence" cloth, folded to four thicknesses, makes a very good mattress, because it is readily washable when washed it should be hung out of doors to dry. A sanitary crib mattress may be made by stuffing bed ticking with excelsior, which can be renewed as often as necessary. Sphagnum moss or straw, can be used in the same way. The mattress cover may be made of bed ticking or heavy unbleached muslin, which can be emptied, washed, and dried in the sun at intervals. In case excelsior or straw is used for the temporary filling, it should be made as level and smooth as possible, and a piece of soft felting or a small comfort should always be placed over the mattress to soften the rough surface. After the baby has learned not to wet the bed at night, an ordinary mattress of hair, felt, or cotton may be used, but it should be protected by oilcloth, rubber sheet-

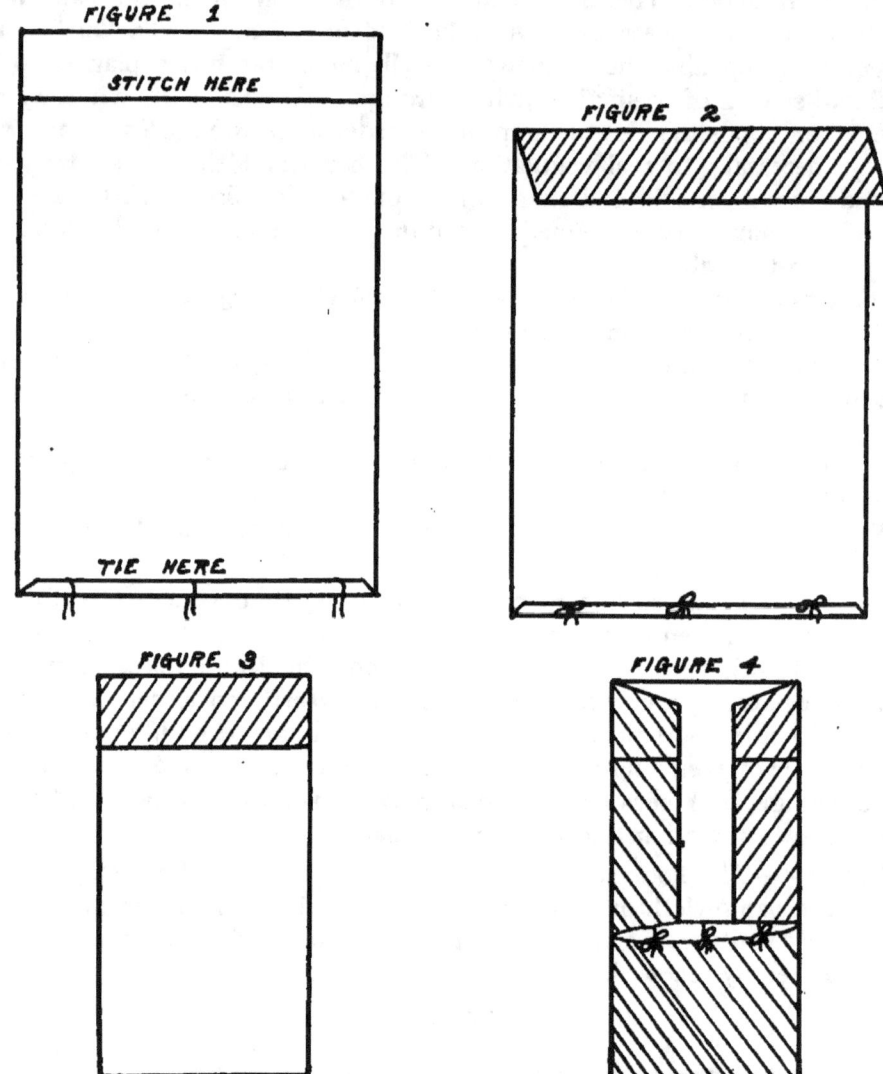

Baby's Night Clothes.

ing, or absorbent paper as an additional precaution. Since a rubber or oilcloth sheet is both hard and cold, a soft pad should always be used directly underneath the baby. Table felting makes excellent pads.

Pillow.—A baby will breathe more easily and take a larger supply of air into the lungs if no pillow is used. If the mother desires, she may place a clean folded napkin or some other clean soft cloth under the baby's head, but it should not be allowed to elevate the head appreciably. Toward the end of the second year a thin hair pillow may be used. Feather or down pillows are unduly heating to the child's head.

Making the Bed.—To make the baby's bed when a metal crib is in use, cover the mattress with the oilcloth or soft rubber sheeting, to each corner of which a strong tape has been sewed. Tie these tapes together under the mattress to hold the rubber smooth. (If desired, the rubber cover may be made like a pillowcase, covering the mattress entirely). Over this place the cotton pad, then cover with a small sheet, which should be tucked under the mattress on all four sides so that the bed is perfectly smooth.

Make a cotton bag the width of a crib blanket and 10 inches longer, closed on three sides like a pillowcase and open at the end, this end to be closed by buttons or tapes. Stitch the case straight across 10 inches below the closed end, thus making a flap. Now put the crib blankets (one or two, according to the temperature) inside this cover. Adjust the blankets smoothly within the cover, tie or button the open end, and turn down the flap at the other end. The object of this flap is to give additional protection to the blanket at the top to save it from being soiled or stained by milk, medicine, or by the material which the baby may vomit.

Then take the blanket thus covered and proceed as follows: Fold the two sides under about 10 inches and turn the bottom up under in the same way about one-third of its length, thus forming what may be described as a sort of loose sleeping bag. (See Figures 3 and 4). Put the baby on his bed and place the cover thus folded over him. The object is to prevent the rigidity of a bed made in the old-fashioned way, with the covers tucked under the mattress, and to give the baby freedom of motion. It is especially adapted to young babies before they are old enough to kick the covers off. Older children will need to have the cover fastened in some way, and in such cases it may be secured by safety pins to the mattress over the baby's shoulders. It is the cover which comes next to the baby and fits in closely around him that keeps him warm, and not an excess of bedclothing piled on top of him. In addition to the top cover, a soft blanket wrapped closely around the baby, especially about the neck and shoulders, should be used in extremely cold weather.

Some of the additional advantages of the blanket cover here described are that it saves trouble in bed making, and especially that it protects the blankets so completely that they will need washing much less frequently than otherwise. The blankets should be well aired and sunned when not in use, and if sewed within clean covers for the summer will be secure from moths.

Other Equipment.

This may include a screen to protect the baby from draughts, a low chair without arms for the mother, baby scales, bathtub, and a basket for the toilet articles. The other furniture of the room should consist of a chiffonier or bureau to hold the baby's clothing and other possessions, and two tables—one for the scales, basket, etc., and the other a low one in which the bathtub may be placed when the baby is being bathed. Later there may be a nursery chair and a high chair. Small rocking chairs are dangerous because they are so easily tipped over.

Clothing.

Clothing should always be adapted to season and climate. A baby is comfortably dressed when his clothing is warm enough without being too warm. If he is too warm, the baby will perspire; if not warm enough, he will have cold

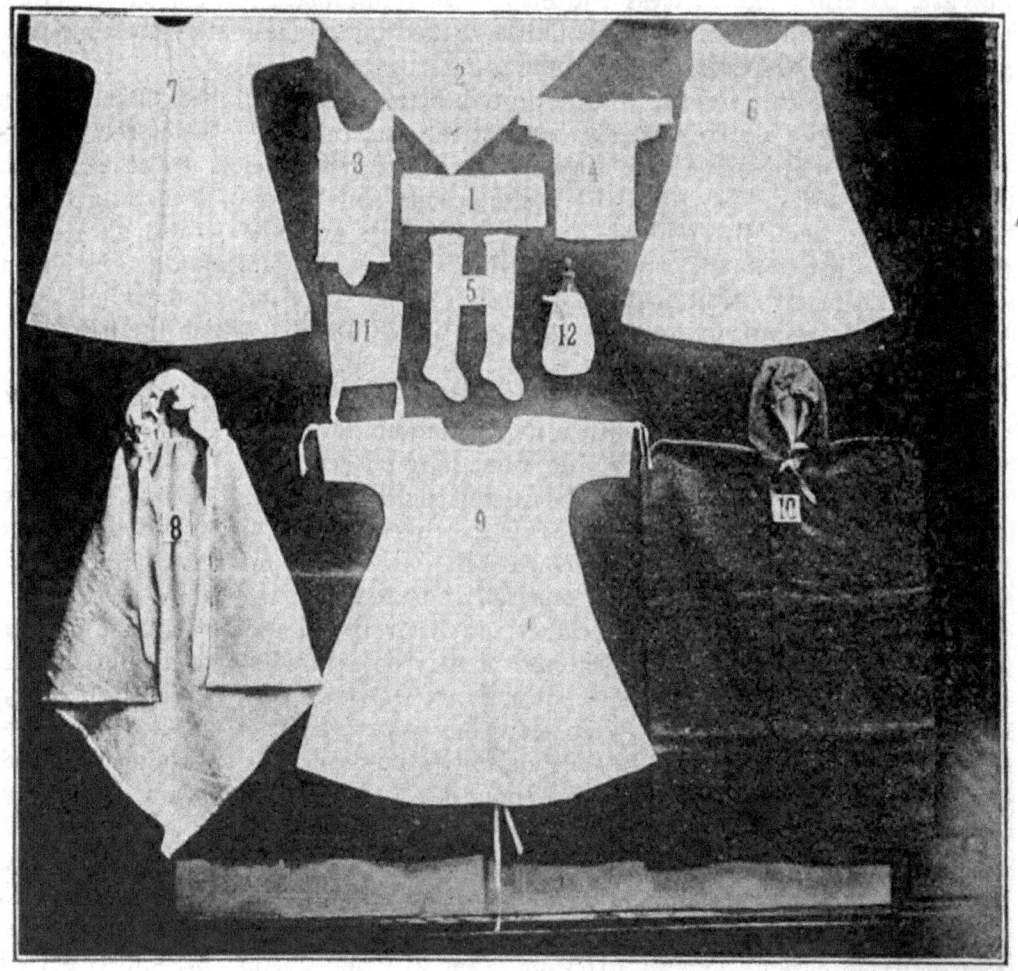

Baby's Clothes.

hands and feet or become blue about the mouth. Little babies need to be kept warm, and gradually accustomed to cooler conditions, but older babies are often overdressed. A baby that is continually dressed in clothing which is too warm becomes pale and languid and is more liable to colds and bowel troubles. The mother should feel the baby's body occasionally, and if she finds it constantly moist the clothing is too warm. In addition, clothing must be loose, so that all the little growing and expanding muscles and organs may have plenty of room to develop. It must be soft and smooth, so that the tender skin will not be irritated, and finally, it must be clean and dry. When these conditions have been secured it does not matter in the least how plain and simple the garments are.

Bands.—Bands are unhemmed strips of flannel, from 6 to 8 inches wide and 18 inches long, and are used to hold the navel dressing in place. The knitted band with shoulder straps should be substituted for the flannel band as soon as the navel has healed. Bands of any sort must never "bind." A band, if drawn tightly about the abdomen, instead of preventing rupture may produce it, especially if the pressure is in the wrong place. The abdominal muscles of a healthy baby need little support, save, perhaps, in the earliest weeks of life; rather they need free play in order to be strengthened in the natural way by the slight exercise the baby can give them.

Shirts.—Baby shirts come in four weights and several sizes. It is well to begin with the second size, as the first is soon outgrown. These shirts, as well as the knitted bands, are made of all wool, or of wool and silk, wool and cotton, or all cotton. Either the all cotton, the cotton-and-wool, or silk-and-wool mixtures are best. The shirts should open all the way down in front.

Many physicians prefer cotton or linen undergarments for children of all ages. They believe that woolen underclothing is responsible for many of the "colds" and similar ailments from which children suffer. Cotton garments do not overheat nor irritate the skin, and at the same time they readily absorb moisture. A summer weight and winter weight should be used, and all other additions to the baby's clothing made according to the temperature. Extra wraps must be used when he is taken out. This rule applies especially to children living in overheated apartments and houses where the indoor temperature resembles that of summer much of the time. A child wearing underclothing that is too warm in such an atmosphere is made unduly sensitive and becomes a ready prey to infection of various kinds. In the North, or in winter, or in case the house can not be easily or sufficiently heated, or for very young or weakly babies, shirts and bands which are part wool are advisable.

Petticoats.—Light-weight part-wool flannel may be used for the petticoats, which for very young babies should not extend more than 10 inches below the feet or 28 inches in full length. They may be made by the "princess" or "Gertrude" model if warmth is desired, but for summer they should be made with a cotton waist, as in the case of older children. Petticoats should always hang from the shoulders.

Slips.—Slips should be made of some very soft material, such as cambric, nainsook, long cloth, or batiste. They should not be more than 28 inches long and should be very simply made. Care must be taken not to have anything about the neck that will scratch or irritate the tender skin, as eczema may be caused in this way. Starch is positively forbidden in a baby's clothes.

Wrappers and Nightgowns.—Wrappers, either flannel or cotton, according to the weather, may be used in the place of slips, and in summer they do away with the need for petticoats as well. The only value of a long petticoat is to provide extra warmth and to make it easier to handle a little baby, while the white slip serves only to keep the petticoat clean and to complete the conventional idea of a baby's toilet; therefore a simple wrapper which opens all the way down the front saves time and trouble for the mother and gives the baby comfort. Besides flannel, other materials may be used, such as challis, nun's veiling, cashmere, henrietta cloth, or any other light, soft material which can be readily washed. Outing flannel may be used, but the fuzzy surface of the cotton flannels is highly inflammable, and great care must be taken not to allow a spark of fire to reach the baby when wearing such a garment. These wrappers may be worn as nightgowns when the baby is older. Nightgowns and wrappers, both short and long, may be bought ready-made, a very satisfactory sort being made of stockinet. At night the nightgown is put on over a clean diaper and the knitted band. No stockings need be worn, for with young babies it is best to use a loose baggy nightgown that closes at the bottom with a drawstring. Drawstrings can also be used on the ends of the sleeves.

Diapers.—The diaper is by far the most troublesome part of the baby's outfit. The ordinary cotton or linen diaper made of "bird's-eye," domett flannel, or terry cloth, is open to objections. In the first place, a large number must

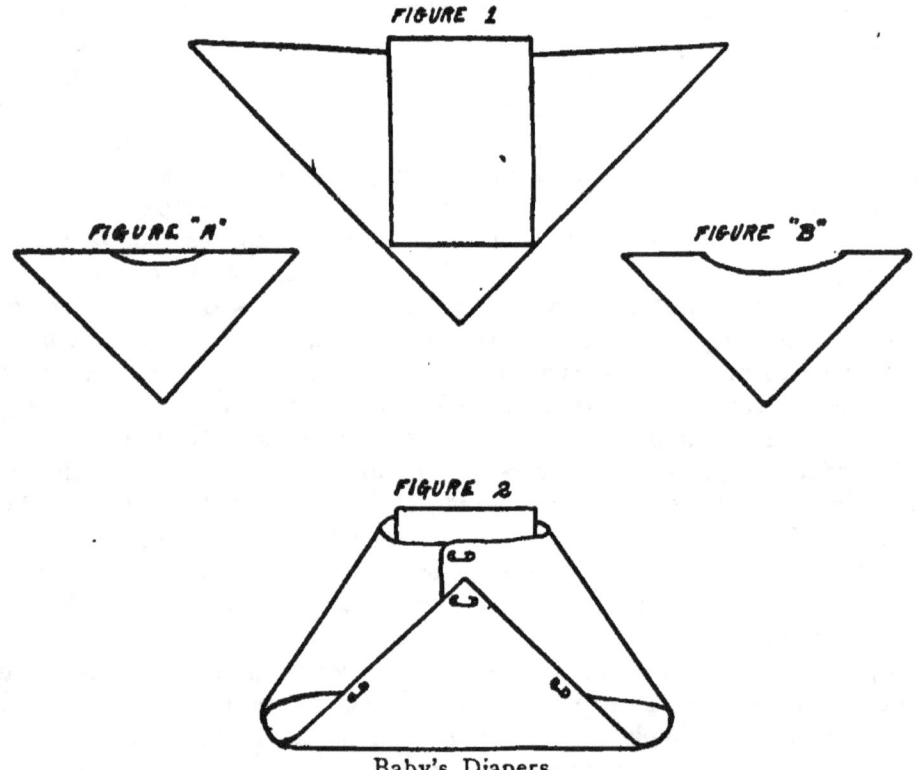

Baby's Diapers.

be provided, which involves a considerable outlay of time and money on the mother's part. Then, as no diaper is fit to use a second time without having been washed and dried, the care of these garments adds to the labor of the household. In addition to these objections the ordinary diaper is hot and clumsy, not to speak of the objectionable odor which clings so persistently to it. There is evidence to show that a wad of thick materials between the legs may deform the thighs to some extent. Besides, unless the diaper is most carefully washed, with soap that contains nothing to irritate the skin (a bland white soap is best), is thoroughly rinsed, and well dried in the open air, there is danger that the baby's flesh may become chafed and sore, especially when hot, nonabsorbent material, such as canton flannel is used.

Pads.—But since diapers are necessary, some practical substitute for those in common use may be found. If an outside diaper is made of cheese-cloth, or some other thin, soft, loosely woven material which is easy to wash, an inside pad may be used to catch the discharges. If this pad is made of something which may be destroyed, the most disagreeable part of the washing will be done away with; but even if the pad must be washed, the time and labor involved in washing pads will be much less than in washing an entire diaper. Washable pads may be made of any soft material at hand, such as old turkish towels or knitted underwear, or other material having a loose texture. Smooth materials, however soft, do not hold the discharges as well. Terry cloth, a material resembling turkish toweling, makes excellent pads after it has been washed a few times to render it more readily absorbent.

How to Put On the Diaper.—The ordinary diaper is a square of material from one-half to three-fourths of a yard wide, folded diagonally and then folded again, making four thicknesses of material. If the inner pad is used, this outer diaper need be folded but once and the extra thickness will be secured in the pad.

Changing the Diaper.—During the mother's waking hours the diaper should be changed as often as it is wet or soiled. In the night it should be changed when the baby is taken up to be fed.

Shoes and Stockings.—It is very important to keep the baby's legs and feet warm. Stockings and diaper should meet, leaving no part of the leg exposed. If the weather is warm the baby will not usually require any covering for his feet, but in cold weather and in all weather when it grows cold toward night it is well for him to wear a pair of merino stockings. These need not be all wool; indeed, if of a mixture of cotton they are much better, as they will not shrink. For an older baby, who is on the floor a great deal, stockings and soft-soled shoes are necessary for comfort, except during the heat of summer. All the shoes from the very first should be chosen to fit the natural shape of the foot, with broad toes and straight soles. Socks may be worn in summer, but in the cooler months the baby's legs should be entirely covered.

Cloaks and Caps.—Since a baby exercises very little when taken out in a carriage, he must be warmly wrapped. Cloaks should either be of warm woolen material or have an interlining of wool, or in cold climates both. For the "runabout" baby additional warmth is secured by the use of leggings, a sweater, overshoes, and mittens. In summer if a wrap is needed it may be of silk or cotton, although a cloak of challis, cashmere, or nun's veiling has more warmth and at the same time is light in weight. Caps should not be thick enough to cause the head to perspire. A silk cap with an interlining of wool wadding or of flannel may be used in winter. In the coldest weather a little hood knitted of woolen yarn, having a cape to come down under the coat collar and protect the neck is excellent. Silk or muslin caps may be worn in the milder months, or the baby may go bareheaded if protected from the sun. No starch should be used in the caps, as stiff strings or ruffles will scratch the delicate skin of the baby and may cause eczema. Cap strings and ribbons should be carefully examined after the child is dressed to see that they are not too tightly tied. Frost-bitten nose or cheeks may result if the circulation is checked by tight ribbons.

Baths and Bathing.

When the mother takes charge of the baby she will find it convenient, usually, to give the bath before the midmorning feeding and after the bowels have moved.

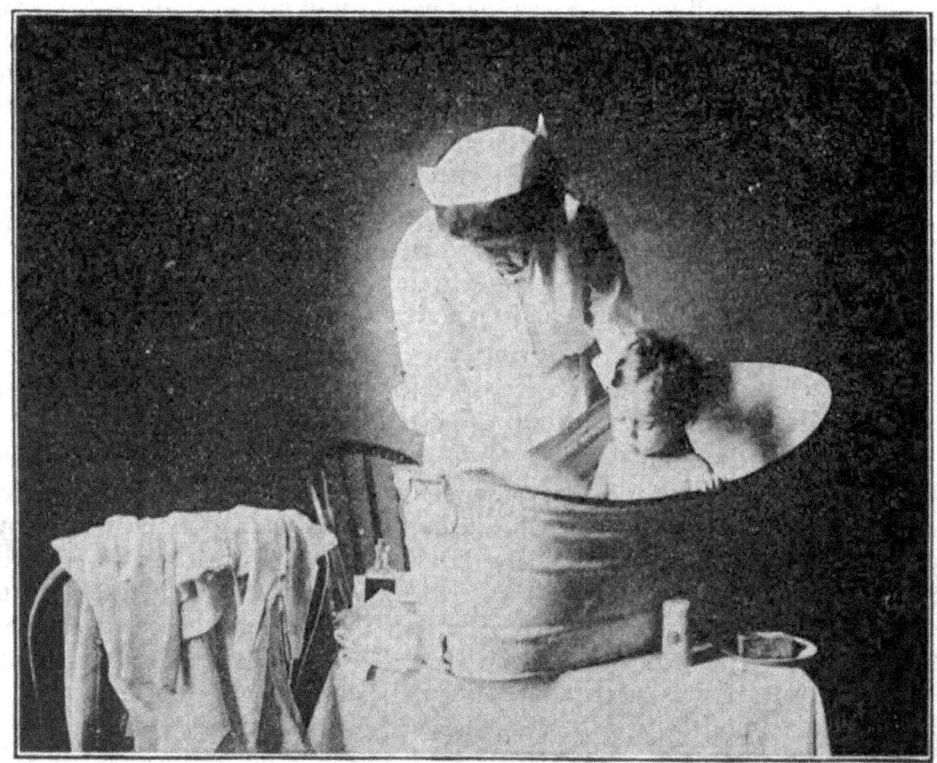

Bathing the Baby.

The room should be comfortably warmed to about 72 degrees. It is not wise to have the room so hot that the baby perspires, as there is grave danger of his being chilled when, the bath over, he is taken into another room where the temperature is lower or when the room itself is rapidly cooled. It is better for the baby to have his bath in a room at ordinary temperature than in a bathroom which is heated by oil or gas. The baby should be protected from drafts by screens or by a shield made by hanging a blanket over the backs of two chairs. The full tub bath may be given as soon as the scar where the navel cord was attached has fully healed. An infant bathtub serves every purpose for the first year of a baby's life or until he has outgrown it. A tiny baby may be bathed in a basin or bowl for some weeks. This basin should always be warmed before it is filled. The water should be at body heat or slightly above: that is, from 98 to 100 degrees. After 6 months, 95 degrees and during the second year, 85 to 80 degrees. A bath thermometer is an inexpensive convenience and should be provided, but if none can be had the mother may test the temperature with

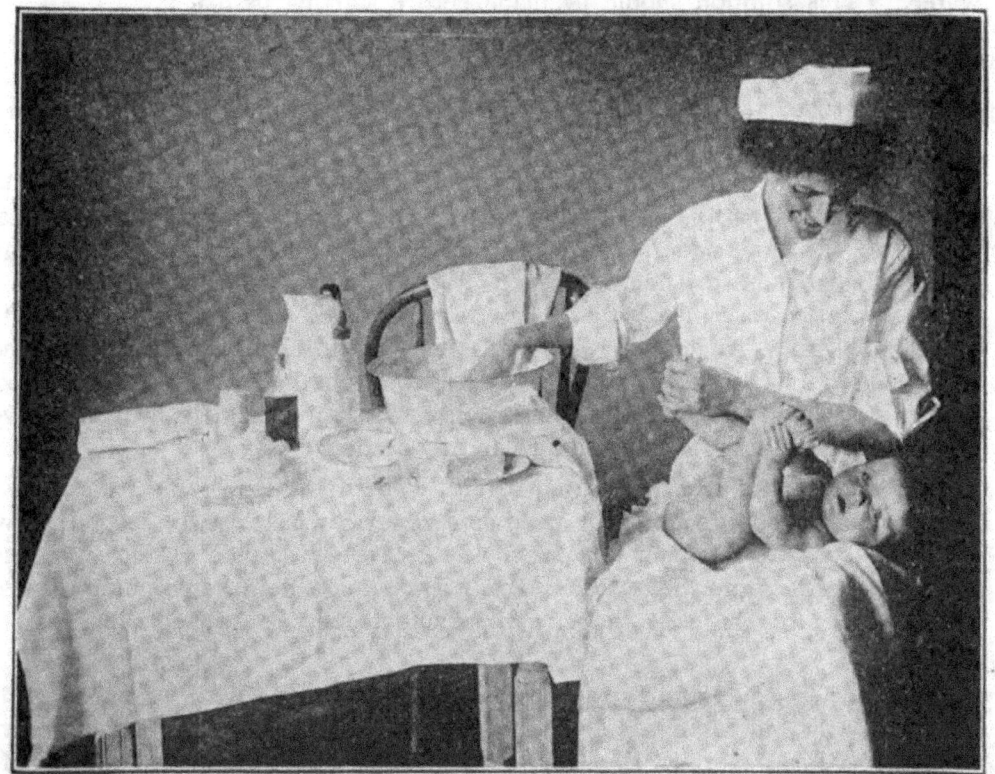

The Sponge Bath.

her elbow. When the water feels neither hot nor cold it will be comfortable for the baby. It should be tested after the baby is undressed and ready to get into the water. Hot water should never be added to the bath while the baby is in the tub. Never leave a young baby alone in the tub. Never put the baby in the bath while the tub is standing on a stove or heater; he might be seriously burned in this way.

No unnecessary exposure or delay should take place, for in cold or cool weather the baby is quickly chilled. To prevent this, all the necessities, such as soap and towels, clothing, bath apron for the mother, tub, water, thermometer, powder, and the like should be placed at hand before undressing the baby. In some cases it may be much more convenient for the mother to give the bath at night, just before the baby's bedtime. Never bathe a baby within an hour after feeding. A baby should always have his own towels and wash cloths. Soft cheese-cloth makes excellent cloths; the towels should be old and soft.

Before the baby is completely undressed his scalp should be washed, the head lowered a little to avoid getting soap in the eyes. Use a pure, bland, white, nontransparent soap. Very little soap is needed for cleaning a baby's skin, and it is most important that the skin be thoroughly rinsed. The eyes, nose, ears and genitals are then cleansed with a fresh piece of absorbent cotton dipped in a bowl of boracic acid and water, a teaspoonful to the pint of boiled water. (This solution should be made before starting bath.)

The mouth should be left alone, not only at the time of the bath, but at all times. The mucous membrane or lining of the mouth is often injured in this way. The baby's mouth will take care of itself and be far better cleansed by its own saliva.

Remove the balance of the clothing and soap the entire body; then place the baby in the bath, holding him with the left forearm under the neck and shoulders, the hand under his arm, lifting the feet and legs with the right hand. Use the right hand to sponge the entire body, then lift the baby out and wrap him at once in a warmed towel. Dry carefully with soft, warm towels, patting the skin gently. Never rub the baby's tender skin with anything less smooth than the palm of the hand. Dress as rapidly as possible if the weather is cold, taking great pains not to expose him unnecessarily. When the weather is very hot in summer, only a slip and diaper are needed.

If the skin is carefully dried after the bath there will be little need for powder, and it should never be used as a cover for careless drying. It is well to use a little pure talcum powder in the creases and folds of the skin, under the arms and around the buttocks, but it should not be used so generally as to fill the pores of the skin and clog them and should be applied only after the skin is dry.

Babies, just like some grown-up folks, do not like a bath. Sometimes this is because the mother has the water either too hot or too cold. If, however, it is just a natural aversion then try to coax him by making a "play game" of it. Toys which float will often divert the baby's attention and make him forget his objections to the water.

But no matter how trying to one's patience, do not resort to force or harsh methods. Such treatment is just as harmful in this case as in regard to other matters in the bringing up of the baby.

When warm days come, in addition to the baby's daily bath, sponge him off two or three times more. It will keep him comfortable and make him better able to endure the heat of the summer.

In putting on the baby's clothes he should lie flat upon the mother's lap or upon the table which is covered with a thick pad of some kind.

The clothes should be drawn over the feet and not over the head. Baby clothes should be changed throughout, once each day at the time of the bath.

Certain Cases When the Bath May or Should be Omitted.

Small thin, emaciated babies often do not stand the bath well. They, of course, are under the care of a physician, and he will recommend a sweet oil rub, or whatever is necessary to take the place of the bath.

Children with eczema or other skin affections are often benefited by omitting the bath. However, I do not believe the bath should be omitted because the child has a cold or a little fever or any other illness too slight to require a physician's attendance. At such times a bath is often restful and quieting, and the child goes off to sleep for the night when he would otherwise have been fretful and restless.

How to Lift the Baby.

To lift a young baby, slip the left hand under the back beneath the shoulders, spreading the fingers in such a way as to support the neck and head, and lift the feet and legs with the right hand. Never lift the child without thus supporting the spine. When a baby has learned to hold up his head and has gained considerable strength in the muscles of the back and neck, he may be lifted by grasping him with outspread fingers under the armpits, the body held firmly, so that the entire strain does not come on the shoulders. A baby should never be lifted by the arms. It is possible to dislocate the shoulder joint by careless lifting.

Care of the Special Organs.

Eyes.—Whether the young baby is awake or asleep, his eyes should always be shielded from strong light, either sunlight or artificial, and from dust and wind. Care should be taken not to allow any soapy water to enter the baby's eyes in bathing. Swelling or redness or any discharge should have medical attention at once.

Mouth.—A healthy baby's mouth needs no cleaning before the teeth come. The saliva is a sterilizing fluid, intended to keep the mouth healthy, and it is possible to injure the delicate tissues by attempting to clean them with a cloth. If the mouth must be washed, a swab made by twisting a piece of sterile absorbent cotton on the end of a clean stick should be used. Dip this in warm boiled water and wipe the gums very carefully. Never put a finger inside the baby's mouth unless in an emergency.

Ears.—Wash the external ear with a soft cloth, but never attempt to introduce any hard instrument inside the ear to clean it. Always dry the ears and creases back of them very carefully.

Nose.—The baby's nose should be cleaned as a part of the daily toilet in the same way as the ears. Use a piece of twisted cotton. When the baby has an infectious cold he should have special attention.

Genital Organs.—These organs in both sexes should be kept scrupulously clean, with as little handling as possible. Boys should be examined by a physician to see whether or not circumcision is needed. The foreskin should frequently be drawn back at bathing time and the organ cleansed. If the mother finds it difficult to retract it, she should not attempt to do this alone, but should ask the doctor to show her how. Perfect cleanliness is the principal treatment required in girl babies. These parts should be carefully washed at the time of the bath with boracic acid. Use a clean piece of cotton for this purpose, never use a wash cloth or soap and water which is used for the bath. It is also necessary to wash the parts toward the rectum so that it will not become contaminated with the matter from the stool. Care should also be taken with the clothes, especially when the girl has become old enough to wear drawers, that they are not too tight so that these parts may be chafed. Occasionally adhesions are found toward the lips of the orifice where they are joined together above. These are apt to cause so-called "reflex symptoms," such as restlessness, nervousness, frequent passing of the urine and often convulsions. Any symptoms of this sort call for an examination by the physician who will separate the adhesions. If at any time the parts look red and irritated the cause should be looked into and proper treatment instituted.

Feeding.

Process of Digestion.—In order to comprehend the principles which underlie the proper feeding of infants, it is well to understand what is involved in the process of digeston and what food elements are needed for the growth, maintenance and repair of the body.

Digestion is the process or series of processes by which the food eaten is changed into the forms in which it can be absorbed by the tissues of the body. This is a most intricate operation, involving the use of many organs and functions, but one which takes place without difficulty in the healthy human body. But since all the complicated machinery necessary for digestion must be started at once, and since, necessarily, the organs of a new-born baby can be but feeble, it stands to reason that the food presented to them must be liquid; also it must contain the five essential elements which the human body requires for growth: namely, the fats, sugars and starches, which furnish the necessary heat and energy; the proteins, or muscle-forming foods; the mineral salts needed for the growth of all tissues; and, lastly, a great amount of water. All these are found in milk, and in no other food which the infant is capable of digesting. Therefore milk is the one proper infant food.

Breast Feeding.—The mother's milk is the only food that was ever meant for a baby during his first year and any other food is at best a poor substitute. Breast milk is the true elixir of life. If we knew how to make it and were able to distribute it in its purity just as it flows from the mother's breast we could save thousands upon thousands of babies' lives each year. Can you imagine a mother so indifferent to her child's life as deliberately to throw away this precious fluid?

Statistics gathered from this country and many others show that breast-fed babies have a much greater chance for life than those who are bottle-fed, and also that the infant illnesses, not only those of the digestive tract but many other varieties, afflict bottle-fed infants much oftener and much more seriously than those who have breast milk. But not only does breast milk protect the nursing baby from illness and increases materially his chance for life, but it practically insures that his development shall proceed in a normal orderly fashion.

The body makes a greater proportional growth during the first year of life than during any other, and the brain increases more in the same time than in all the rest of the years of life put together. It is therefore of the utmost importance to the whole existence of each individual that during this most critical period the baby be surrounded with all possible conditions for perfect health. The most important of these conditions is breast milk. Food is the one question of overwhelming importance to the baby.

Nursing Mother.—The majority of mothers can nurse their babies, at least in part, if they have suitable care and advice. What is chiefly required is that this conviction should enter the mind of the mother and abide there; for the fear that she will not be able to perform this function, or that the milk will not or does not agree with her child has more to do with the supposed inability to nurse than any other one factor. The gland which secretes maternal milk is a wonderful and delicate mechanism. So intimate is the connection of the mammary nerves with the mind that the mental states of the mother are readily reflected in their function. Fear, anger, or worry may serve to check the secretion of the milk, or to change its quality so much that, for the time being, it is unfit for use, while, on the other hand, a calm mind, joy, laughter, and delight in life, coupled with the desire and intention to nurse the baby, will make it possible to do so. Failing this spirit, all other measures may prove futile.

The secretion of milk is induced by the efforts of the baby to nurse, and therefore he should be put to the breast regularly for at least two weeks after birth, even if only a very little milk is secreted. This patient effort, with proper food and care, coupled with the determination to succeed, will usually result in a good supply of milk, and no physician or nurse who appreciates the value of breast milk for the baby will counsel another course. It is rarely true that the mother's milk does not agree with the baby. It is much more often deficient in quantity than in quality. The return of menstruation may lead to a slight temporary disturbance, but is not a sufficient cause for weaning.

Diet.—A nursing mother should have a light, abundant, and appetizing diet, and such a one as causes her no indigestion. Disturbances in the digestive tract of the mother are quickly reflected in the baby's condition, and therefore the mother should refrain from eating or drinking those things which she knows from experience she cannot digest. As a rule, indigestion in the mother, which shows itself in constipation, eructations of gas, headache, diarrhea, and the like, is caused by such foods as heavy puddings or underdone pastry, doughnuts, fried food soaked in fat; made dishes such as croquettes and fritters; pickles, mincemeat, baked beans, pork and cabbage, and other heavy or poorly cooked foods; but people differ greatly in their power of digestion, and what will suit one person may upset the next. Overeating may be a cause of indigestion.

A mixed diet of such digestible and nutritious foods as are readily available, is desirable for the nursing mother. All foods are milk-making foods. The foods selected will differ widely according to circumstances, but will usually include vegetables, ripe fruits, meat, poultry and fish, with oysters and the like, eggs, milk, cheese, farinaceous foods of all kinds (cereals, flour, meals, etc.), breads, especially graham, whole wheat, corn meal, and bran, and simple desserts. Occasionally acid fruits, vegetables, and spices eaten by the mother may cause some disturbance in the baby, and in such cases they should be avoided.

Constipation is to be most carefully avoided by eating bran bread and other laxative foods. Drugs should be taken as little as possible, and only on the doctor's advice. Tea and coffee may be taken in moderation, not more than one cup of each, a day. Alcohol drinks of all sorts are better avoided. One quart of milk should be taken each day. Six to eight glasses of good drinking water a day are required, one or two of which should be taken on rising to encourage the action of the bowels.

Exercise.

In order that a healthy nursing mother may be able to eat and digest a generous supply of food materials, exercise in the fresh air is indispensable. A vigorous walk is one of the best of tonics, because of its effect both on the body and on the mind. Worries take flight when treated to sunshine and fresh air and leave the nervous system free to perform its normal functions. The woman who has a garden to look after or other interests which take her out of doors a good deal in the course of a day gets her exercise in the most natural way, but she will need to be on guard against overtaxing herself. No exercise should be carried to the point of weariness, because then the nutriment which should go to make milk for the baby will be used to renew the mother's worn-out tissues.

Sleep.

An abundance of sleep is essential. The nursing mother should have at least eight hours of sleep every night and an hour in the daytime. A mother soon learns to rest herself whenever the baby nurses, and these brief periods of relaxation help greatly to keep her in good condition.

Bathing.

A daily bath is desirable, should be taken whenever possible. It is especially important to remove the odors of perspiration or old milk from the mother's body and clothing, as the baby may refuse to nurse when an unpleasant odor is forced upon him.

Amusements and Recreation.

A conscientious young mother is very apt to defeat her own ends by staying at home too constantly and watching over her baby so incessantly that she grows pale and nervous and begins to worry, a condition which often results in depletion of the milk and corresponding disturbance in the baby. Healthy babies are better off with a judicious amount of "letting alone," and there is no reason why a mother should not be absent some part of every day if there is a responsible person to be left in charge. Out-of-door life, pleasant recreation which is not exhausting, visiting, and other diversions are essential to every nursing mother if she is to keep up an abundant supply of milk. The family, especially the husband, should realize how important it is to shield the nursing mother from unnecessary work and worry, and to provide her at intervals with the opportunity for rest and recreation. However, a healthy mother should not regard herself nor permit her family to regard her as in any sense an invalid at this time. She is much more likely to succeed in nursing if she goes about ordinary duties as usual and fills her life with normal interests.

Technique of Nursing.

The first secretion of the breasts is called colostrum, and while not a true milk, is adapted to the baby's needs in the first hours of his life. He should therefore be put to the breast as soon after birth as the mother is able to bear it. This early nursing is important to the mother because it helps to contract the uterus, and to the baby for various reasons, one of which is that he needs to learn how to draw his food before the breast fills with milk and becomes less pliant and more painful.

The mother holds the baby on her arm, drawing him to the breast in such a way that his head is comfortably supported, turning slightly toward the side she wishes to present and drawing the baby's feet and legs against her body. A pillow under the opposite shoulder is a welcome support. The baby should be able to grasp the nipple squarely. If his head is too low, the milk may flow back in his throat, making him cough and choke; but the head must be low enough so that the nostrils are not covered by the breast. It is impossible for the baby to suck properly unless he can breathe freely, and the mother should hold the breast away from his nostrils with the fingers of her free hand. When the breasts have filled, if the milk flows too fast, as sometimes happens, she may control the flow by taking the breast in her hand so that one finger is above and one below the nipple and by pressing it gently at the base. If the baby's efforts to nurse make the mother's nipples sore, they should be washed with plain boiled water or boric acid solution, before and after each nursing and may be anointed with lanolin at night, covering them with gauze or clean linen. If a crack should appear, the greatest care should be taken to prevent infecting the breast, as if this happens a painful breast abscess may result. A doctor should always be consulted. The cracked nipple should be kept constantly clean by washing it with boiled water. A glass nipple shield should be used, care being taken that it is always perfectly clean and made sterile by boiling. The shield will not materially increase the difficulty of nursing for the baby and will safeguard the mother. If the breasts become engorged, they may be relieved by using a breast pump, if necessary, or by gentle massage; but all manipulation only serves to stimulate the breast to greater activity and the less handling it can have the better. Hot or cold applications, according to the patient's preference, are useful, and a breast binder is often a great relief, but should be applied by a physician or nurse. Usually the matter rights itself without difficulty as soon as the relation between the supply and demand is established. If the mother has received the proper care during pregnancy and the breasts and nipples have received due attention, which is part of a doctor's duty, the nursing period will be shorn of much of its pain and trouble. In general, the nipples should be kept as clean and as dry as possible and should be washed before each nursing.

Regularity in Nursing.

The baby should be nursed regularly, by the clock, from the very first and should have nothing between meals save water to drink. It takes from one and one-half hours to three hours for a baby's stomach to empty itself after a full meal of breast milk and considerably longer for the process of digestion to be completed in the intestines.

The baby should not ordinarily be allowed to remain at the breast over 20 minutes in any case, and the nipple should be withdrawn several times during the nursing, so that he will not take the food too rapidly with consequent regurgitation and indigestion. If the milk is plentiful, the breasts should be nursed alternately, but it may be necessary to give both breasts at one feeding, in order to satisfy the baby. Do not let the baby go to sleep while nursing.

When to Feed.

The first and second day every 6 hours or 4 times in 24 hours, beginning at 6 a. m. After the third day when the milk is established, every 2 hours during the day and once at night, usually at 2 a. m. This feeding may be discontinued after the fourth month. From the fourth month to the ninth month 6 feedings in 24 hours: 6, 9, 12, 3, 6, 9. Some babies thrive well when fed every 4 hours: 6, 10, 2, 6, 10.

In order to find out whether the baby is gaining in weight, he should be weighed before and after feeding, not changing the clothing.

A baby should be weighed at least every week throughout the first year. The average baby weighs about seven or seven and one-half pound. He doubles his weight at six months, triples it at one year. There is usually a loss during the first week of from four to eight ounces; after this a healthy baby should gain from four to eight ounces a week up to about 6 months. From 6 to 12 months the gain is less, usually from two to four ounces per week. If, however, baby does not show a steady and consistent gain, or if he begins to lose weight, it is a sign that something is wrong. If the mother is nursing the baby, it may mean that she has not enough milk, or that she is not well, therefore her milk is disagreeing with the baby. In some cases it signifies that the quality of the mother's milk has changed.

If the latter is the case the mother should consult her physician who can advise her what to do to keep her milk in good condition.

Artificial Feeding.

Artificial feeding is the method of feeding which must be employed when a baby is, for any reason, denied breast milk.

If the breast is not sufficient in quantity or quality to satisfy the baby there is no objection to feeding him at night, in order not to disturb the mother's rest. If the mother has only milk enough for 2 or 3 nursings a day, this should be continued so long as the milk agrees with the baby. Even a small amount of good breast milk greatly improves a child's nutrition.

Milk.

Wide experience has shown that fresh cows' milk is the best substitute for breast milk. This milk should be the purest and cleanest possible; it should be the product of a tuberculin-tested herd, one that is healthy, well fed, properly housed and cared for, and milked by clean milkers into sterilized utensils. The milk should be bottled and cooled at the dairy and delivered to consumer in sealed bottles. The milk commonly sold from open cans, known as "loose" or "dipped" milk, should never be given to a baby.

Certified Milk.—In certain places it is possible to obtain what is known as "certified" milk, which is fresh, clean, pure, normal milk of uniform composition and highest quality obtained from healthy cows and produced and handled under the supervision of a medical milk commission, with special sanitary precautions. Although the amount of certified milk is as yet far too small, the demand for it is steadily increasing. As soon as mothers become convinced of the infinite advantage of having a supply of raw milk whose quality is guaranteed they are quite ready to pay the additional cost. There can be no doubt that the use of certified milk has been a great factor in the reduction of deaths from infantile diarrhea in recent years. The American Association of Milk Commissions publishes literature on the subject. The secretary may be addressed at the Ortz Building, Cincinnati, Ohio.

Heating or Cooking Milk.—When certified milk can not be had, or some other milk known to be clean, it is safer to heat that which is used. Bad milk may look clean and may taste and smell sweet, since disease germs do not reveal their presence by the ordinary tests. It is very difficult to insure the cleanliness of the general milk supply, and since it seems impossible to be certain that the milk is always perfectly clean, it is necessary to kill these germs by some process of heating before using the milk for young babies, or for any babies, in the heat of summer. These processes, however, do not make good milk out of bad, nor clean milk out of that which is dirty; they merely make a poor thing a little less dangerous, and emphasize the necessity for raising the standard of local milk production.

Care of the Milk.—One of the reasons why cows' milk is not always a safe food is that it is very readily infected with germs, some of which may make the baby sick. These germs multiply with astonishing rapidity when the milk is allowed to stand for any length of time at a moderate temperature. but do not flourish if the milk is kept very cold. The milk should never be left standing on the doorstep in the sun, nor in a warm kitchen, but should be put in the ice-box as soon as it is delivered. It must be kept covered, protected from dust and flies, not left standing in shallow, open pans nor put into the refrigerator in pitchers or open dishes, as it is very readily contaminated by other foods. Milk should be kept in glass jars or bottles, which are made sterile by boiling before being filled. If the milk is sour, or shows a sediment in the bottom of the bottle, it is not fit to give to the baby.

How to Feed the Baby.

What to Feed.—Leading authorities differ so widely on various points connected with this subject that no directions can be given which will meet with general agreement. A few of the fundamental points are given here, but whenever possible the mother should confer with a good doctor regarding an artificially fed infant.

The only proper artificial food is cows' milk, suitably modified to suit the child's age and development. Some babies have peculiarities, and with them rules can not be closely followed; but with most, if proper rules are followed from the outset, there will be comparatively little trouble. The advice of a good doctor should be sought and followed. It is most unwise for the mother to experiment with different foods or different mixtures, or to try to feed her baby by the advice of her neighbors.

Whenever there are signs of indigestion, such as vomiting or frequent loose stools, the mother should dilute the food, or omit it altogether, giving nothing but a little plain boiled water until the doctor sees the baby.

Formulae for modified milk and any additional food for babies under a year should be prescribed by a physician at least once every month.

The following directions for feeding the baby have been prepared by a committee of the American Medical Association:

Beginning on the third day, the average baby should be given 3 ounces of milk daily, diluted with 7 ounces of water. To this should be added 1 tablespoonful of limewater and 2 level teaspoonfuls of sugar. This should be given in seven feedings.

At one week the average child requires 5 ounces of milk daily, which should be diluted with 10 ounces of water. To this should be added 1½ even tablespoonfuls of sugar and 1 ounce of limewater. This should be given in seven feedings. The milk should be increased by one-half ounce about every four days. The water should be increased by one-half ounce every eight days.

At 3 months the average child requires 16 ounces of milk daily, which should be diluted with 16 ounces of water. To this should be added 3 tablespoonfuls of sugar and 2 ounces of limewater. This should be given in six feedings. The milk should be increased by one-half ounce every six days. The water should be reduced by one-half ounce about every two weeks.

At 6 months the average child requires 24 ounces of milk daily, which should be diluted with 12 ounces of water. To this should be added 2 ounces of limewater and 3 even tablespoonfuls of sugar. This should be given in five feedings. The amount of milk should be increased by one-half ounce every week. The milk should be increased only if the child is hungry and digesting his food well. It should not be increased unless he is hungry, nor if he is suffering from indigestion even though he seems hungry.

At 9 months the average child requires 30 ounces of milk daily, which should be diluted with 10 ounces of water. To this should be added 2 even tablespoonfuls of sugar and 2 ounces of limewater. This should be given in five feedings. The sugar added may be milk sugar or if this can not be obtained cane (granulated) sugar or maltose (malt sugar). At first plain water should be used to dilute the milk.

At 3 months, sometimes earlier, a weak barley water, or oatmeal water may be used in the place of plain water. ·Oatmeal water: Take 2 heaping tablespoonfuls of Rolled Avena or 2 even tablespoonfuls of chopped oats or oat

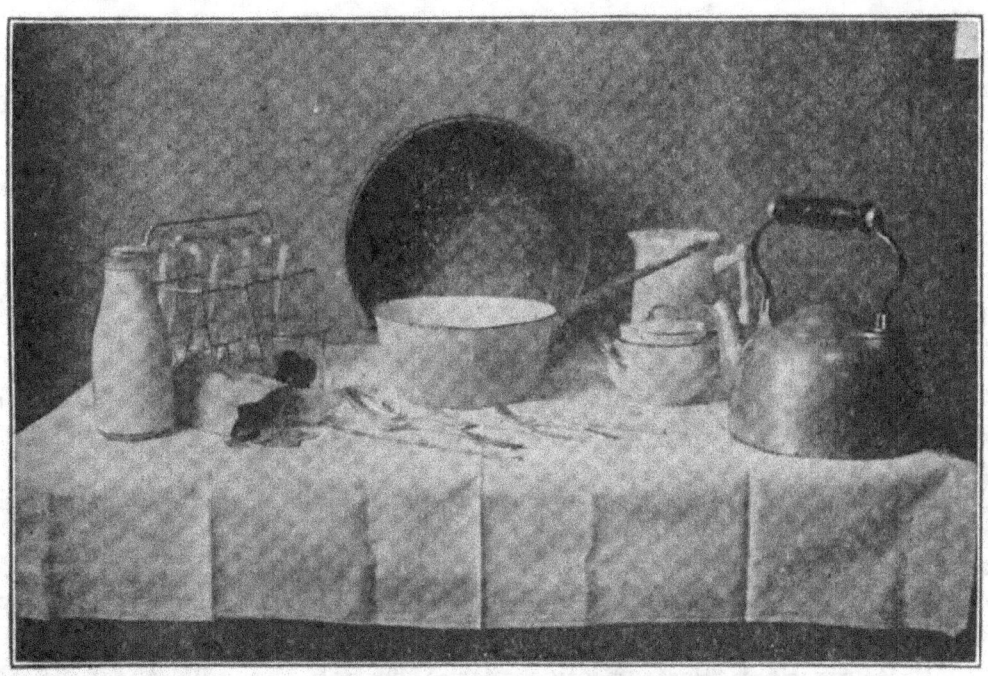

Utensils Necessary in Preparation of the Baby's Food.

flour; add 1 quart of cold water and boil down to one pint in about 30 minutes and pour through a clean sieve or cheese-cloth. If the oatmeal water is to. be given without milk dilute half with water, as otherwise it will be too thick. Barley water: Take 2 even tablespoonfuls of barley flour, add one quart of water and boil down to one pint in about 30 minutes and pour through clean sieve or cheese-cloth. If the barley water is to be given without milk dilute half with water, as otherwise it will be too thick. If pearl barley is used take 1 heaping tablespoonful to 1 pint of water and soak over night or for 4 or 5 hours; then boil for 4 hours, always adding enough water to keep the quantity up to the pint, then pour through clean sieve or cheese-cloth.

Sugar is added to the food not to sweeten it but to furnish a necessary foodstuff. Physicians differ as to the best sugar for use in infant feeding. Malt sugar gives very good results, and several preparations which contain dextrin as well as maltose are on the market, but are expensive. Milk sugar is also expensive, and some physicians believe that it has a greater tendency to upset the baby. Cane sugar is the cheapest form of sugar, and many babies seem to digest it very well. One objection to the use of cane sugar is that the baby quickly becomes accustomed to the sweet taste, making it difficult lafer to induce him to eat unsweetened foods.

Preparation of the Food.

Modification.—(a) Modification means the changing of the milk by dilution and by the addition of various substances to meet the needs of the individual infant.

(b) **Utensils Necessary.**—

(1) A graduated measuring dish which can be purchased at any drug store.

(2) A mixing pitcher which holds from one to two quarts.

(3) One teaspoon and one tablespoon of correct size for measuring and stirring.

(4) As many nursing bottles as the child is to have feedings in twenty-four hours.

(5) Non-absorbent cotton or caps for stoppering.

(c) **Method of Modification.**—First measure out the sugar and the diluent (i. e., water, oatmeal water, barley water, and the like) and see that all of the sugar (i. e., cane sugar, milk sugar, malt sugar, and the like) is dissolved. Pour this mixture into the mixing pitcher and add the other ingredients to the contents of the pitcher in the quantities ordered by your physician. Mix well and pour, while stirring, the required amounts into the number of bottles ordered. Now stopper the bottles and pasteurize and cool the milk in the following manner.

Pasteurization.—Pasteurization means heating the milk to about 150 degrees F. for 30 minutes and then rapidly cooling it. Milk for the baby should always be pasteurized in the feeding bottles. It may be done as follows: The milk should be mixed and poured into the clean feeding bottles, which should then be stoppered with clean, non-absorbent cotton or caps. It is then ready for pasteurization. While a number of satisfactory pasteurizers may be bought in the shops, a home-made pasteurizer can be easily constructed.

Take a wire basket that will hold all the nursing bottles used in 24 hours and place this basket containing the bottles in a vessel of cold water filled to a point a little above the level of the milk. Heat the water and allow it to boil for five minutes. Then run cold water into the vessel until the milk is cooled to the temperature of the running water. The milk is then put into the ice chest, which should be not warmer than 50 degrees F.

Bottles.—The best nursing bottle is the one which affords the least harbor for germs. An 8-ounce cylindrical bottle having the scale in ounces blown in the side is most convenient, as it fits readily into the ice box and the pasteurizer. Such a bottle should have a short neck which slopes gradually into the shoulder. It is difficult, if not impossible, to clean a long-necked bottle having a sharp angle below. It should be possible to reach every part of the inside with the bottle brush. New bottles should be annealed by placing them on the stove in a dishpan of cold water and leaving them to boil for 20 minutes. Allow them to stay in the water until it is cold. Bottles thus treated will not readily break when filled with boiling water or when the food is being cooked in them.

Each bottle should be emptied as soon as the baby has finished nursing, then rinsed with cold water and left standing, filled with water, until the bottles for one day's feedings have all been used.

Nipples.—A conical nipple is best, since it can be readily turned inside out to be cleaned. Nipples attached to long rubber tubes should never be used, as it is impossible to clean them. They are so dangerous to infant health and life that the sale of them ought to be prohibited by law. The hole in the nipple should be just large enough so that when the filled bottle is held upside down the milk drops rapidly. If the hole is large enough so that the milk runs in a stream, the baby will take his food too fast.

Care of Nipples.—Nipples need special care. If allowed to soak in water when not in use the rubber quickly becomes spongy and disintegrates, the hole grows larger and larger, and the nipple is soon unfit for use.

Immediately after the feeding remove the nipple and rinse with cold or warm (not hot) water. Rub the outside with a little common salt to remove the milk, turn the nipple inside out, rinse, and rub with salt; rinse again and boil for five minutes. The nipple will dry at once when removed from the boiling water. Place in a dry glass jar which has been boiled and screw the cover on tight. Keep from the light. The nipples should be rinsed in boiled water just before using.

It is wise always to have extra nipples prepared, as they are subject to many accidents.

How to Give the Baby the Bottle.

When it is time to feed the baby take the cold bottle from the ice; do not pour out the milk, but place the bottle, still corked, in a vessel of warm water, having the water cover the bottle above the milk line, and allow the water to heat. Do not allow the water to boil, as that will make the milk too hot. To test the temperature of the milk, open the bottle and drop a little milk on the inner surface of the arm. If it feels comfortably warm to the mother's skin it will be right for the baby. If it has been made too hot cool the bottle under running water. The mother should never put the nipple in her own mouth to test the temperature of the milk, as an infection, such as a "cold," might easily be conveyed in this way from mother to baby. Put on one of the sterile nipples from the jar.

Hold the baby on the left arm in the same position as for breast feeding. The bottle should be held by the mother or nurse throughout the feeding. It must be presented to the baby at such an angle that the neck of the bottle is kept continually filled and the baby is able to grasp the nipple squarely. If he is sleepy, keep him awake until the bottle is finished. If, in spite of this, he falls asleep, remove the bottle and do not give another until the next feeding time.

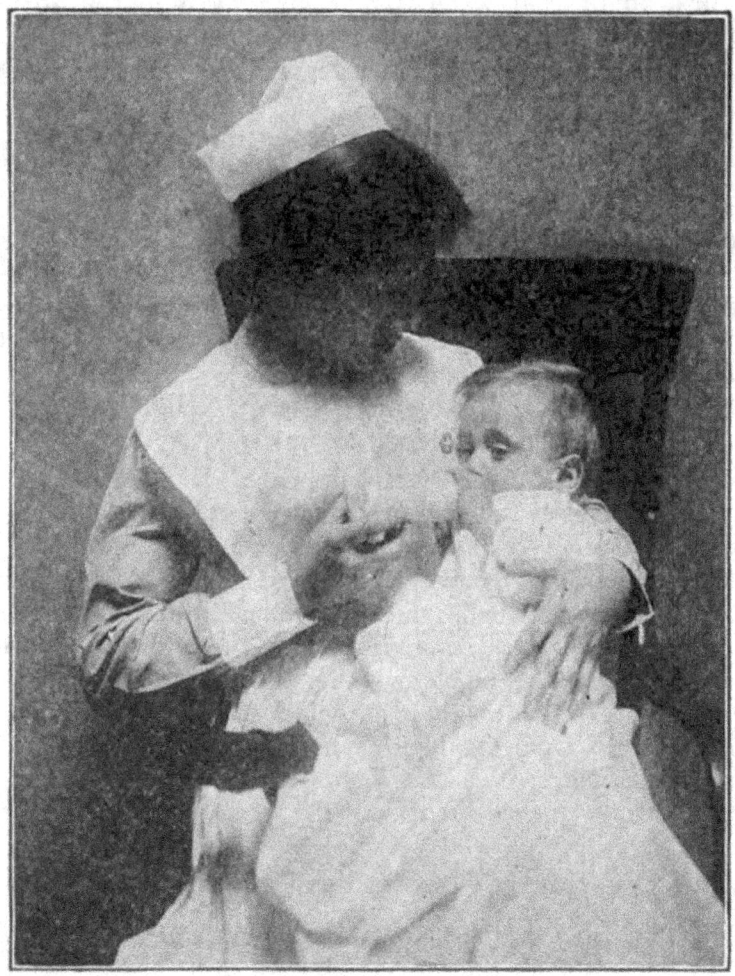

Proper Way of Holding the Baby and the Bottle when Feeding.

Normal Feeding.

If the baby has been breast fed for a while and is then put on cows' milk, it is wise, until he has become somewhat accustomed to the new food, to use a weaker mixture at first than the one indicated for that age. The food can be strengthened every few days if necessary until it suits his age. If the baby shows any signs of disturbed digestion it is wise to return at once to the weaker food until he is quite well again; if he seems satisfied, is gaining from 4 to 6 ounces a week, does not vomit, and has normal stools, it is reasonably certain that the food is of the right strength and quantity.

Underfeeding.

As a rule, babies are overfed rather than underfed. But if the baby cries as soon as the bottle is taken away, and again before the next feeding time, a careful increase may be made day by day toward a stronger mixture, stopping at a point where he is satisfied.

Overfeeding.

If he sleeps restlessly, vomits his food, or has loose bowel movements, it usually indicates that he is being fed too much, too often, or that his food is stronger than he can digest. If the baby is breast fed, the interval between nursing should be lengthened to 4 hours, as a first measure. It is wise to see the doctor, when possible. For bottle-fed babies the amount of the day's feeding may be decreased by using one-half of the usual contents of each bottle until the disturbance has subsided.

Drinking Water.

The baby needs plenty of cool, unsweetened water to drink. It is safe to boil all the drinking water for a baby, which should be given to a young baby lukewarm, never ice cold. Never put sugar or anything else in it. Offer it to the baby between feedings; in summer especially he needs to drink frequently. A "runabout" baby is constantly exercising while awake and requires a great deal of water. Fretful babies, especially those who are cutting teeth, are often quieted by a cool drink.

Infant Stools.

The first passages from a newborn baby's bowels are known as meconium. The excretion is black or nearly so, and is thick, of a tarlike consistency, with little or no odor. This soon changes to the normal yellow stool of the healthy infant as the baby begins to feed at his mother's breast. The stools are then of a dull yellow or orange color without disagreeable odor and soft and mushy in appearance. They are passed from one to three times a day, averaging twice a day in most breast-fed babies until 6 months of age, when one stool a day is usual. When there is a long interval between feedings the number of stools is usually lessened, being only one a day, and sometimes only one in 36 hours. Artificially fed infants usually pass but one stool a day, and the color and odor vary with the character of the food. With breast-fed babies the stool is a mass, while with those fed on the bottle there is more tendency to a "formed" stool.

When there is a greatly marked difference in the character of the stools, especially when the number increases, the mother should have a doctor see the baby, meanwhile decreasing the food or, better, withdrawing it altogether for some hours, giving water instead.

In order to do away with the need for diapers as early in life as possible, the baby should be taught to use the chamber. This training may be begun by the third month, or even earlier in some cases. It should be carried out with the utmost gentleness, since scolding and punishment will serve only to frighten the child and to destroy the natural impulses, wild laughter will tend to relax the muscles and to promote an easy movement. In order to be effective, the chamber must be presented to the baby at the same hour every day, usually just before the morning bath, and it must be presented persistently each day until the habit is formed. Much time and patience will be required on the part of the mother, but in the end the habit thus formed will be a great saving of trouble to her and of untold value to the child, not only in babyhood, but throughout the whole of life.

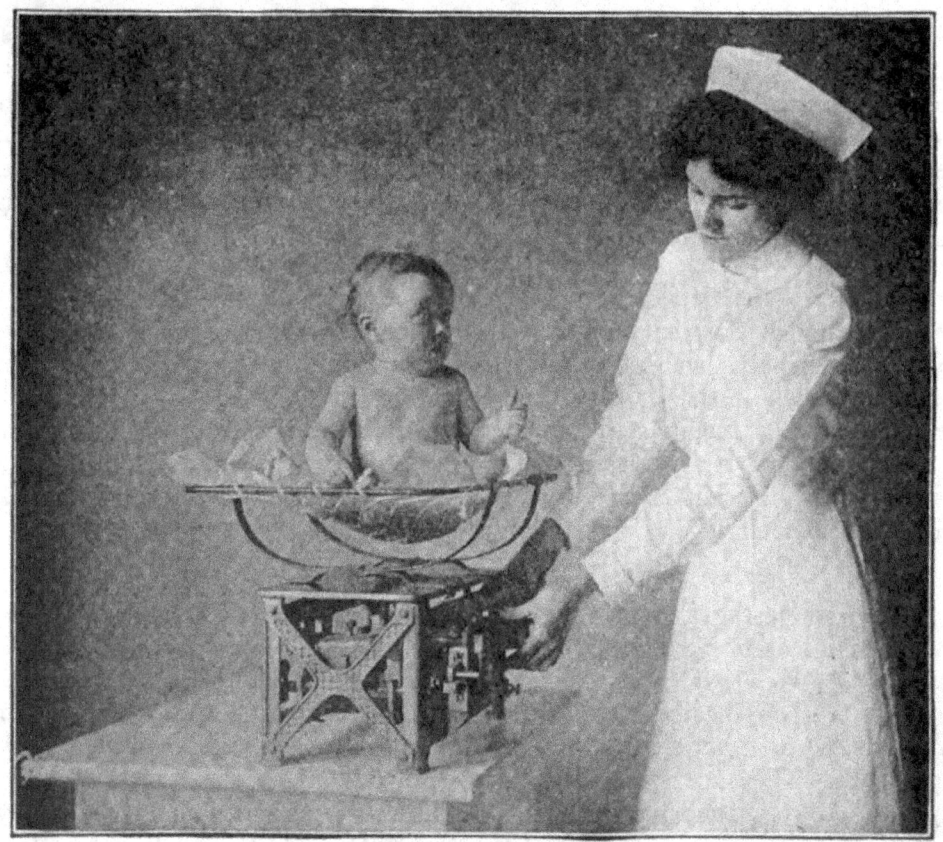

Weighing the Baby.

Experience has shown that an ordinary porcelain cuspidor is an excellent vessel to use for a young baby. It should be kept scrupulously clean and in cold weather must be warmed before being used. The mother takes the vessel in her lap, seating the baby upon it with his back toward her breast, so that she may support him in a comfortable position. If the movement does not come within a few minutes the better course is to wait until the next day. A little observation on the mother's part will lead her to know at what hour the baby's bowels are ready to move, and she should choose that moment for the trial. If the baby has a tendency to be constipated, it may be well to introduce a well-oiled soap stick for a moment before beginning, in order to start the movement and to indicate to the baby what is wanted.

Development.

Many an inexperienced mother does not know the signs whereby she can tell if her baby is developing properly. The following are the leading characteristics of a normal, healthy better baby:

Clean skin, bright eyes, steady gain in weight, good appetite, regular bowel movements, absence of vomiting after feeding, alert, springy muscles, sound sleep at the proper periods, and a steady growth in stature and intelligence.

The soft spot in the top of baby's head will begin to close at the fourteenth month and will be entirely closed by the time he is two years old.

About the fourth month he should begin to hold up his head and by the sixth month to reach for his toys. By the time a normal baby is eight months old he usually can sit erect and hold the spine upright, while at the ninth or tenth month he will make his first attempts to bear his weight on the feet.

A few words generally can be spoken when baby is one year old, and by the fifteenth or sixteenth month he can walk alone.

Teeth.

The embryonic teeth begin to develop at least six months before birth. It is probable that a nutritious diet for the prospective mother lays the foundation for healthy teeth in the baby and that lack of proper food for the mother may deprive both her own and the baby's teeth of some part of their normal vigor. Every child has two sets of teeth. The first set, known as the deciduous or "milk" teeth are replaced, beginning at about the sixth year, with the permanent or "second" teeth. Nearly all so-called "teething" troubles belong to the first period, as a disturbance is rarely connected with the coming of the permanent set.

The two central lower teeth are usually the first to appear, and come from the fifth to the ninth month; next are the four upper central teeth, which come from the eighth to the twelfth month. The other two lower central teeth and the four front double teeth come from the twelfth to the eighteenth month. Then follow the four canine teeth and the two upper ones, being known as the "eye" teeth, and the lower as the "stomach" teeth; they generally come between the eighteenth and the twenty-fourth month. The four back double teeth, which complete the first set come between the twenty-fourth and the thirtieth month.

Growth.—During the second year the baby should have more or less dry hard foods on which to chew. There is sometimes a tendency to keep a baby too long on an exclusively soft diet for fear that solid food will upset him, but it is important to the development of strong, healthy teeth that they shall have exercise in biting and chewing. Begin by giving the baby of about a year of age some dry, hard crust or toast, or hard crackers, at the end of a regular meal. During the second year, other kinds of food requiring chewing may be gradually added to the diet list and taken as part of the regular meals.

Care.—It is generally believed that much of the health of the second teeth depends upon the care that is given to the first set. As soon as the molars make their appearance they should be gently cleaned each day with a soft brush. As the baby grows into childhood he should be taught the daily care of his own teeth.

Ailments of Teething.—Altogether teething is a natural process and is not alone responsible for all the illness attributed to it, nevertheless there is no doubt that many babies suffer severely while cutting their teeth. When the gums are red and swollen it sometimes affords relief if they are lanced, and it may be well to have a doctor examine the baby's mouth to see if the operation is needed. The process of teething is occasionally associated with digestive disturbances. The number of stools may increase and vomiting may occur. The baby may be restless and fretful and try continually to bite on something. In all these cases the quantity and strength of the food should be reduced and drinking water should be offered at frequent intervals. No teething lotions nor medicines of any kind should be given for the relief of the pain of teething. If they do relieve it, it is probably because they contain opium in some form or other narcotic drugs.

There is a dangerous tendency to attribute to teething many ailments which are due to other causes. The teeth begin to appear at about the same time that the baby is being weaned and new foods are being tried. Disturbances of the digestive tract are very likely to occur for these reasons. If the baby cuts his teeth in the summer, his illness may be due to excessive heat, to improper feeding or overfeeding, and to the pain of cutting the teeth, and it would be difficult to say which factor is chiefly responsible. In any case, careful feeding is of the utmost importance.

The baby should not be expected to gain in weight during these periods of painful eruption of the teeth, but the weight may remain stationary for two or three weeks without harm. The baby should not be urged to eat when he has no appetite, merely for the sake of the desired increase in weight. After the disturbance has passed he will be hungry and will soon regain the lost ground. On the other hand, if the baby is coaxed to take more food than he wants, his digestion is sure to be upset, and this, added to the pain of teething, may result in serious illness. The "second summer" has gained reputation for being the most critical period of the baby's life, but, as a matter of fact, statistics show that the first summer is a much more hazardous time, and if properly fed and cared for a healthy baby should be brought through the second summer in perfect condition:

Weaning.

Weaning is the process whereby baby is gradually deprived of breast milk. It should proceed slowly, one bottle feeding being substituted for one breast feeding during the day for some time, then two bottles, and so on until all breast feeding has been done away with and the baby is entirely weaned. In order that this change may be accomplished with as little disturbance as possible, one bottle feeding may be given to the baby in 24 hours as early as the fifth or sixth month. This will hardly be sufficient to upset the baby's digestion and yet will serve to accustom him to the taste of strange food and to the use of the bottle and to begin educating the stomach in dealing with new materials.

When to Wean.—In most cases the baby should be weaned by the end of the first year, and in some cases from one to three months earlier, depending largely upon the health of the baby, the amount and quality of the breast milk, and upon the time of the year. It is unwise to wean the baby in the heat of summer or when infant illness of any sort is epidemic. It has been proved over and over again that breast milk will save a sick baby's life and restore him to health after the strain of a long hot summer, and that often there is no other food that can be relied upon to accomplish the same result. Therefore, even though the breast

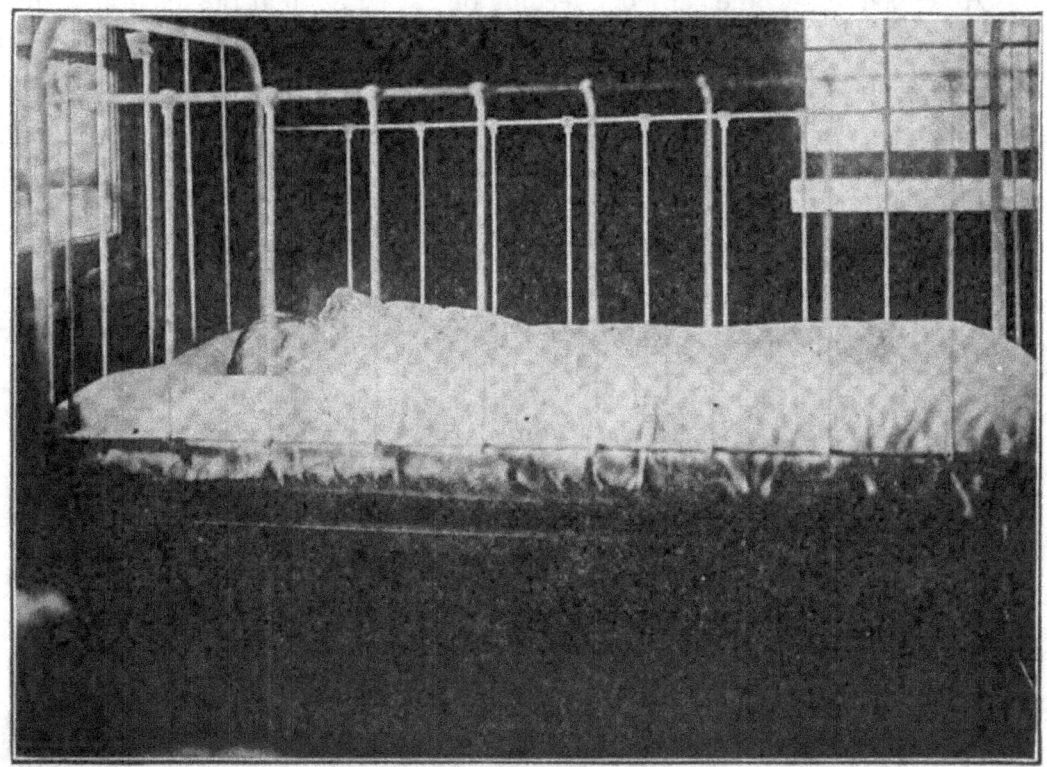

Baby's Bed.

milk must be supplemented with one or several bottles, it is wise to nurse the baby through the summer so that breasts will not cease entirely to secrete and may be called on in an emergency.

If drinking water has been given by means of a nursing bottle during much of the first year, the baby will take his food in the same way the more readily. A healthy infant weaned at 9 months should begin with the food for an infant of 4 or 5 months. If he digests this mixture well, the strength can be increased until within two or three weeks he is taking the food full strength. Increase in the diet should be made with special caution at the beginning of summer or during the heat, when there is great danger of inducing diarrhea. It is far better to keep the baby on rather a low diet, even without increasing his weight, than to upset the intestinal tract by overfeeding. If, after trying a new food, vomiting occurs or the stools show that there is indigestion, it is always best to return to the weaker food until the disturbance has subsided.

Weaning from the Bottle.—An artificially fed infant is weaned from the bottle by beginning at 10 months to substitute one feeding a day from the spoon or cup for one bottle feeding, gradually increasing the number of such feedings until the baby is weaned, usually by the thirteenth month. The mother will find it a convenience to continue the bottle for the night feedings as long as necessary.

It is good to give the baby one feeding of Farina Soup at the noon meal in place of the bottle. This may be given about the eighth or ninth month in addition to the bottle. FARINA SOUP: To one pint of meat broth, gradually add while stirring 1 to 1½ tablespoonfuls of farina and boil down to one cup (¼ pint) in about 20 minutes. It is a good plan to boil the farina from 15 to 20 minutes before adding it to the broth, then broth and farina need be boiled together but 10 minutes.

Sleep.

The infant brain increases its size two and one-half times in the first year, a greater growth than takes place during all the remaining years of life. At the same time this enormous brain development is taking place the other organs of the little body are growing rapidly. During sleep the body tissues are re-created and the energy and materials needed for the activity of the waking hours are stored up. It is manifest, therefore, that the baby must have a correspondingly large allowance of sleep. He should always sleep in a bed by himself, and whenever possible in a room by himself, where he need not be disturbed by the presence of other persons, and where light, warmth, and ventilation may be adjusted to his particular needs. Not a few young babies are smothered while lying in the bed with an older person, some part of whose body is thrown over the baby's face during heavy sleep.

Amount.—A young baby sleeps 18 or 20 hours out of 24. At 6 months of age a baby sleeps about 16 hours, at 1 year about 14 hours, and at 2 years at least 12 hours. Daytime naps should be continued as long as possible

General Care.

The mother who wants her babe to be a "Better Baby" will begin early to instruct it in good habits. By establishing the habit of regularity from the very beginning, the care of baby, if it is healthy, can be reduced to a system that will save the mother a great amount of time.

Regular habits regarding the physical functions of an infant, such as eating, sleeping and bowel movements, should begin at birth, for they are of the utmost importance in keeping baby well.

Much of the fussing and fretting of young babies is really due to physical causes. A baby that is kept clean and comfortable, that is properly fed, receives plenty of sleep and fresh air, has no reason to "act up."

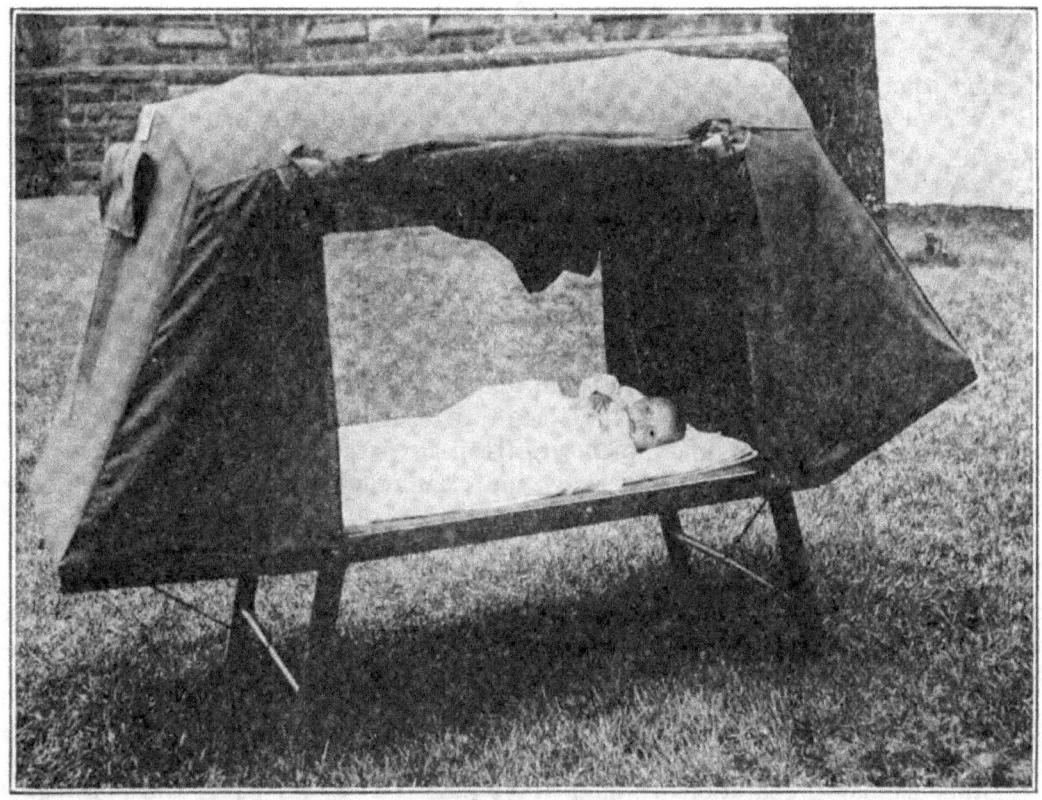

Sleeping out-of-doors.

The following is suggested as a system that most mothers will find profitable to follow:

6 a. m.—Baby's first feeding.

Breakfast for other members of the family.

9 a. m.—Bathe baby and give him his second feeding.

Let baby sleep until noon.

12 to 12:30—Baby's midday feeding.

Airing in fresh air followed by nap.

3 p. m.—Baby's afternoon feeding.

Play or a waking period.

6 p. m.—Undress ready for bed, then his 6 o'clock feeding.

For the first few months he will be fed again at 9 p. m. but after that he should not be taken up.

He must be made comfortable in every way, the light should be put out, the window opened, his covers adapted to the temperature, but after the mother has assured herself that everything essential to his comfort has been attended to, should not go to him when he cries, if he is a perfectly healthy baby. A few nights of this training will result in entire comfort for the baby and the family, while the opposite conditions will make the baby a tyrant who ruthlessly spoils the comfort of the entire household.

Disturbed Sleep.

If the baby sleeps lightly, wakens often, and seems uncomfortable it may be that something is disturbing him which can be remedied.

He may be nervous from having been tickled, played with, or tossed about in the latter part of the day. Overstimulation is to be avoided at all times, no matter what its source nor what the age of the baby.

He may be too warm, too cold, or wet; there may be something scratching him, or there may be wrinkles in the bedclothing; he may be lying in a cramped position, or the band or diaper may be too tight.

Or, more likely, he has been overfed, or has had something unsuitable to eat, or is hungry or thirsty.

The room may be too hot, too cold, too light, too noisy, or not sufficiently aired. The conditions which make sleep a delight to older persons affect the baby in the same way, namely, plenty of fresh air passing in a constant current through the room, quiet, a clean body, and clean, comfortable clothing, a good bed, and suitable coverings.

A cool bath or a warm one, according to the temperature, will help to induce quiet sleep. In the summer, when the baby is fretful and sleeps restlessly, a tub bath at bedtime will help to relieve him. A little baby should be turned over once or twice in the course of a long nap.

Medicines.

Never give a baby any sort of medicine to induce sleep. All soothing syrups or other similar preparations contain drugs that are bad for baby, and many of them are exceedingly dangerous. Many babies die every year from being given such medicines. The baby should never be allowed to go to sleep with anything in the nature of a pacifier in his mouth. Thumb and finger sucking babies will rebel fiercely at being deprived of this comfort when they are going to sleep, but this must be done if the habit is to be broken. The baby ought to have a quiet place in which to sleep, but he should be taught to sleep through the ordinary household noises, unless they are unduly disturbing. It should not be necessary to walk on tiptoe and talk in whispers while the baby sleeps, provided he has a room to himself during his daytime naps.

Habits, Training, and Discipline.

Habits are the result of repeated actions. A properly trained baby is not allowed to learn bad habits which must be unlearned later at great cost of time and patience to both mother and babe. The wise mother strives to start the baby right.

One common fault in caring for babies is permitting them to be violently rocked or jumped up and down on the knee. Constant, violent motion of this kind upsets a baby's stomach and disturbs the nervous system. This does not mean that it should not be "mothered." But proper "mothering" means holding baby quietly in one's arms and soothing it. Change the position frequently so that no one set of the infant's muscles becomes strained from remaining too long in the same position.

Mothers should not kiss them on the mouth nor permit other people to do so, for infections of various kinds can easily be transmitted to an infant in this way.

Bad Habits.

"Pacifiers" or "Comforts."—The extremely bad habit of sucking on a rubber teat, or a sugar ball, or a bread ball, or any other similar article, is one for which some one else is entirely responsible. The baby does not teach himself this disgusting habit, and he should not have to suffer for it. The pacifier is never clean and may readily carry the germs of disease into the baby's mouth; and last and least, it is a habit which is particularly disfiguring to the baby's appearance.

Thumb or Finger Sucking.—This is another habit leading to the same results as the use of pacifiers, but one which the baby may acquire for himself, although it is frequently taught to him. To break up either habit requires resolution and patience on the part of the mother. The thumb or finger must be persistently and constantly removed from the mouth and the baby's attention diverted to something else. The sleeve may be pinned or sewed down over the fingers of the offending hand for several days and nights, or the hand may be put in a cotton mitten. Ill-tasting applications have very little effect. There are patent articles for holding the hand from the mouth sold in the stores, but the persistent covering of the hand often works very well. The baby's hands should be set free now and then, especially if he is old enough to use his hands for his toys, and at meal times, to save as much unnecessary strain on his nerves as possible, but with the approach of sleeping time the hand must be covered.

Bed Wetting.—It requires great patience and persistence on the mother's part to teach the baby to control the bladder. Some babies may be taught to do this during the day by the end of the first year, but it is ordinarily not until some time during the second year that this is accomplished. It is necessary to put the baby on the chamber at frequent intervals during the day. Bed wetting may be due to some physical weakness if it persists in children 3 years old and over. A doctor should be consulted. In ordinary cases, it may suffice if no liquid food is given in the late afternoon and if the baby is taken up the last thing before the mother retires.

Masturbation.—This injurious practice must be eradicated as soon as discovered, if at all, as it easily grows beyond control. It is more common in girls than in boys. If the mother discovers the baby rubbing its thighs together or rocking backward and forward with its legs crossed, she should divert him at once to some other interest. Nursemaids sometimes ignorantly rub the genital organs of babies thinking that it quiets them, but nothing could be more deplorable than this. Mothers cannot be too watchful of nursemaids and the methods they employ to quiet or amuse a baby. Children are sometimes wrecked for life by habits learned from vicious nursemaids, and mothers cannot guard too strictly against this evil. Another way in which this habit is learned is by means of playthings which rub upon the sensitive parts, such as rocking horses, swings, teeter boards and the like. The habit may also be due to some local irritation, and it is wise to consult the doctor at the first evidence of the trouble.

In the case of babies the treatment consists in mechanical restraints. A thick towel or pad may be used to keep the thighs apart, or at night the hands may have to be restrained by pinning the nightgown sleeves to the bed, or the feet may be tied one to either side of the crib. Wet or soiled diapers should be removed at once. Cleanliness of the parts is of great importance.

Punishment.

. Harsh punishment has no place in the proper upbringing of the baby. A baby knows nothing of right or wrong, but follows his natural inclinations. If these lead him in the wrong direction the mother must be at hand to guide him in another and better one and to divert his eager interest and his energy into wholesome and normal directions. This is the golden rule in the training of babies and one which applies to the training of children of all ages. Many parents conceive that their whole duty is to thwart and forbid, enforcing their prohibitions with penalties of varying degrees of severity, forgetting that they are dealing with sensitive beings endowed with all the desires, inclinations, and tendencies that they themselves have, and that if these natural feelings are continually suppressed and thwarted they are sure to seek and find some outlet for themselves. A child who is often punished may be so dominated by fear of his parents that the natural expression of his vital interests being denied him, he becomes sullen and morose as he grows older.

Early Training.

The training in the use of individual judgment can be begun even in infancy; the child should early be taught to choose certain paths of action for himself; and if he is continually and absolutely forbidden to do this or that he is sometimes seriously handicapped later, because he does not know how to use his own reasoning faculties in making these choices. On the other hand, obedience is one of the most necessary lessons for children to learn. A wise mother will not abuse her privilege in this respect by a too-exacting practice. For the most part she can exert her control otherwise than by commands, and if she does so her authority when exercised will have greater force and instant obedience will be more readily given.

How to Keep the Baby Well.

Many mothers are so situated as to be unable to command the services of a physician at once, and since in any case there may be a delay in his arrival, it is well for the mother to understand something of the symptoms of illness and be prepared to deal intelligently with the emergencies that may arise in connection with the care of her children. In all cases of illness, the discretion and self-control of the mother are of infinite assistance to the doctor, and when the physician's services are not immediately available the life of the child may depend on the coolness and wisdom of the mother.

The old and most pernicious idea that a certain amount of illness is the necessary accompaniment of infant life is happily fast dying. With the constant increase in the knowledge of the conditions that lead to sickness among children, it is seen that a very large proportion of such illnesses and deaths are preventable by the application of the well-established rules for the proper care of babies. It should therefore be the aim of all intelligent mothers to learn how to save her children from needless illness.

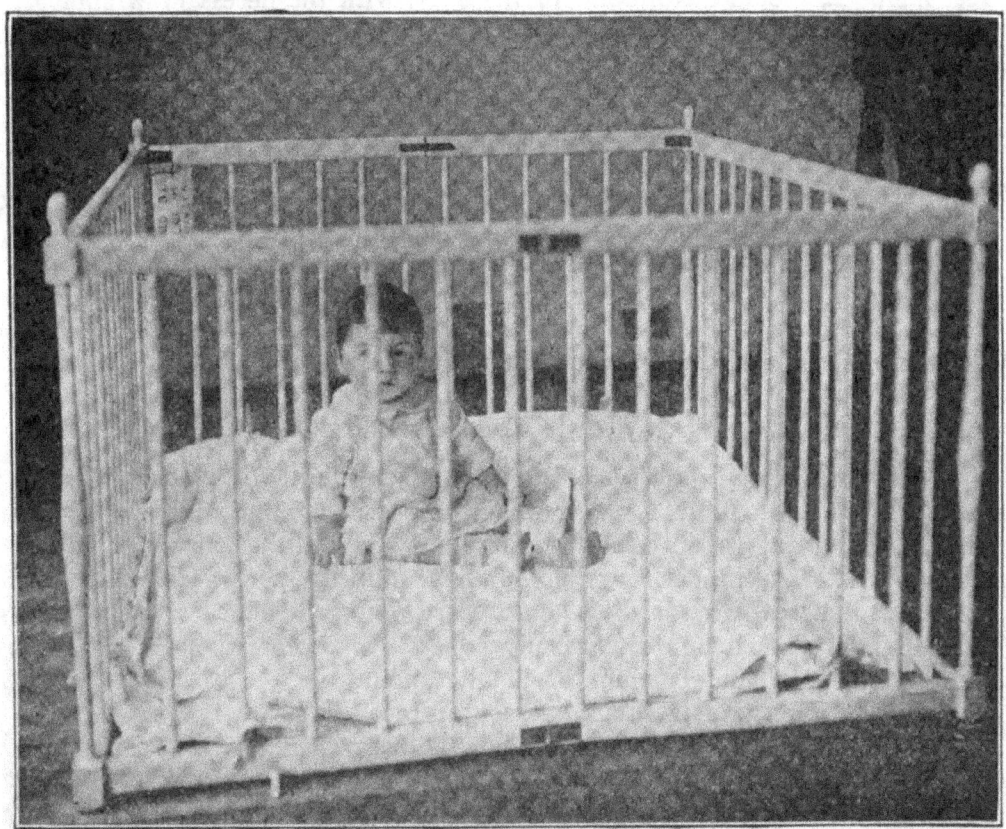

Baby's Pen.

It is said that nine-tenths of all infant illness is due to improper feeding. Whether this is the exact proportion or not, it is quite certain that many babies suffer unnecessarily from mistakes in diet, and it is in this field that the intelligence of the mother is of the greatest value. Babies are usually born healthy and if they are fed at the breast, or, when this is not possible, with strict regard to the rules for proper artificial feeding, and if they are given hygienic care in other respects and allowed to develop in a natural, normal way, there is little reason why they should be sick, and the responsibility for this rests upon the parents.

Vehicles.

The choice of a vehicle for the baby is a matter of great importance. The folding cart, which may be taken on the street cars, permits mother and baby to go out many times when it would not otherwise be possible. The great convenience of this cart cannot be denied, but such carts should be used only for the purpose for which they are intended, namely, to convey the baby short distances, and not as pleasure vehicles, nor should the baby be left to sit fastened in one of these small carts for any great length of time.

The best vehicle for ordinary use about the home is one which is at least 2 feet high. It should have room for the baby, with the necessary wrappings, in any position, and a cover that can be readily adjusted to secure the needed protections; it should have strong, well-balanced springs and stand squarely on four wheels. A safety strap which fastens about the baby's waist gives greater protection than the ordinary carriage strap.

Some of the go-carts of the present day are so small, so stiff, and so ill adapted to the baby's anatomy that they can hardly be recommended even for temporary use. Also they are so close to the ground that the child is propelled through only the lower and colder air currents, which fling an unending stream of germ-laden dust off the street into his face. They frequently have no cover with which to shield the baby from heat or cold, or sun or wind, and in cold weather it is impossible to keep a baby sufficiently warm in one of them.

When Not to Take the Baby Out.

When the weather is very cold, as in winter in the North, when the snow is melting, or when there is a heavy storm in progress or a high wind blowing quantities of dust about, it will be best to give the baby his airing indoors or on a protected porch. Dress him as for going out, open all the windows wide, and let him remain in the fresh air for some time. Very young or delicate babies require much heat and must be very warmly covered to protect them against being chilled, and baby under 3 months of age should not be taken out in severe weather; but plenty of fresh air is essential to all babies.

When the weather is excessively hot the baby should be taken out early in the day and then kept indoors until the late afternoon. From that time on until the rooms have cooled in the evening he should be kept out, being well protected from mosquitoes. If a screened porch is available, the health and comfort of the baby will be greatly increased.

Caution.

A word of caution should be given as to the danger of young children climbing up to open windows and falling out. If the windows have screens, they should be so carefully fastened in that there is no possibility of pushing them out. When screens are not in use, the windows should either be lowered from the top or thin wooden slats should be used to protect the lower sash. Similar precautions must be used if the baby is put to sleep on the fire escape. Sleeping porches are usually well protected.

The baby's eyes and head should always be carefully shielded from the direct sunlight. This is just as important while he is asleep as while awake. Do not allow the baby to lie staring up into the sky, even when the sun is not shining.

Great care should be taken to protect the baby from flies and mosquitoes. If the house is not provided with screens, the baby's bed, crib, or carriage should be covered with netting suspended over a pole or two clotheslines in the form of a tent, so as not to shut off the air. Never lay a netting directly over the baby's face.

Toys.

Since a baby wants to put everything in his mouth, his toys must be those that can safely be used in this way. They should be washable and should have no sharp points nor corners to hurt the eyes. Painted articles and hairy and woolly toys are unsafe, as are also objects small enough to be swallowed, and those having loose parts, such as bells and the like.

A child should never have so many toys at one time as to distract his interest. He will be quite satisfied with a few things for the time being, and a handful of clothespins, for example, will often please just as much as an expensive doll or other toy. It is an excellent plan to have a box or basket in which to keep empty spools and other household objects which the baby may play with.

Common Ailments.

Diarrhea.—The normal, healthy baby usually has one or two stools a day. If the number increases to four or more the mother should be on her guard against diarrhea. Diarrhea is a symptom of nearly all the disturbances of digestion in infancy, both of the mild and of the severe types. The doctor should be consulted at once if possible, for even a slight attack of diarrhea, unless correctly treated, may lead to a severe disturbance such as cholera infantum. Diarrhea is far more frequent in summer than in winter. This is chiefly because the baby is directly affected by the hot weather so that he is more easily upset by his food. Therefore in hot summer weather all babies, and especially bottle-fed babies, should receive especial care. They should be kept as cool as possible. They should be outdoors except when it is cooler indoors; all unnecessary clothes should be removed, a band and diaper being sufficient clothing; frequent cool sponge baths should be given, and the amount of food on especially hot days should be reduced to two-thirds of the ordinary amount, large quantities of water being given in addition.

The disease is more frequent in bottle-fed babies. If it occurs in a nursing baby it is usually because the baby has been nursed too often or at irregular intervals, or has been given food other than milk. Extend the nursing interval and allow the baby to nurse only 5 or 10 minutes. If the trouble continues, withhold the breast altogether for some hours until there is an improvement. Give a little water to drink now and then.

For bottle-fed babies, if the disturbance is slight, the amount of milk used in the feedings should be reduced by half, skimmed, and all sugar omitted. If the trouble is more severe, all food should be stopped, only plain boiled water should be given, and a physician should be consulted at once.

A baby takes some time to get back to full vigor after even a slight digestive disturbance, and the return to food must be gradual. It will take from 10 days to 2 weeks to restore the normal condition of the digestive tract. A second attack of illness occurs much more readily than the original one.

Constipation.—A nursing baby often responds to this condition in the mother. The mother should have a free evacuation of the bowels each day. If she is regular and the baby is still constipated, he must be held over the chamber at exactly the same hour every day in the effort to induce regular movements. Persistence in the establishment of a regular bowel habit in the baby prevents much of this trouble. Orange juice may be given once a day an hour before his midmorning feeding after the baby is 6 months old. Other remedies are suggested in connection with the treatment of the bottle-fed baby.

Constipation in a bottle-fed baby is more difficult to relieve. After the baby is 5 or 6 months old, oatmeal gruel may be found useful in this condition, and fruit juices as well. Orange juice may be given at 5 or 6 months and the strained pulp of prunes or baked apple in the second year. Massage of the abdomen may be tried. Just before holding the baby over the chamber, undress him as much as necessary and let him lie on his back. Moisten the hand in warm olive oil, albolene, or vaseline, and gently massage the abdomen, using a light circular movement and very little pressure. Begin just above the right groin, carry the hand to the ribs, then across the body and down on the left side. Keep this up for 5 or 10 minutes, but do not let the baby become chilled.

If the baby is constipated, a soap stick or a gluten suppository may be tried. Take a piece of firm white soap half an inch thick and about 2 inches long and shave it down toward one end until the point is about one-quarter of an inch thick and perfectly smooth. Wet the soap stick or dip it in vaseline before using it. Hold the stick by the thick end, insert the other end in the anus, and allow it to remain in one or two minutes. Gluten suppositories may be purchased at a drug store and are accompanied by directions for their use.

Hiccough.—This is a spasm of the diaphragm. In infants it is usually due to an irritation of the stomach caused by overfilling the stomach or by swallowing air with the food. In some cases it may be brought on as the result of a sudden exposure to cold. Care should be taken to avoid these causes. When the trouble is in progress, gentle massage of the abdomen or placing the baby face downward across the mother's lap will sometimes afford relief. A few drops of water to drink may help.

Colic.—This is caused by indigestion due to overfeeding, improper feeding, or too frequent feeding. The bowel is distended by gas, giving rise to severe pain. The baby cries sharply, alternately drawing its legs up to the body, then kicking them away. One of the best means of relief is a small enema of warm water, which will serve to relieve the pain by driving out the gas from the intestine. The feet and legs should be kept very warm, and the abdomen may be massaged with warm oil. Do not feed the baby while the attack lasts. Though the introduction of warm milk into the stomach may quiet the baby temporarily, the pain will return with greater intensity. Warm water may be given if the baby will swallow it. Colic is peculiarly an ailment of young babies and usually disappears by the third or fourth month. It is also very common in breast-fed babies. Constipated babies are more liable to it than others, and attention should be given to remedying this condition as a method of prevent-ing colic. Colic is also caused by cold, and if the baby has been chilled in any way it is well to place him in a warm bath for 5 or 10 minutes, wrapping him warmly after taking him out of the water. The temperature of the bath should be about 100 degrees.

Cold in the Head (Coryza).—This ailment is particularly annoying to babies, because the obstruction of the nasal passages, making breathing difficult, greatly interferes with the ease of nursing. Serious complications may also follow a bad cold. If the baby becomes infected, a few drops of albolene placed in each nostril by means of a medicine dropper will relieve the baby very much. The bowels should be kept open, and if there is fever the food should be reduced. Babies who live out of doors, who are fed properly and not too heavily dressed, are much less liable to colds than others. It is wise to keep careful watch over a baby thus affected, as certain contagious diseases appear first as a cold in the head.

Prickly Heat.—This disease is due to the heat of summer, or to unduly heavy underclothing. It manifests itself in a fine red rash which comes when the baby is overheated and fades away under cooler conditions. The rash often shows itself first on the back of the neck and spreads over the head and shoulders. It is a very annoying trouble and makes the baby fretful and restless.

If the rash appears in cold weather, the baby is too warmly dressed. Heavy flannels are to be avoided, and a thin cotton or silk garment should be worn next to the skin. When it is caused by summer heat, the baby should be made as cool as possible, dressed in the thinnest clothing, and frequently bathed in cool water. Soap should never be used on an inflamed skin, but a starch, bran, or soda bath will help to relieve the intense itching. Ointments are not so soothing in this condition as powders. A satisfactory powder is made by mixing 1 ounce each of powdered starch and powdered oxide of zinc with 60 grains of boric acid. Any druggist will make this up, and it should be used freely over the inflamed spots.

Chafing.—A fat baby is very apt to become chafed in the folds and creases of the skin, especially about the buttocks, where it is due to wet diapers or to those which have been washed with some irritating soap powder or not thoroughly rinsed. Chafed flesh should not have soap used upon it. Starch or bran water may be tried. Keep the skin clean and use the powder above recom-mended. In obstinate cases, clean with fresh olive oil only, using no water.

Eczema.—This is one of the most persistent and annoying afflictions of babyhood. It is characterized by a swollen, reddened skin, often covered with tiny pimples or crusts, sometimes having a watery discharge; at other times dry and scaly. Some babies have a predisposition to the disease, and in them a slight cause is sufficient to produce it. A baby's skin is very delicate, and any irritation such as chapping from exposure to cold wind or the use of hard water or strong soap, may lead to eczema, or it may be caused by woolen underclothing, starched bonnets, and strings, or unclean diapers. The disease is also caused by digestive troubles due to overfeeding, and often appears in constipated babies. These causes suggest the measures needed for its prevention.

The disease should be treated by a physician, as it is very persistent and must have careful and constant attention. Neither soap nor plain water should be used on the affected parts, which are usually the head and face. Bran or starch water may be used if necessary.

All liquors should be excluded from the diet of a nursing mother, the amount of meat reduced, and her out-of-door exercise increased. For babies fed on cows' milk the diet should be much reduced, both in quantity and strength, and in older children the starchy foods restricted, potatoes and oatmeal being forbidden. It is of the greatest importance that the child have a free bowel movement every day.

To allay the itching, grease the surfaces with an application made of, equal parts of limewater and sweet almond oil, or cover them with a starch and boric-acid powder. It is most important that the baby shall not scratch the inflamed skin, and to prevent it pasteboard splints may be bound lightly about the baby's elbows with strips of cotton. It will thus be impossible for him to get his hands to his face, while having their free use for other purposes. A doctor's help and advice are greatly needed in this disease.

Milk Crust.—Yellowish, scaly patches sometimes form on a baby's scalp. To remove, anoint with oil or vaseline at night and wash with warm water and pure soap in the morning, but do not attempt to force the crust away. If it does not all come off, repeat the operation as many times as needed, but on no account use a comb or any hard instrument to remove it, as it is very easy to start eczema in such a way if the skin is broken.

EMERGENCY DEPARTMENT.

Webster defines an emergency as "an unforeseen occurrence, or combination of circumstances, which calls for immediate action or remedy."

In arranging the material for this department, we have tried to bear in mind the need, and state the simple remedies which may be found helpful and efficacious in time of such emergency. Very much of the material has been copied verbatim from various authorities on the subject. For convenience, the department has, as far as practicable, been alphabetically arranged.

APOPLEXY.

Apoplexy is due to the bursting of a blood vessel or hemorrhage of the brain. Whether the hemorrhage is slight or severe can be determined from the symptoms.

Symptoms.—In case of slight hemorrhage of the brain, the patient often remains conscious. The face has a flushed appearance, the head is hot, there is a throbbing of the veins and arteries of the neck and temples, dimness of sight and dizziness. These symptoms are accompanied by loud snoring, usually slow respiration.

In case of severe hemorrhage of the brain, the patient usually becomes wholly unconscious, with a local or general paralysis of one side of the body. The face is dark or flushed and the head is hot.

First Aid Treatment.

Elevate the head slightly to arrest further escape of blood within the head.

Apply an ice bag to the head.

Keep the patient lying on the paralyzed side and as quiet as possible.

Do not give medicine but send for a physician at once.

BANDAGING.

Bandages are used for the following purposes: to hold dressings in position; to check hemorrhage; to reduce swelling; to support and render immovable different parts of the body, the two kinds most commonly used being the roller and the triangular bandage.

The Roller Bandage.

The roller bandage is usually made of linen, flannel, gauze or muslin. It should be from four to eight yards long and from one-half to six inches wide, depending on the part of the body to which it is applied. For bandaging the finger, use one-half or one-inch bandage, two to three yards long; for the upper extremities, three-inch bandage, six yards long; for the lower extremities, four-inch bandage, six yards long; for the chest and abdomen, five- or six-inch bandage, six to eight yards long.

In applying a roller bandage always place the outer surface of the bandage **next to** the skin and fix the end by a couple of turns around the bandaged

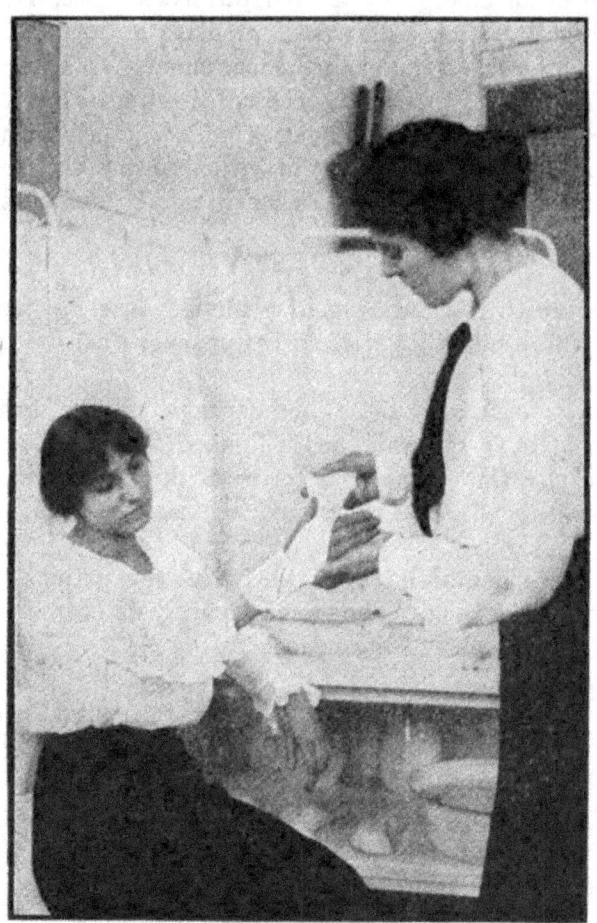

Bandaging the Hand—First Operation.

part. In case the bandage is used for pressure or support, it may begin at the extremity of the limb and be wound toward the body; otherwise if the bandage is drawn rather tight, there is considerable danger of inflammation or congestion because of the interference with the circulation. The extremities, fingers or toes, are usually left exposed and watched closely in order to note whether or not the circulation is being retarded. If the extremities become blue, cold or swollen the bandage should be loosened.

While bandaging, the part should be held in the position in which it is to remain after bandaging. If the bandage is used to support a dressing, it can be begun any place. The dressing underneath will prevent any serious interference with the circulation if the bandage is not applied too tight. Each turn of the bandage should overlap two-thirds of the preceding turn. After the part has been bandaged, the end may be secured by means of adhesive tape or safety pins, always being secured so as to avoid pressure over the wound. The roller bandage may be applied in three ways—the spiral, spiral reverse and .the figure eight.

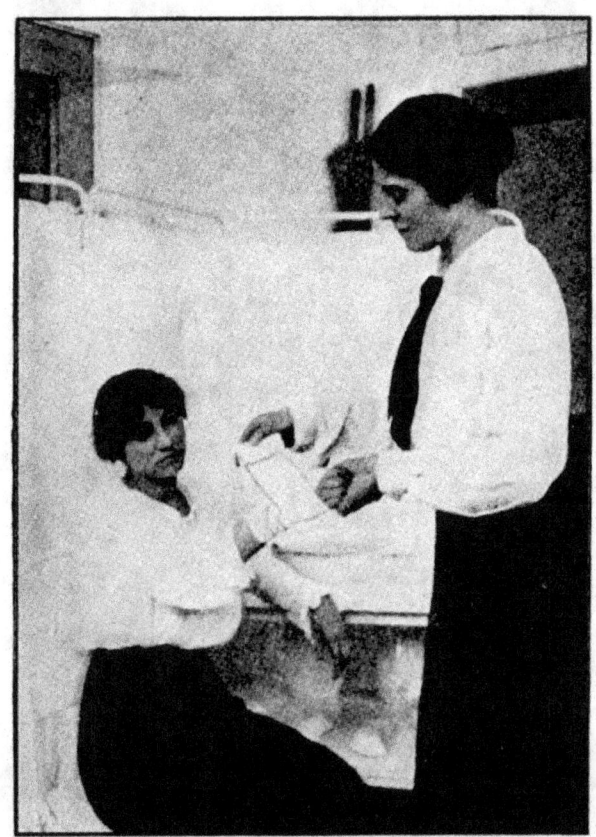

Bandaging the Hand—Second Operation.

The Spiral.—This is the simplest form and should be used whenever possible. It is used where there is fairly uniform circumference of the part bandaged. It consists of a succession of spiral turns from below upwards, each turn overlapping the preceding turn by one-third of its width.

Spiral Reverse.—When the diameter of the limb is uneven—increasing or decreasing in size, the spiral reverse bandage should be applied. It consists of the ordinary spiral bandage with reverses. The reverse is made by placing the thumb of the left hand at the point where the reverse is to be made and doubling the bandage back on itself as shown in the accompanying illustration.

Figure Eight.—This is the one generally used about joints or where any abrupt enlargement occurs. It consists of a series of oblique turns which cross at the joint, that is, the middle of the figure eight is at the joint or median line of the part bandaged; each turn overlaps the preceding one by one-half or two-thirds its width and alternately ascends and descends.

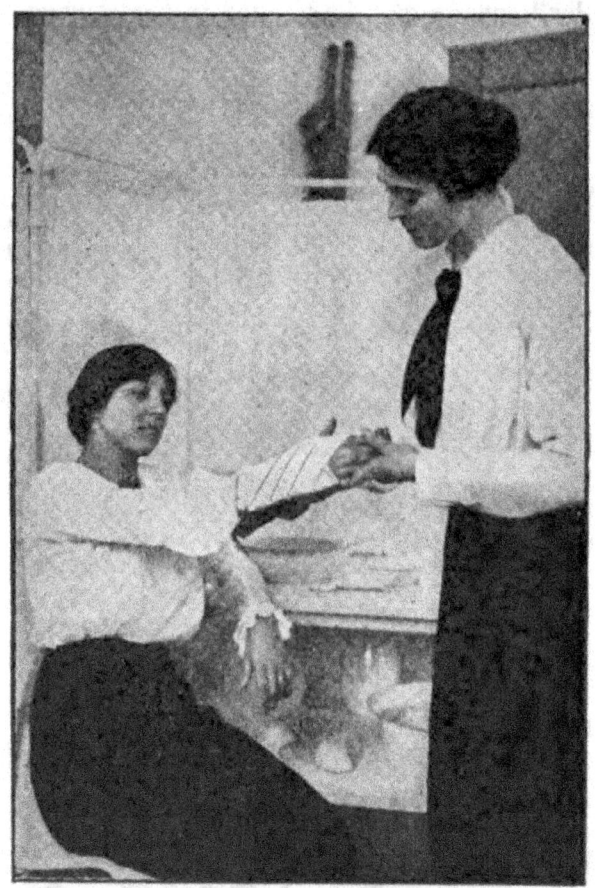

Bandaging the Hand—Completed Operation.

The Triangular Bandage.

The triangular bandage which may be substituted for the roller bandage in many cases where uniform pressure is not necessary is generally used for bandaging the head, shoulders, chest, hands, and often as an arm sling. (The size is determined by the part of the body to be bandaged and the size of the patient). This is often called the handkerchief bandage, as the handkerchief is frequently used in case of emergency. It is easily made by taking a square piece of muslin, folding it diagonally and cutting it along the fold. The long lower border (b) is called the base, the opposite point (a), the apex, and the other two points (c and d), the basal ends.

Application of Triangular Bandage.—(From American Red Cross Text Book on First Aid).

Arm Sling.—Place one end of bandage over shoulder of uninjured side. Allow length of bandage to hang down in front of chest so that point of triangle will be behind elbow of injured arm. Bend elbow of injured arm to a right angle. This will bring forearm across middle of bandage. Then carry lower end of the bandage over the shoulder of the injured side and tie to the

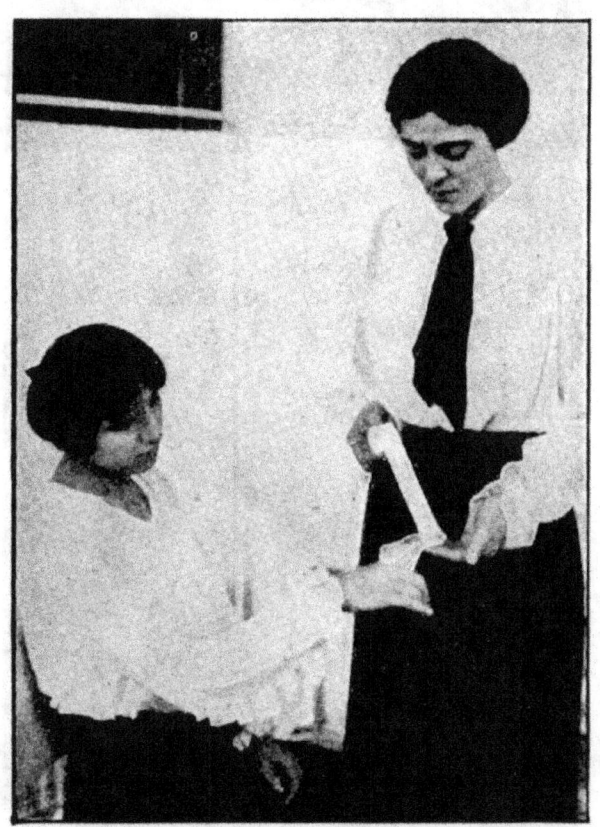

Bandaging the Finger—First Operation.

upper end behind the neck. Bring the point of the bandage at the elbow forward to the front and pin there so that bandage is snug but does not pull.

This makes an excellent arm sling, but even without a bandage a good sling may be made for the arm by pinning the sleeve or the skirt of the coat to the front of the coat. The skirt may be used in the same way.

Foot Bandage.—Spread out bandage. Place foot in center with toes toward point. Raise point over toes to instep in front. Bring both ends forward, cross them over instep and tie them round the ankle.

This bandage has but a limited range of usefulness.

Hand Bandage.—This is applied exactly like the foot bandage. The bandage is spread out. The hand is placed on it, palm down, with the fingers toward the point (if desired the hand may be closed), and the wrist is at the long side. The point is then brought over the back of the hand to the back of the wrist and the two ends are crossed over the wrist and tied.

This bandage will be found useful more often than the preceding one.

Head Bandage.—First, fold a hem about one and one-half inches wide at the long side of the unfolded triangular bandage. Place the bandage so that

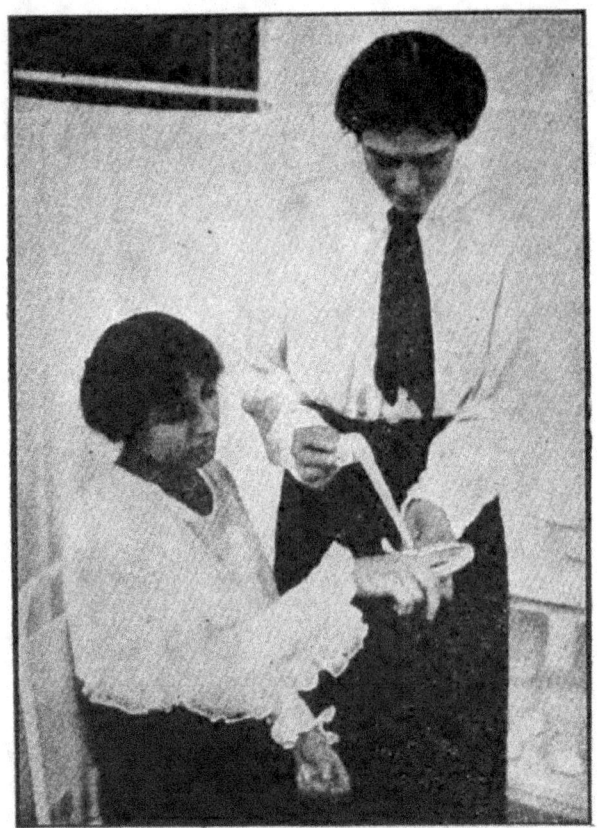

Bandaging the Finger—Second Operation.

the hem lies squarely across the forehead just above the eyes and the bandage is over the head with the point hanging down the back. Carry the two ends around the head above the ears, cross at the back and tie them across the forehead. Draw the point down tight, turn it up and pin it at the top of the head with a safety pin.

This is a useful bandage.

Cravat Bandage.—The triangular bandage folded, is sometimes called the cravat bandage, and in practice by folding the cravat is made wider or narrower as required. As may readily be seen, a cravat may be made of use in any part of the body. It is especially useful to hold splints, dressings, etc., in place, and to check bleeding when applied snugly so as to compress the bleeding point.

The following are good examples of the use of the **folded** triangular bandage or cravat.

Eye Bandage.—Place the center of the cravat over the injured eye, bring the ends to the back of the head and tie.

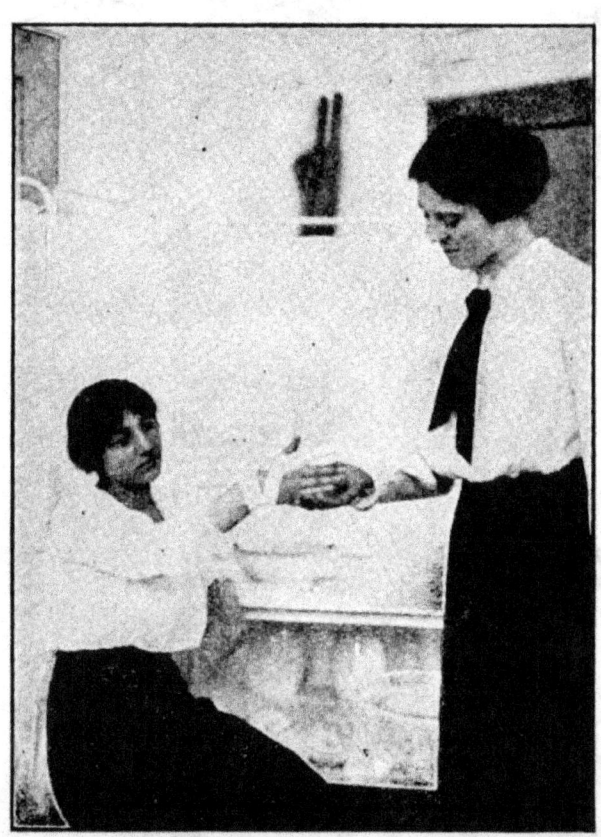

Bandaging the Finger—Completed Operation.

Jaw Bandage.—For this, two cravats are necessary. Apply the centre of the first across the chin in front, bring the ends to the back of the neck and tie. Place the center of the second cravat under the chin, cross the ends over the top of the head, bring them down and tie under the chin.

Neck Bandage.—The center of the cravat is placed over the injured place and the ends are carried around the neck and tied as convenient. This bandage may sometimes be improved by the use of a cardboard support which is held firmly in place between the layers of the bandage.

Bandage for Palm of Hand.—Place the center of the cravat on the palm of the hand, cross the ends at the back of the hand and again at the front of the wrist and tie at the back of the wrist.

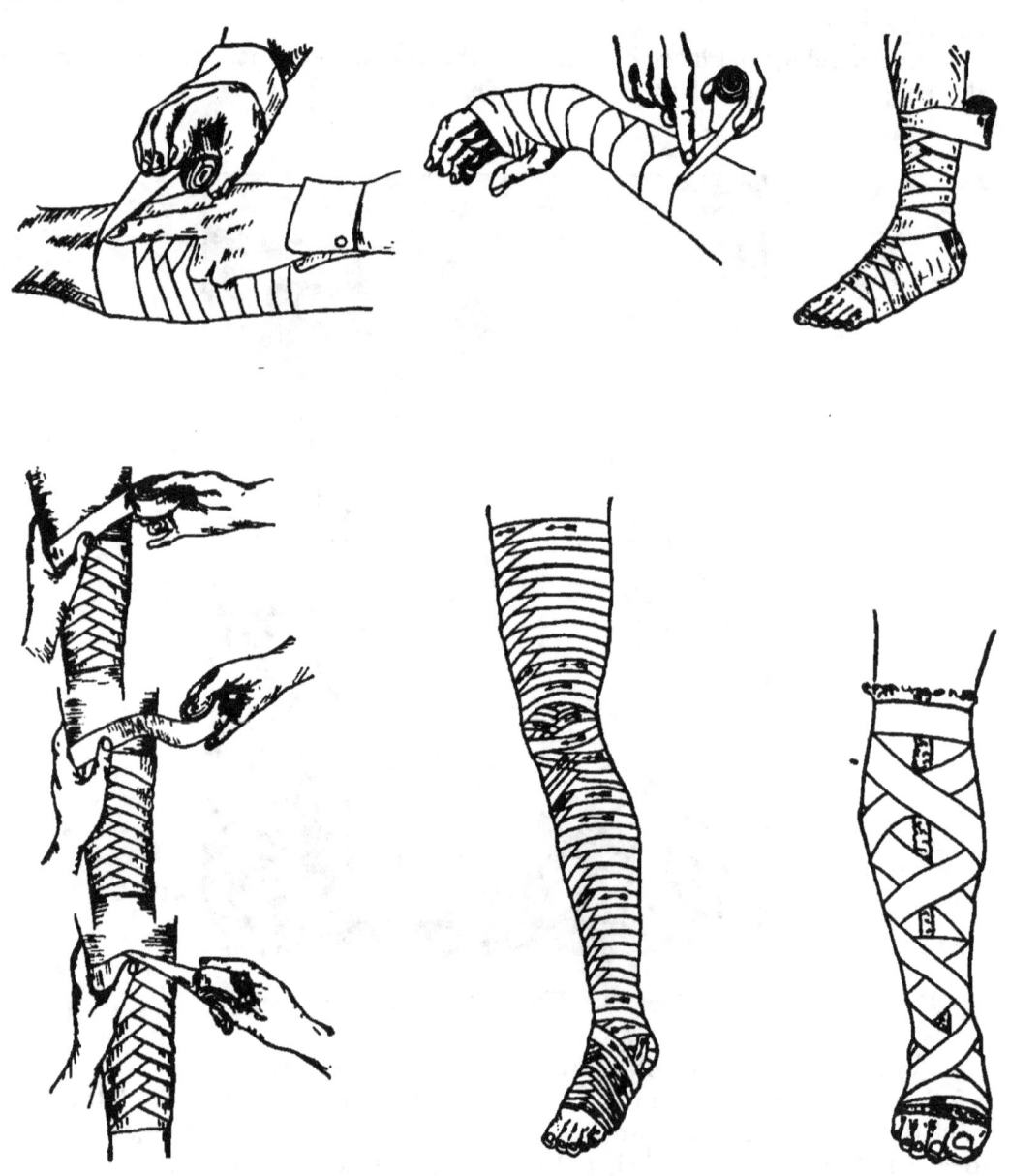

Methods of using the Roller Bandage.

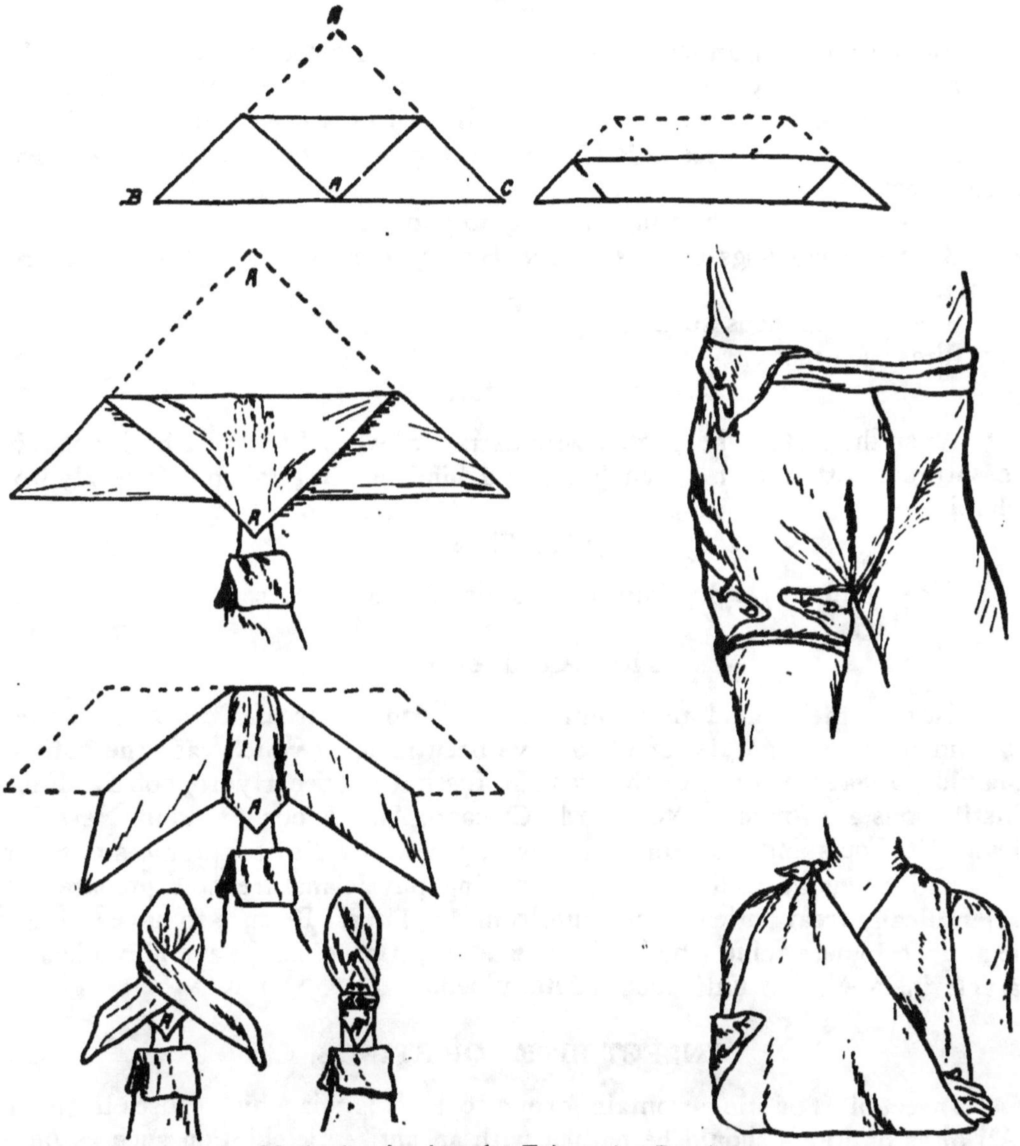

Methods of using the Triangular Bandage.

Sling.—The cravat may also be used for an arm sling. For this purpose it is employed in the form of a loop which encircles the forearm, bent at a right-angle, and the neck. When the cravat is used to hold splints or dressings in place on an extremity it is simply carried around the splint or dressing, and the limb, and is tied at the most suitable point. Of course, the number of cravats employed for this purpose is dependent on the size of the special splint or dressing.

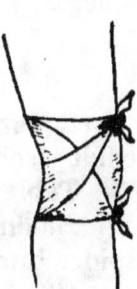

Four-Tail Knee Bandage.

BITES.

The bites of men, animals or snakes produce jagged, dirty, contuse wounds, which are not unlike other jagged wounds, except as noted below. The fact that such wounds are jagged, torn and dirty makes them slow to heal and often serious. The causes noted below need special attention because of their serious aspect:

Bites of persons suffering from hydrophobia.

Bites of mad dogs or cats. (See Hydrophobia—Special Disease Department).

Bites of poisonous snakes.

Bites of insects.

Cat Bites.

Wash the wound thoroughly with extract of witch hazel or a better plan is to saturate cotton with witch hazel and bind on the wound. (See Hydrophobia).

Dog Bites.

When bitten by a dog immediate action is very necessary.

First Aid Treatment.

Cleanse the wound thoroughly with warm water and treat as another wound unless the dog is found to have been mad, in which case the patient should be taken at once to the Pasteur Institute. (See Hydrophobia). Such institutions are found at New York, Chicago, Ann Arbor, St. Paul, New Orleans, St. Louis and Houston. However, practically all health offices in cities or small towns as well as many practicing physicians are now prepared to scientifically treat patients suffering from dog bites. Be sure to have the dog examined to determine whether he is mad, or, if necessary, have him taken to a veterinary surgeon until such is determined.

INSECT BITES OR STINGS.

Insect bites or stings contain formic acid. It is this which causes the pain. All bites or stings should be bathed with an antiseptic solution such as pure vinegar, hydrogen peroxide, or a hot normal salt solution.

First Aid Treatment.

Common Baking Soda.—Dampen and place on the affected part common baking soda, which will give relief.

Table Salt.—Common table salt as an antiseptic will kill the poison.

Baking Soda and Salt.—Equal parts of baking soda and salt applied to spider bites will aid in relieving pain and reduce swelling.

Witch Hazel.—Witch hazel applied freely will give quick relief.

Olive Oil.—This is also good to apply, as it is soothing in its effects.

Arnica.—Arnica may also be applied for bites or stings.

Plantain Leaves.—Plantain leaves crushed and applied as a poultice are very beneficial.

Coal Oil.—Coal oil may also be used, but as the skin of the patient may be easily blistered, the dressing should be removed as soon as the skin becomes reddened.

HORNET OR BEE STING.

For hornet or bee sting, first pull out the "sting," then apply an antiseptic dressing.

Mud Poultice.—A poultice made of clay and applied to the affected part is an excellent thing to relieve pain and keep down the swelling. There is some danger, however, of infection from the clay.

Raw Onion.—Raw onion made into a poultice and kept on for three or four hours will kill the poison from a sting or bite.

BRUISES.

A **bruise** or **contusion** is an injury due to a crushing of the tissues and blood vessels beneath the skin. It is usually the result of a blow from a blunt instrument, a fall or severe pressure.

The blackness of a bruise is caused by the blood escaping from the injured blood vessels into the surrounding tissues.

Symptoms.—At first the color of the injured area is red, then dark blue or black, and as absorption of the blood takes place, a yellow or greenish color develops which gradually fades and as the injured tissues heal, the color becomes normal and the pain is dull and aching, but rarely lasts long.

First Aid Treatment.

For severe bruises, four things are of great importance:
1. To stop the escape of blood into the tissues.
2. To counteract the pain, inflammation and shock which follows.
3. To preserve the vitality of the part, if this is possible.
4. To assist in the absorption of the blood which has escaped.

The affected parts should be elevated.

Hot or Cold Packs.—To prevent further escape of blood in the tissues, use hot or cold applications. Hot applications should be applied if the patient is old or the tissues badly destroyed, as in such cases the tissues have very little vitality, therefore circulation needs stimulation which is accomplished by the hot application. In this case use hot water bags, bags of hot bran, or any form of dry heat. Otherwise cloths wrung out of very cold water, ice bags or ice caps are more effective. Treatment should only be continued for a short period, half to three-fourths of an hour. Repeat if necessary.

Salt Water.—The application of hot saline solution will give much relief.

Vinegar.—Apply cloths wet in hot, diluted vinegar. This will greatly relieve the pain and soreness.

Witch Hazel.—Applications of tincture of witch hazel and cold water, equal parts, will help remove the discoloration resulting from a bruise.

Lemon Juice.—Bathe the parts with lemon juice or apply a slice of lemon. The lemon should be held in place with a bandage.

Hot Water.—Bathe the parts with hot water for fifteen or twenty minutes.

Salt Butter.—Apply salty butter at once, as this will keep the parts from becoming black.

Plantain Leaves.—Crush fresh plantain leaves and apply to the bruise. This kind of poultice will be found very effective.

BULLET WOUNDS.

The bullet should not be removed except by a physician or under his direction. In case of a flesh wound, it may be treated as a punctured wound. (See Punctured Wounds). If the wound is in a vital part of the body as the abdomen, chest or head, simply protect the opening from dirt or dust by covering with a soft cloth. Remove the patient immediately to the hospital or doctor's office.

BURNS.

A burn is an injury to the tissues produced by dry heat, acids or alkalies. It may be a surface or slight burn, it may be deep seated and severe. Burns are classified according to the cause and depth of injury to the tissues, and may be taken under the following classes:

Sunburn.—A sunburn is often very severe and painful, especially if covering a large part of the body. The treatment consists mainly in protection from the air. It should be treated as any other burn. The clothing should not be allowed to irritate the surface.

First Aid Treatment.

Soda.—Soak a piece of clean gauze or cotton in a solution of soda water made by dissolving a teaspoonful of baking soda in a cup of water, and apply to the affected area.

Olive Oil.—A cloth dipped in olive oil placed over the burn is good.

Vaseline or Cold Cream.—Apply vaseline or cold cream to the affected parts.

Alkali Burns.—These burns are caused by lime, caustic potash or caustic soda coming in contact with the tissues. They should be treated by neutralizing the alkali. This is done by the application of a weak acid solution, such as lemon juice or vinegar; then treat as any other burn.

Acid Burns.—Some of the acids from which burns are most commonly caused are nitric, hydrochloric and sulphuric acids, or those known as the concentrated acids. Some alkali, such as limewater, solution of washing soda, soap or chalk should be used to neutralize the acid. Then treat as any burn.

If the eye has been burned, wash it with a weak solution of bicarbonate of soda, after which apply a few drops of olive or sweet oil to the eye.

Slight Burns.—The burn coming in contact with air causes the pain, therefore exclude the air from the burn. The following simple remedies are suggested.

First Aid Treatment.

White of Egg.—Apply immediately and liberally the white of an egg, giving the burn two or three coats which will thoroughly shut out the air and relieve the suffering.

Raw Potato.—Raw potato scraped and applied to a burn will relieve the pain.

Raw Linseed Oil.—Apply raw linseed oil and apply loose dressing.

Baking Soda.—When the skin is only reddened, apply over the burned parts a cloth which has been dipped in water in which baking soda has been dissolved. This will keep out the air and reduce the inflammation.

Carron Oil.—If the skin is blistered, pour oil over the part, then cover with a soft cloth soaked in the oil. A good oil for this is the carron oil made of equal parts of linseed oil and limewater.

White of Egg and Olive Oil.—White of egg and olive oil or clean lard thoroughly mixed and applied is an excellent remedy for burns.

Mentholatum or Carbolated Vaseline.—Apply freely and dress with clean linen. These may be purchased at any drug store.

Cold Sweet Milk.—If possible, immerse the part in cold sweet milk or apply a cloth wet in milk, this dressing should be changed frequently.

SEVERE BURNS.

In severe burns, the clothing should be removed very carefully, either by cutting or ripping the seams, then remove the adherent parts with oil or warm water. When the tissues are badly destroyed a weak antiseptic dressing should be used, and the vesicles punctured by a sterilized needle. Apply and remove dressing in small portions so as not to expose much of the surface to the air at once. Deep burns are very serious and should be treated by a physician even though a small surface has been burned. If a large part of the body is burned, place the body, clothes and all, into a tub of water. If only water has been used no harm has been done, and yet the patient has been eased. If other applications have been made, they may delay the doctor's plans. Call a physician at once.

CARBOLIC BURNS.

If carbolic acid should be spilled on the hands or any part of the body, pour alcohol over it immediately. If this cannot be procured at once, immerse the injured part in soap and water till alcohol can be procured. If there is danger of poisoning from the acid, watch the urine carefully, as one of the earliest symptoms is a dark green color of the urine. Headache and nausea follow. Give Epsom or Glauber salts in large doses, raw eggs, castor oil or sweet oil (See Carbolic Acid Poisoning.)

CHOKING.

Choking may be caused by such foreign bodies as coins, needles, fish bones, pins, false teeth, or particles of food becoming lodged in the throat. Symptoms of suffocation very often are present, the face becomes blue, the patient gasps for breath and violent fits of coughing ensues, etc.

First Aid Treatment.

Sometimes the object may be easily expelled by passing the finger into the throat, or by slapping the person on the back between the shoulders. If the patient is a young child, raise the arms as high as possible above the head, or place the child, stomach downward, over the knees, bend the head low, and slap it hard on the back between the shoulders. This will often remove the foreign body.

If only a small object has lodged in the throat it may cause less harm to allow it to go through the body. Do not give castor oil, but plenty of bread and potatoes, which will carry the object through.

Lemon Juice.—If a fish bone has been swallowed, slowly sip the juice of a lemon, as this will dissolve the bone.

Vomiting.—Give an emetic of warm mustard water which will cause vomiting and often expel the object. If there is any difficulty in disposing of the foreign body, call a physician at once, as delay frequently causes serious symptoms to develop.

COLLAPSE.

Collapse is an extreme degree of shock, and is generally due to disease, while shock is the result of an accident or operation. The treatment is the same as for shock. (See Shock).

COMPRESS.—(Red Cross First-Aid).

A compress is simply something which is used to press on or, in other words, to cover an open wound. It should always be sufficient in size to do so with a lap of at least one and one-half inches on all sides. Compresses should preferably be made of gauze or cheese-cloth.

Above everything else they should be safe to apply to wounds. That is to say, they must have been properly disinfected in the first place, and in the second, they must not be contaminated by the fingers or anything else in the handling necessary to apply them. This is the great advantage of the Red Cross first-aid outfit, which is so prepared by the manufacturers that it is safe to put in direct contact with a wound and is then protected from accidental contamination by being enclosed in a sealed metal box. Moreover, the compress is so attached to its bandage that only gross carelessness in applying it will contaminate it then. A number of other first-aid packets are on the market which contain compresses that may be safely applied to a wound, though none is quite so easy to handle without accidental contamination as the Red Cross outfit. Each has printed directions on the box or container which must be carefully followed. If a first-aid packet can be procured it should always be used in preference to anything else to dress a wound. The next choice should be sterile or antiseptic gauze. Small packages of such gauze suitable for compresses may be bought in most drug stores, and are found in emergency outfits. (Sterile gauze is ordinary gauze in which the germs have been destroyed by heat, and antiseptic gauze is ordinary gauze in which germs have been destroyed by an antiseptic, usually bichloride of mercury.) In a city, therefore, or if an emergency outfit is available, one may easily procure a safe compress and all he need do is to handle it so that he will not contaminate it. This may be accomplished by holding it not with the fingers, but by the paper which covers it, allowing only the inner surface of this paper to come in contact with the gauze and never removing part of the paper until it has served this purpose. If, by chance, the gauze is touched by the hand great care should be taken to drop the untouched part on the wound and to place the gauze which has come in contact with the hand as near the outer layer of the dressing as possible.

Unless a safe gauze can be procured it is much safer to leave a wound exposed to the air than to cover it, but this will not always prove practicable. It is especially in localities where no gauze can be procured that circumstances render it necessary to cover wounds. In such localities it may be hours before the service of a doctor can be procured, so an uncovered wound will be exposed for a long time to accidental contamination, which will be almost inevitable from the hands or clothing of the patient who must perhaps be moved. A compress, too, affords an excellent means of checking bleeding, being often all that is required for this purpose. Under such circumstances, therefore, it will be necessary to make a compress, which, if not as safe as is desirable, is, at least, as good as can be procured. First, as surgically clean cloth for the compress as can be obtained should be used. This will be found in a towel, a handkerchief or other cloth of the same kind which has recently been laundered and has not been used since it was washed. Preferably, this cloth should be boiled for ten minutes or soaked in a solution of 1-1,000 bichloride of mercury (corrosive sublimate) for an equal length of time. This process recommended will give a compress which is safe to use, but an important practical difficulty is presented in applying such a compress to a wound. It will, of course, be so wet that it will not be possible to put it on the wound without squeezing some of the water out of it. To do this the compress must necessarily be handled and, as will be explained, pus germs exist in countless millions on the hands. If possible, therefore, the hands must be cleaned surgically, which means they should be freed of germs. This should be done by active scrubbing for five minutes with hot water, soap and a nail brush, paying special attention to the nails. Preferably the hands should be washed under a tap instead of in a basin, and if a basin is used the water had best be changed two or three times. As a further precaution, when corrosive sublimate is procurable, the hands after being washed should be soaked in a 1-1,000 solution of that chemical for a period of five minutes. The hands must not be wiped and they must not touch anything except the compress. The piece of cloth which is intended for a compress may now be taken from the vessel in which it has been boiled or disinfected, but in so doing the operator should be very careful not to allow his hands to come in contact with that part of the compress which he intends to put on the wound. On the contrary, he should pick up the piece of cloth by its outer surface and, holding it at all times by this, squeeze the water from it until it is comparatively dry and then put it on the wound without delay. If a fairly large piece is taken for the compress and if, previous to boiling, or disinfection, it is folded so as to fit the wound it will be handled much more easily and safely.

When no facilities are available for washing and disinfecting the hands, naturally this must be omitted, but the same precautions should be taken in handling the compress. Suppose, however, that in addition the compress cannot be boiled or disinfected, and yet it is absolutely necessary to have one. In this case one should again take a towel, handkerchief, etc., which has just been laundered, and without unnecessary handling apply its inner surface to the wound. Towels, handkerchiefs, etc., which have been used or handled, though they may look clean, are never so in the surgical sense and are therefore particularly dangerous to use as compresses.

No attempt should be made to wash or to disinfect a wound. These are matters for the surgeon, and for him only in favorable surroundings and conditions. It is as unjustifiable for a student of first-aid to wash or to attempt to disinfect a wound as it would be to probe it. If he leaves the wound undisturbed and untouched except with the safest compress that can be procured, he will have done his best and the patient should be greatly his debtor. If he goes further than this he may be solely responsible for much unnecessary suffering and perhaps even for an unnecessary death.

COMPRESSION OF THE BRAIN.

Compression of the brain is due to an injury to the skull, a tumor or blood clot from an artery which has been ruptured, or some other pressure on the brain.

Symptoms.—In compression, the stupor is more profound than in concussion, pulse is slow, breathing slow and labored.

First Aid Treatment.

Summon a physician, put the patient to bed with head elevated a little, and an ice bag placed to it. The room should be darkened.

CONCUSSION OF THE BRAIN.

Concussion of the brain is due to a blow or fall on the head, or a great jarring of the head.

Symptoms.—In concussion the symptoms are, partial stupor, feeble pulse, contracted or dilated pupils. The skin is cold; restlessness and vomiting are present.

First Aid Treatment.

Treat the patient quickly with head elevated and cold applications on the head and warm ones at the feet. Let patient have plenty of rest. Call a physician at once.

CONVULSIONS.

Convulsions in infants are not uncommon and seldom leave permanent results. They are generally due to disturbances of digestion, local irritation such as burns, tight foreskin, teething or worms. Whooping-cough is often accompanied by convulsions. They sometimes usher in scarlet fever. Convulsions occur most frequently between the fifth and twelfth months, but may occur as late as the fifth year.

Symptoms.—Convulsions come on without warning, but restlessness and fever usually precede. The child is unconscious, the eyes vacant and fixed, hands clenched, forehead cold and clammy, the lips and finger tips may turn blue. The body may become rigid for a few moments followed by stupor. The convulsions may last a few seconds or many minutes and one is apt to follow another.

First Aid Treatment.

Find and remove the cause. If undigested food is the cause, give an emetic such as warm water and mustard. If teething is the cause, have the gums lanced. In any case the physician should be called. Place the patient in a warm bath. Dissolve 2 tablespoonsful of mustard in a cup and add this to a small tub of hot water 100° F. in which place the child for five or ten minutes while you gently rub the limbs and body. Before placing in the bath apply a cold compress to the head. After the bath, and when the muscles have become relaxed, empty the bowels by giving a soapsuds enema, after the enema the child should be placed in bed, wrapped in warm blankets. Apply heat if necessary. A good dose of castor oil may be given in preference to the enema if conditions are acute.

CRAMPS.

Sometimes brought about by disorder of some abdominal organ. If this is the cause, have a physician attend the patient at once.

First Aid Treatment.

Peppermint.—Give 8 or 10 drops of spirits of peppermint in a little hot water.

Hot Water Bottle.—Put a hot water bottle at the feet and back and keep the patient in bed for the first 24 hours, if possible.

Hot Ginger Tea.—A drink of hot ginger tea is good.

Keep the bowels open.

Mustard Plaster.—For cramps in stomach, make a mustard plaster using the white of egg instead of water, and apply to the pit of the stomach.

Blackberry Roots.—Make a tea from blackberry roots and give a tablespoonful every half hour till relieved.

Turpentine.—Cramps in the limbs may be relieved by applying a cloth dipped in turpentine.

Red Pepper Tea.—Red pepper tea applied will relieve cramps in the neck or legs.

Stone Root.—An infusion or poultice made from steeped stone root is good for cramps.

CROUP.—(See "Disease Department").

CUTS AND LACERATIONS.

Lacerations differ from cuts in that the wounds are ragged tears and often consist of masses of torn tissues. Lacerations may be the result of tearing by blunt instruments. They are harder to deal with than cuts.

First Aid Treatment.

Cuts and lacerations should be thoroughly cleaned since lacerations especially are apt to become infected.

Allow to bleed freely. This is the best way of cleansing wounds. The loss of ½ pint of blood in an adult does no harm.

Even if they are not bleeding, be sure to tie large torn vessels. Cleanse thoroughly with warm water and dress with a clean compress or piece of cloth. If all slivers or foreign bodies have been removed from the wound, keeping the wound clean and covered with a clean dressing, usually is all that will be necessary. However, if the laceration or cut is severe after the first aid treatments have been followed, the patient should consult a physician.

Cold Compresses.—If it is advisable to stop the bleeding, cold compresses applied to the injury with slight pressure will stop moderate bleeding.

Lemon Juice.—A cloth soaked in lemon juice and bound around the cut will assist in stopping the flow of blood.

DEATH.

When the patient has ceased breathing, the nurse or attendant should close the eyes by gently pressing down the lids with the fingers, and close the lips. If the patient has false teeth, they should be placed in the mouth before closing. Place a roll of some material, towel or napkin, under the chin to keep the mouth closed. Straighten out the limbs, and fold in some natural position, then wash the body with soap and water and some disinfectant. The rectum and vagina must be packed with cotton to prevent any discharge. Sometimes it is necessary to pack the nostrils and mouth too. Put a napkin, drawers, undervest, nightgown and stockings on the body. Comb and dress the hair in the way it was usually worn. Clean the nails. If there are any wounds, fresh dressing should be applied. Place a wide bandage around the knees and ankles to keep the limbs together.

Remove all appliances used during the illness, and put the room in order. Keep the room cool and the house quiet.

DISLOCATION.

Dislocation is a complete displacement of an articular bone. It may be caused by violence or by great muscular action. Dislocations are usually of ball and socket joints or other free motion joints, such as the shoulder, hip, etc.

Symptoms.—Great pain usually accompanies dislocations since the ligaments about the joints are torn and wrenched. Swelling soon appears; the shape of the joint is different; the direction of the limb is changed; a flattened appearance at the joint is observed, and an abnormal projection of the bone.

Dislocation of the Jaw.—The jaw may be dislocated by a blow or caused by yawning or laughing.

First Aid Treatment.

A severe dislocation should be treated by a physician, although a person of good judgment and nerve control may perform the operation of location quite effectively. Seat the patient in a comfortable chair, and have another person stand behind the patient holding the head firmly, while the first person having bandaged the thumbs well, places them on the patient's lower teeth, seizes the jaw firmly but gently with both hands and moves it downward and backward at the same time pulling the chin upward. With these movements the jaw will usually return to its proper position, making a snapping noise, which unless expected, is rather startling to the operator and patient.

Dislocation of the Shoulder.—Shoulder dislocation is usually caused by a blow or fall. This is a very common dislocation. The arm is held rigidly, the elbow stands off from the body and cannot be placed at the side, as can the normal arm. There is pain and great swelling at the place of injury, and a marked depression at the injured point of the shoulder.

First Aid Treatment.

Cold applications as ice bags, or hot applications of cloths wrung from hot water should be placed on the shoulder in order to prevent swelling, until a surgeon can be called. The injured member should be carefully supported by a pillow or sling until the doctor arrives.

Dislocation of the Finger.—The second joint of the thumb is more difficult to set when dislocated and should be taken to a physician. Grasp the finger firmly and pull away from the hand, then place in splints and bandage firmly, but not too tight.

DROWNING.

This is a condition of suffocation caused by the air passages of the lungs becoming filled with water. The body does not need to sink in order to cause drowning. The nose and mouth only need to remain under water for several minutes. For this reason the greatest care should be taken to guard against small children getting into vessels or puddles of water, as they may drown in a very small amount of water.

First Aid Treatment.

In case of drowning loosen the clothing from the neck and chest, free the nose and throat from any obstruction. Gently draw the tongue out, having some one hold the tongue, and twist a handkerchief around it, fastening the ends around the neck, if possible.

Artificial Respiration.—Artificial respiration must be used in different cases, such as in drowning, after an electrical shock, in suffocation, in anaesthesia and on the new born; though drowning is probably the most frequent occasion for its use.

In drowning the following precautions should precede the use of artificial respiration. See that all clothing is loosened and that all water has been expelled from the lungs. This may be done by laying the body on its stomach and lifting it at the center so that the head hangs down, and then jerking the body several times. After this turn it over and perform artificial respiration.

Several methods have been proven successful in restoring respiration. The following is a very simple method. Place the patient on his back with the head lower than the feet if possible, then place a folded blanket under the shoulders and allow the head to fall back. If three persons are near, have one stand at the head of the patient, carefully watching that nothing hinders the breathing. The other two should be at either side and grasp the arms at the wrist and elbow, raise the arms evenly and regularly over the head and down even with the body, then return to the side again. Then fold the forearms over the chest and gently lean your weight upon the body, thus expelling all the air from the lungs. Repeat many times. The persons at the sides should act together until the patient begins to breath, or until thoroughly convinced that no life remains. The arm movements should be regulated by the breathing of the chief man or someone giving a signal or count.

DRUGS AND POISONS.

There are certain drugs which are very valuable in the treatment of diseases and injuries but which are deadly poison when improperly used. This is often the result of leaving them where children can get hold of them, or they may be taken by mistake or for attempts at self-destruction.

These poisons are of three kinds: narcotics, irritants and corrosives.

Narcotics.—Narcotics are used to produce a soothing effect or sleep, and when taken improperly the symptoms are those of stupor, delirum, insensibility, hard breathing and sleepiness.

Irritants and Corrosives.—These are used for their local effect, also for their constitutional effect. Their improper use is apparent by the marked irritation and corrosive effect they produce in the tissues which they touch—generally the lips, mouth and throat. They also produce intense pain in the stomach and bowels, severe vomiting and symptoms of shock when taken internally.

In the **treatment** of cases of **poisoning**, there are three things which should be done: **Remove** all the **poison** possible at once, **neutralize** whatever cannot be removed and **counteract** the ill effects which have already been produced. Poisons may be **removed** from the stomach by means of **emetics** (causing vomiting), by the use of the **stomach pump** and by means of **cathartics.** They may be **neutralized** by means of **antidotes.** After the poison has been removed or neutralized, the effects produced on the system must be treated.

Whatever is done must be done **at once** as poisons act very quickly and there is seldom time to secure medical aid. However, a physician should be summoned immediately and in the meantime everything done to remove the poison, counteract its further effect and give relief to the patient.

Emetics.—An emetic is an agent which acting directly on the nerves of the stomach causes vomiting. Emetics are used in case of poisoning, thus removing the poison from the stomach. Under this heading may also be included the putting of the finger or a feather back in the throat and causing the patient to vomit by the tickling sensation.

Mustard.—Add one tablespoonful of mustard to a pint of warm water and give to the patient suffering with poisoning. It is one of the most simple and valuable emetics which can be given, as it not only will invariably cause vomiting, but it has a stimulating effect and is for this reason valuable in narcotic poisoning.

Salt (Sodium of Chloride).—Add two tablespoonfuls to half a pint of warm water. Have the patient drink this while warm. Salt is a remedy, always at hand, but somewhat less effective than the mustard emetic.

Alum.—Add one tablespoonful to half a pint of warm water. This also acts as an emetic.

Siphonage.—This is a good way to remove the contents of the stomach and can be performed without much trouble. Take a small rubber tube about five or six feet long, oil thoroughly and pass one end of it down the throat into the stomach (being very careful that the tube is not passed into the windpipe instead of the oesophagus). The tongue should be pressed down and the end of the tube passed back as far as possible and then turned downward. Then attach a funnel to the end projecting from the mouth and pour gradually two **pints of tepid water** into the funnel allowing it to pass beween the thumb and finger and lowered below the level of the stomach, a basin should be in readiness to receive the contents. As soon as the thumb and finger are removed the tube will act as a siphon and draw off the contents of the stomach, providing the stomach does not contain too much indigested food. It is often well to place a large cork or a spool of thread between the teeth so that the tube will not be bitten in two. The rubber or metal end may be cut off the tube of the ordinary fountain syringe thus making it a good instrument for this purpose.

The siphon or stomach pump should never be used in case of **carbolic acid poisoning** or in **corrosive poisoning** as the tissues, burned by the carbolic acid or corrosive would be injured by the introduction of any foreign material or instrument.

Stimulants.—It is often necessary to give a stimulant because of the depressing effect of some poisons; this is most apt to be the case in **narcotic poisoning**—those drugs which produce stupor or sleep.

Strong Coffee.—One of the commonest and best stimulants, is ordinary strong coffee. This is especially good in narcotic poisoning. It can be administered either by mouth or rectum. All stimulants given by rectum should be given in much larger doses than when given by mouth. Stimulants may be diluted with warm water or milk when given by mouth. Stimulants may also be administered by inhalation. When given this way there should be a few drops placed on a cloth or handkerchief and applied to the nose. Do not hold the bottle to the nose as it may be spilled and the patient get too large a dose.

When the patient is suffering from a corrosive poisoning, stimulants given by inhalation should be given with great care because of the inflammation of the tissues.

Ammonia.—This is one of the commonest stimulants administered by inhalation. It is, however, very strong and should be given with much care.

Strychnine.—Strychnine is a valuable stimulant and is only administered hypodermically and should be done by a physician.

Caution.—Accidents are largely the result of carlessness. Keep all bottles or boxes containing drugs well labeled, especially those containing poisons. Keep them out of the reach of children, and those not responsible for their actions. Have the simple remedies noted below at hand. Don't get excited. Keep cool and apply them at once.

Aconite—Monk's-hood—Wolf's-bane.

Tincture of aconite may be mistaken for sherry wine which it resembles in appearance. It is found in neuralgia cures, ointments, liniments and fever mixtures. It is very poisonous.

Symptoms.—There is tingling sensation in the lips, mouth, throat and limbs. Slow and weak pulse, eyes are fixed and pupils dilated; mind is clear. Convulsions may result.

Emetic.—Give strong mustard water or other emetic promptly or use stomach pump.

Antidote.—No antidote.

Treatment.—Place in a reclining position with the head low and feet elevated slightly, apply heat to the extremities. Keep the patient very quiet for movements may cause collapse. Apply mustard to the heart and calves of legs. Strong coffee as stimulant may be given by rectum. Use artificial respiration.

Alcohol.

Alcohol taken into the system by accident causes poisoning similar to that of its prolonged use. It should not be confused with apoplexy or skull fracture. Total unconsciousness is characteristic of apoplexy or skull fracture, while the person with alcohol poisoning can be aroused to answer questions.

Symptoms.—The person with alcohol poisoning lies in a stupor, has an odor of alcohol on breathing and pupils of eye are dilated.

Emetic.—Give mustard and warm water if the patient is exhausted.

Antidote.—No antidote.

Treatment.—Allow the patient to rest and sleep, cover warmly and apply heat to limbs. If the pulse is weak give stimulants such as strong coffee by mouth or rectum if necessary.

Antimony.

Such compounds of antimony as tartar emetic act as irritants, but the chloride, or butter of antimony, acts as a corrosive. Antimony is found as a metal or a mineral.

Symptoms.—There is a marked depression, metallic taste in the mouth; violent vomiting; purging; diarrhea; and finally collapse; cold and moist skin.

Emetics.—Use the stomach pump to remove the contents of the stomach.

Antidote.—Tannic or gallic acid is the antidote.

Treatment.—Maintain the prone position, give soothing drinks, apply heat and stimulate.

Arsenic.

Arsenic is often found in colored candies, painted toys, etc. Medically it is used in the form of Fowler's solution. Compounds of arsenic and copper compose Paris green.

Symptoms.—Abdominal pains, vomiting, intense thirst, bloody and offensive stools, puffiness of eyelids.

Emetics.—Cause vomiting at once by giving warm mustard water, warm salt solution, or by tickling the throat with a feather.

Antidote.—Raw eggs beaten, hydrated oxide of iron.

Treatment.—Give plenty of milk to drink, olive oil or castor oil. Stimulate if necessary.

Belladonna—Deadly Nightshade.

Found in cough mixtures, liniments, plasters, and eye lotions.

Symptoms.—Inability to swallow, headache, eyes brilliant, pupils dilated, vision often doubled, flushed face, dizziness follows, and rapid pulse.

Emetic.—Warm mustard or salt water, or alum.

Antidote.—No chemical antidote.

Treatment.—Apply heat to the extremities. and use stimulants. Use artificial respiration if necessary.

Bichloride of Mercury—Corrosive Sublimate.

Bichloride of mercury occurs in the form of white crystals, and is a powerful germicide, used as a disinfectant in the form of a solution. It is very poisonous when taken into the system.

Symptoms.—The lips and tongue are stained white, cramps, cold and moist skin, vomiting of blood and mucus, diminishing urine and finally convulsions and collapse.

Emetic.—An emetic of strong salt water may be given.

Antidote.—Albumen or white of egg in water should be given as an antidote.

Treatment.—Mucilaginous drinks, milk and flour paste, full doses of potassium iodide, stimulants if necessary.

Blue Vitriol—Sulphate of Copper.

Very poisonous in large quantities. Food cooked in copper vessels may produce this poisoning. Also canned fruit contaminated with copper salts.

Symptoms.—Burning sensation in the stomach, vomitus colored green, abdominal pains, diarrhea, great thirst and weakness.

Emetic.—Warm mustard or salt water.

Antidote.—Potassium ferrocyanide.

Treatment.—Great amount of warm water, white of eggs, linseed oil, sweet oil, flour and water, milk. Stimulants.

Camphor.

Taken in the form of spirits of camphor or gum camphor. Found in cough mixtures and many liniments.

Symptoms.—Noise in the ears, skin is cold and clammy, headache, odor of camphor on the breath, burning pain in the stomach, delirium may occur.

Emetic.—Any common emetic such as alum or warm water with mustard or salt.

Antidote.—No chemical antidote.

Treatment.—Apply heat to the extremities and stimulate. Hot and cold douches.

Cantharides, Spanish Fly, or Blister Beetle.

Cantharides is the powdered bodies of certain beetles, obtained in the form of a plaster or a solution. It is a powerful counter irritant.

Symptoms.—Intense burning and pain in the mouth, vomiting and purging, irritation of the urinary organs, bloody urine, delirium and convulsions.

Emetic.—Give warm lard.

Antidote.—There is no antidote.

Treatment.—Give flour and water, milk and raw eggs, or flaxseed tea.

Carbolic Acid—Phenol.

Carbolic acid poisoning acts very rapidly, and is very deadly in effect.

Symptoms.—Odor of carbolic acid on the breath, abdominal pains, cold skin, irregular pulse, great swelling of the tissues, smoky urine, the urine greatly decreased.

Emetic.—No emetic.

Antidote.—Epsom or Glauber salts.

Treatment.—White of egg, castor oil may be given after the antidote.

Chloral Hydrate—Chloral.

An ingredient in sleeping medicines, liniments, and cough mixtures. Odor similar to bananas or pears.

Symptoms.—Skin cold, irregular pulse, face congested, difficult breathing, contracted then dilated pupils, finally sinking into a deep stupor and unconsciousness.

Emetic.—Any common emetic if the poison has just been taken.

Antidote.—No antidote.

Treatment.—Stimulate, keep patient in reclining position with head low, give hot coffee by rectum, apply mustard over the heart and calves of legs, artificial respiration.

Chloroform and Ether.

It is an ingredient of cough mixtures and liniments. May be taken internally in form of spirits or water of chloroform.

Symptoms.—Odor of chloroform on the breath. Burning sensation of mouth, lips, and stomach; dizziness and unconsciousness. When chloroform or ether is inhaled, pulse is weak and irregular, face pale, pupils dilated.

Emetics.—One tablespoonful of mustard in warm water.

Antidote.—No antidote.

Treatment.—Give bicarbonate of soda and water. If inhaled, place patient in a recumbent position, keep the head low and feet raised, pull tongue well forward, and perform artificial respiration. Slap with a wet towel in order to arouse. Give plenty of fresh air.

Croton Oil.

May be taken by mistake for castor oil, since it is of a pale yellow color resembling castor oil.   It is a strong irritant.

Symptoms.—Vomiting and purging, abdominal pains, cold and clammy skin.

Emetic.—Give warm mustard water, or salt water promptly.

Antidote.—No antidote.

Treatment.—Give whites of eggs, or milk and flour, stimulants as coffee.

Digitalis—Foxglove.

Digitalis is used as a heart stimulant.

Symptoms.—Slow and irregular pulse, out of proportion to the heart beat, headache, face pale and great prostration, vomiting and convulsions may follow, eyes staring and prominent.

Emetic.—Give an emetic if the poison has been taken in one large dose.

Antidote.—Tannic acid is the chemical antidote.

Treatment.—Keep the patient in a reclining position, place mustard over the heart and to the calves of the legs, give strong tea or oakbark as a stimulant.

Fungi.—(See Mushrooms).

Holly Berries.

Birds and animals may eat them without injury but human beings may not.

Symptoms.—Cramps, colic, vomiting, purging, unconsciousness may follow.

Emetics.—Give some common emetic as mustard or warm salt water.

Antidote.—No antidote.

Treatment.—Apply heat to extremities and stimulate if necessary.

Hydrochloric, Nitric, Sulphuric Acids.

These are corrosive acids, very destructive to the tissues. Do not give emetics or use stomach pump.

Symptoms.—Vomiting, swelling of the tissues, great burning, stupor, abdominal pains, cold skin, irregular pulse, later there may be convulsions.   Nitric acid leaves yellow stains in the mouth and lips, sulphuric leaves a black color.

Emetics.—Give no emetic and do not use stomach pump.

Antidote.—Soda, lime water, chalk, magnesium, alkalies, or soap, given immediately.

Treatment.—Give oil, milk, albumen, external heat, stimulants.

Iodine.

Iodine is generally found in the form of tincture of iodine; a reddish brown fluid.

Symptoms.—Mucous membrane of the mouth is colored yellow, burning sensation in the throat, vomiting bluish colored matter.

Emetic.—Give strong salt water or other emetic.

Antidote.—The antidote is starch.

Treatment.—Give thin boiled starch paste and follow with stimulants and white of egg beaten in milk. Chalk or magnesia also is good.

Iodoform.

Iodoform is used as an antiseptic in dressing wounds, and susceptible persons often become poisoned after prolonged use of it.

Symptoms.—In some cases there is severe irritation of stomach and intestines, while quite mild in other cases, with only headache and nausea. An eruption or inflammation appears on the skin. Sleeplessness, loss of memory, hallucination, vomiting, retention of the urine.

Emetic.—No emetic.

Antidote.—No antidote.

Treatment.—Do not use the drug longer. Sponge the patient with warm water and wrap in hot blankets to produce sweating.

Ivy Poison.

Very common poison.

Symptoms.—Intense itching, swelling, large blebs and blisters form on the skin. If the poison is inward, it produces drowsiness and stupor.

Treatment.—Solution of baking soda, or strong soapsuds, sugar of lead, dry starch dusted over the affected parts.

Laudanum.—(See Opium.)

Lead.

Painters often get lead poisoning, however, acute lead poisoning is due to taking internally paints, sugar of lead, white or red lead.

Symptoms.—Severe colic, colored lines on the gums, muscles of forearms paralyzed, purging, vomiting milk white matter.

Emetic.—Give warm lard or other common emetic if vomiting has already taken place.

Antidote.—Epsom or Glauber salts, white of egg and milk.

Treatment.—Apply heat, give milk and flour paste, strong coffee as a stimulant, mucilaginous drinks.

Lunar Caustic.—(See Silver Nitrate).

Lye.

Lye is an alkali, similar in properties to caustic potash and soda lime and other caustic alkalies.

Symptoms.—Great pain and swelling of lips and mouth. Later burning in throat and abdomen, difficult breathing, vomiting, irregular pulse, cold, moist skin.

Emetic.—Do not give emetic or use a stomach pump.

Antidote.—Weak acids such as vinegar, lemon juice, orange juice, hard cider, diluted, are antidotes for alkalies.

Treatment.—Raw eggs, olive oil, castor oil, flour and water, barley water, or milk. Give stimulants freely.

Mushrooms—Fungus.

Great caution should be used in the selection if mushrooms since very harmful results occur from mistaking the poisonous for the edible variety.

Symptoms.—Nausea, vomiting, cold and moist skin, colic, diarrhea, dilated pupils, muscular weakness.

Emetic.—Mustard or salt water.

Antidote.—There is no antidote.

Treatment.—Give castor oil, apply heat, give stimulants.

(Mushrooms may prove poisonous if heated a second time.)

Nitric Acid.—(See Hydrochloric Acid).

Opium.

Opium is present in morphine, paregoric, laudanum, many soothing syrups, and sleeping drugs.

Symptoms.—Contentment, drowsiness and finally a profound sleep from which the patient can scarcely be aroused, moist and pale skin, very slow and noisy respiration, pupils of the eye contracted as small as pin heads at times.

Emetic.—Warm mustard water or salt water.

Antidote.—Potassium permanganate.

Treatment.—Wash the stomach with potassium permanganate solution 1:6,000 and give strong coffee as stimulant. If unconscious, give stimulant by rectum. Keep the patient awake by slapping with a wet towel or walking about, but keep him awake.

Oxalic Acid.—(See Vegetable Acid).

Phosphorus.

Poisoning often results from sucking or swallowing the heads of matches. Rat pastes contain phosphorus.

Symptoms.—The symptoms are not all evident at the same time. The breath has an odor of phosphorus and there is a taste as of garlic in the mouth. There is a burning sensation in the stomach followed by vomiting. The vomited matter is tinged with blood and is luminous in the dark. Pulse weak and the pupils of the eyes are dilated headache and later there may be hemorrhages from the nose and stomach.

Emetic.—Give warm lard, warm mustard water or alum.

Antidote.—Give water containing small amount of oil of turpentine. Do not give other oils as they hasten the absorption of the poison.

Treatment.—Mucilaginous drinks, white of egg, milk and flour paste. Give Epsom or Glauber salts to move the bowels.

Poke Berries.

Since the berry is large, red, and juicy it is very attractive to children and a very common poison among them.

Symptoms.—They act as irritants when taken in small doses, but have a narcotic action when taken in large doses.

Emetic.—Give mustard or salt water.

Antidote.—No antidote.

Treatment.—Give castor oil, mucilaginous drinks such as egg in water and oily drinks.

Ptomaine Poisoning.

Ptomaine poisoning occurs from eating tainted ice cream, cheese, fish, tomatoes canned in tin, canned meats, etc.

Symptoms.—Nausea several hours after eating, abdominal pains, faintness, weak pulse, cold moist skin, sometimes red rash, and vomiting.

Emetic.—Give strong salt water or strong mustard water at once.

Antidote.—No antidote.

Treatment.—After the stomach has been emptied, give a large dose of castor oil, and fluid foods, and light diets. Apply heat to abdomen and feet.

Prussic Acid.

Very deadly poison found in the peach and cherry pits.

Symptoms.—First, a tightening about the throat, giddiness, then unconsciousness follows, open staring eyes, fixed jaws, vomiting and convulsions, involuntary discharge of feces and urine. Death may occur immediately.

Emetic.—An emetic of strong salt water may be given. Mustard water is also good. If there is time an emetic should be given or the stomach pump used immediately.

Antidote.—There is no chemical antidote.

Treatment.—Stimulants should be given by hypodermic injection, especially strychnine, use artificial respiration and give inhalations of ammonia.

Silver Nitrate—Lunar Caustic.

It may be received from sticks of silver nitrate during cauterization of the throat.

Symptoms.—Burning and pain in the throat and abdomen, white stain in the mouth. Abdominal irritation.

Emetic.—Give any common emetic.

Antidote.—Salt.

Treatment.—Give plenty of salt and water.

Paris Green.—(See Arsenic).

Paregoric.—-(See Opium).

Strychnine.

Strychnine is found in the St. Ignatius bean, and is the active element in nux vomica. Strychnine poisoning resembles lockjaw or tetanus in that it affects the jaws, but it can be detected from lockjaw easily by observing that the locking of the jaws is the first symptom while in strychnine poisoning, it comes late. In strychnine poisoning the upper extremities are affected while in lockjaw they are only affected slightly in the most severe cases.

Symptoms.—Twitching of the muscles followed by severe convulsion in less than a half hour, the convulsions occur at intervals, the body takes the form of a bow because of the contraction of the great muscles of the back, open and staring eyes, the patient has an appearance of laughing, difficulty in breathing.

Emetic.—Give strong emetic of warm mustard water if the case is taken before convulsions occur.

Antidote.—Give tannin or charcoal as an antidote if the case is taken early before convulsions begin.

Treatment.—Give strong tea or an infusion of oakbark. Follow with artificial respiration, if necessary.

Sugar of Lead.—(See Lead).

Tobacco—Nicotine.

It will produce poisoning immediately if taken internally, and will also cause poisoning by prolonged use.

Symptoms.—Burning in the mouth and throat and abdominal disorder, nausea, vomiting, pulse feeble but rapid, difficult breathing, contracted pupils.

Emetic.—Give some strong emetic or use the stomach pump.

Antidote.—Tannic acid in some form.

Treatment.—Keep patient in reclining position, apply heat to abdomen and feet, use artificial respiration, if necessary.

Tartar Emetic.   (See Antimony).

Tartar emetic is an irritant and a compound of antimony.

Symptoms.—Vomiting and purging, skin cold and moist, profuse per-spiration, streaks of blood in vomited matter, great thirst.

Emetic.—Use stomach pump if all contents have not been expelled.

Antidote.—Mixtures of tannic acid act as an antidote.

Treatment.—Use warm water, white oak bark, strong tea. Stimulate.

Tartaric Acid.—(See Vegetable Acids).

Vegetable Acids.

Such acids as Oxalic, Tartaric, Acetic are found in vegetables and also crystal forms—Oxalic acid in the crystal forms is sometimes mistaken for Epsom salts. It is used for cleaning boilers, etc., and may get into the food by accident.

Symptoms.—Burning pain in the mouth and a feeling of the throat being bound.

Emetic.—No emetic.

Antidote.—Alkalies are antidotes for acids. In case of oxalic acid, use only chalk or limewater. In case of tartaric or acetic, use limewater, baking soda, chalk, soap, or white wash.

Treatment.—Magnesia or lime in some form should be administered. Castor oil or sweet oil should be given.

Salt of Lemon and Sorrel.

Poisoning should be treated as oxalic.

Electrical Burns.

Electrical burns are usually deep seated and very severe, resulting in immediate death if the current is strong enough. Otherwise, they should be treated as severe burns. (See Burns)

Electrical Injuries.

When a person receives an electric shock, the result may not be fatal, but causes the person to become stunned or to cease breathing for a time, when artificial respiration will usually restore life if resorted to in time. In case the shock is received from a live wire and the person appears dead, observe the following precautions:

Separate the body from the live wire by using a dry coat, rope or board to remove the body or the wire so that the contact will be broken.

Do not use metal or any moist material.

Do not touch the soles or heels of the shoes, for these are transmitters of the current.

Use rubber gloves or dry cloths over the hands if obliged to touch the body, and use but one hand if possible. As soon as the victim is freed from contact with the live wire, examine the mouth and throat carefully to ascertain whether or not the patient may have swallowed gum, tobacco, false teeth, or any other foreign body. Then begin artificial respiration at once; every moment of delay is serious. If the shock is the result of stroke of lightning, keep warm and use artificial respiration as described above or as in the following manner:

Artificial Respiration.—Lay the subject on his belly, with arms extended as straight forward as possible, and with face to one side, so that the nose and mouth are free for breathing (Illustrations Page 172). Let a helper draw forward the subject's tongue.

If possible, avoid so laying the subject that any burned places are pressed upon.

Do not permit bystanders to crowd about and shut off fresh air.

Kneel, straddling the subject's hips and facing his head; rest the palms of your hands on the loins (the muscles of the small of the back), with thumbs nearly touching each other, and with fingers spread over the lowest ribs.

With arms held straight, swing forward slowly so that the weight of your body is gradually brought to bear upon the subject (see Figure 1). This operation which should take from two to three seconds, must not be violent—internal organs may be injured. The lower part of the chest and also the abdomen are thus compressed, and air forced out of the lungs.

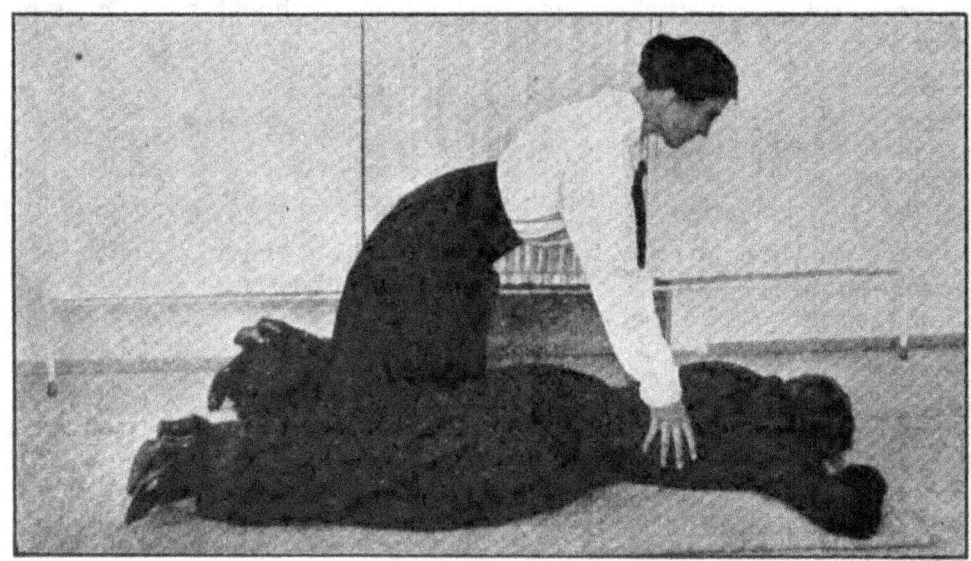

Fig. 1. Pressure Applied.

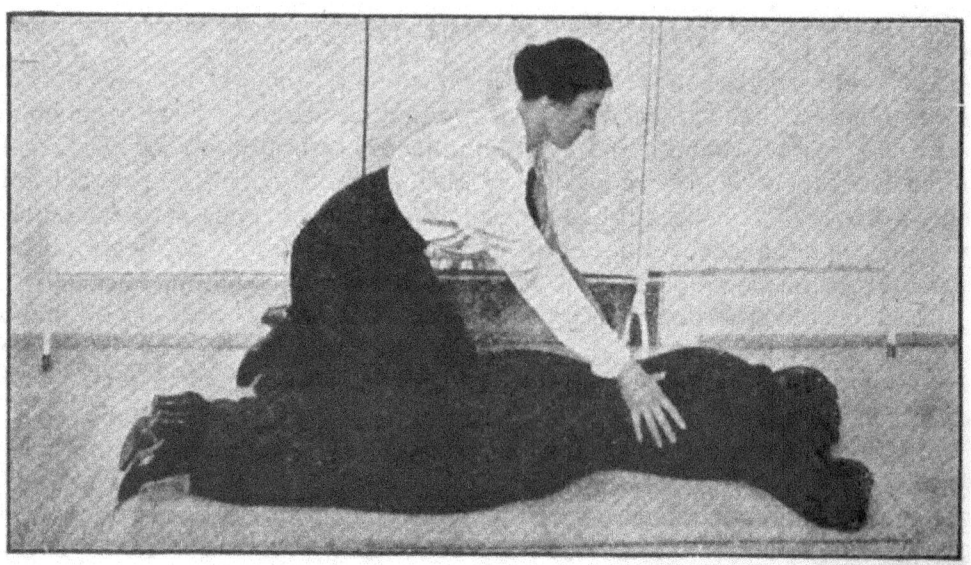

Fig. 2. Pressure Released.
Performing Artificial Respiration.

Now immediately swing backward so as to remove the pressure, but leave your hands in place, thus returning to the position shown in Figure 2. Through their elasticity, the chest walls spring out and the lungs are thus supplied with fresh air.

After two seconds swing forward again. Thus repeat deliberately the double movement of compression and release twelve to fifteen times a minute—a complete respiration in four or five seconds. If a watch or clock is not visible follow the natural rate of your own deep breathing, swinging forward with each expiration, and backward with each inspiration. While this is being done a helper should loosen any tight clothing about the neck, chest or waist.

Continue artificial respiration (if necessary, at least an hour), without interruption, until natural breathing is restored, or until a physician arrives. Even after natural breathing is restored, carefully watch that it continues. If it stops begin artificial respiration again. During the period of operation, keep the victim warm by applying bags filled with hot water. The attention to keeping the patient's body warm should be given by an assistant or assistants.

Do not give any liquids whatever by mouth until the patient is fully conscious.

EPILEPSY.

Epilepsy is a nervous disease with loss of consciousness accompanied by convulsions. The frequency or severity of the attacks varies in each individual thus afflicted.

Symptoms.—The person affected usually utters a piercing cry and becomes unconscious. Convulsions generally follow. The eyes are open, upturned with the pupils dilated. The frothy saliva may be blood-tinged usually due to biting of the tongue.

First Aid Treatment.

First put something between the back teeth, such as a piece of wood, cork or knotted handkerchief, to prevent biting the tongue. Do not pry the teeth open, as by so doing, they may be broken. Wait until the muscles of the jaw become relaxed, then quietly slip in some protector, being careful your own hand is not caught between the teeth, as may be in the case of another spasm or convulsion.

Loosen the clothing and make the patient comfortable. He should be watched carefully as he may become violent. Quiet and rest are the best medicine for the patient. ·

FAINTING—SYNCOPE.

Fainting is a temporary unconsciousness associated with a diminution of blood in the brain caused by a sudden weakening of the heart's action. Fainting may be the result of hemorrhage, heart disease, severe pain, fright, grief, joy, hot and vile air in crowded halls, exhaustion, certain drugs, etc.

Symptoms.—Face becomes pale, pulse weak, respirations rapid, extremities cold and clammy.

First Aid Treatment.

The head should be lowered and the feet raised. Give plenty of fresh air, loosen clothing and dash cold water into the face. Do not hold strong smelling salts too close to the nose. This is irritating. Rub arms and legs toward the heart. If the patient does not revive, a stimulant given by way of rectum, with a mustard plaster over the heart may be necessary.

Shock and fainting may be confused, but in shock the patient is more or less conscious, while in fainting he is unconscious. Frequent attacks, indicate need of advice from a physician.

FIRE.

The chief of the fire department in one of our large cities says: "The fire department is usually called too late. If you smell smoke and suspect fire do not waste time in trying to find it. Call the Fire Department at once. Do not try to put out the fire before calling in aid. If the fire is out before the Fire Department arrives, so much the better."

Where Fire Exists.—Close doors and windows to prevent draft. The air near the floor is fairly free from smoke. A wet cloth tied over the mouth and nose is at times useful.

If the clothing catches fire, do not let the sufferer walk or run about, as it fans the flames. Have him lie down on the floor immediately and cover with coat or blanket.

To Extinguish Fire from Clothing.—In attempting to rescue a person whose clothing is in flames, if necessary throw the patient on the floor, snatch a rug, blanket or coat, and placing one edge of it under your foot, stand at the head of the patient and cast the blanket over the body toward the feet so that the flames will be driven toward the feet instead of the face of the patient and also away from the rescuer. Wrap the covering closely about the body especially at the neck to keep the flames from the face.

FISH BONES IN THE THROAT.

By passing a finger into the throat the bone may be felt and removed. The patient may be stood on his head in the hope of dislodging the bone. Give lemon juice to dissolve the bone. Give dry bread to eat and water to drink. Slap the patient on the back between shoulders. If asphyxia is to be feared, call a physician and perform artificial respiration till he arrives.

FISH HOOKS.

If a fish hook has become caught in the flesh, push the point on through the skin. Cut off the back end of the hook close to the skin and pull the remainder through by the point. For treatment of wound see Punctured Wounds.

FITS.

Take care that the person does not injure himself. Loosen all tight clothing and leave him alone. Send for a doctor. (See Epilepsy.)

FOREIGN BODIES IN THROAT, EAR, EYE, AND NOSE.

Throat.—(See Choking).

Ear.—Great caution and care should be used in removing any foreign body from the ear. The organs of the ears are very delicate and easily injured.

If the foreign body has just entered the ear, often a cough, sneeze or blowing the nose which should be held firmly closed will remove it quickly. Picking and probing by the unskilled will invariably force the body farther into the ear and make it very difficult to be removed, even by a surgeon.

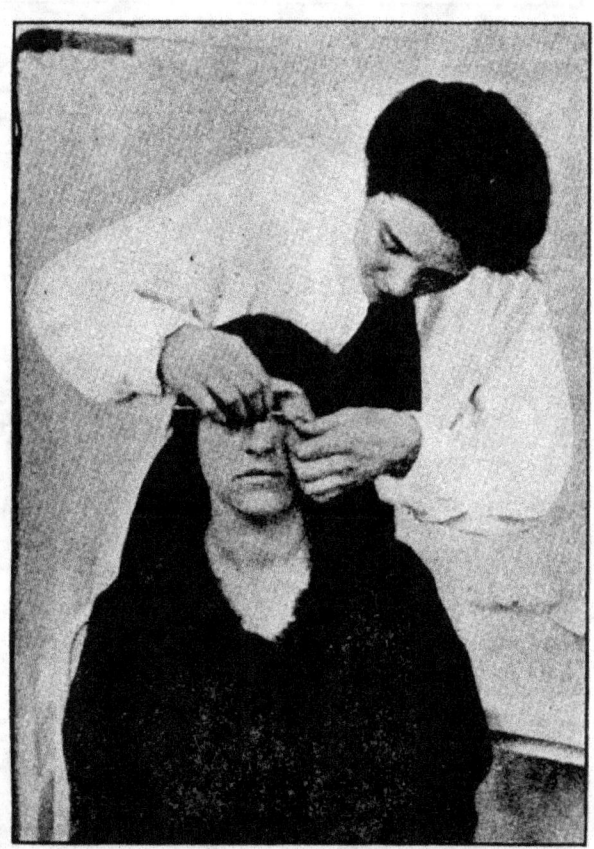

Removing Particles from the Upper Lid.
First Operation.

If an insect or a bug has entered the ear it may be removed readily by carefully syringing the ear with warm water, or filling it with olive oil. If the body be a bean or pea or other body likely to swell, do not syringe or put water into the ear, but go at once to the physician.

Toothpicks, button-hooks, and other similar instruments, should never be put into the ear.

In case of seeds, a little alcohol may be used, since it causes the seed to shrink. However, the wisest and safest procedure is to go at once to the doctor and allow him to care for the patient.

Eye.—The eye is the organ of sight and extremely delicate in construction, therefore, all handling of it should be gently done. The hands should be thoroughly scrubbed before touching the patient, and all dressings or solutions used be perfectly clean. To remove foreign bodies is often difficult, but may be done in the following ways:

Tears may be made to collect by holding the eyelid away from the ball and blowing the nose vigorously, and the particle may be washed out, or close the eye

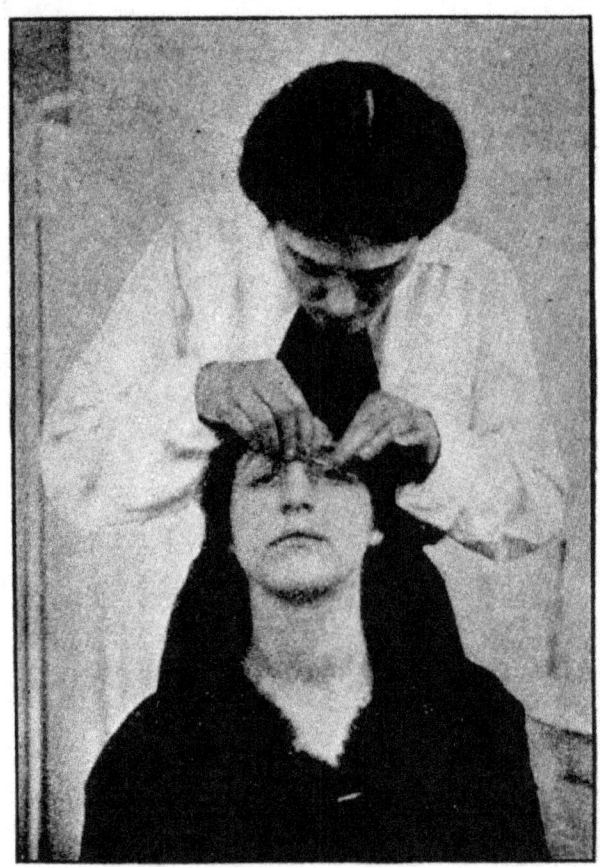

Removing Particles from the Upper Lid.
Second Operation.

for a minute and allow tears to collect. Do not rub the eye. If the object is not removed by tears, draw the upper lid down over the lower carefully. This will generally remove particles on the upper lid. If this does not remove the object, seat the patient with his face to the light and stand behind his chair with head bent back over the chair and with a swab (toothpick wrapped with cotton wet with a mild antiseptic solution) carefully attempt to remove the object, or place a pencil or match on upper part of lid about one-half inch from edge and carefully turn the lid over it and the particle may be dislodged. Wash the eye with boracic acid water.

If glass or steel has become lodged in the ball see a physician at once. The pain and inflammation may be relieved by applications of warm water or rose water.

Nose.—Foreign bodies will not remain long in the nose, for the presence of the body will cause violent sneezing and coughing and thus expel it. Encourage sneezing and blowing from the nostrils which will in most instances dislodge the object. Should the object still remain, consult a physician. Do not probe or pick the nose.

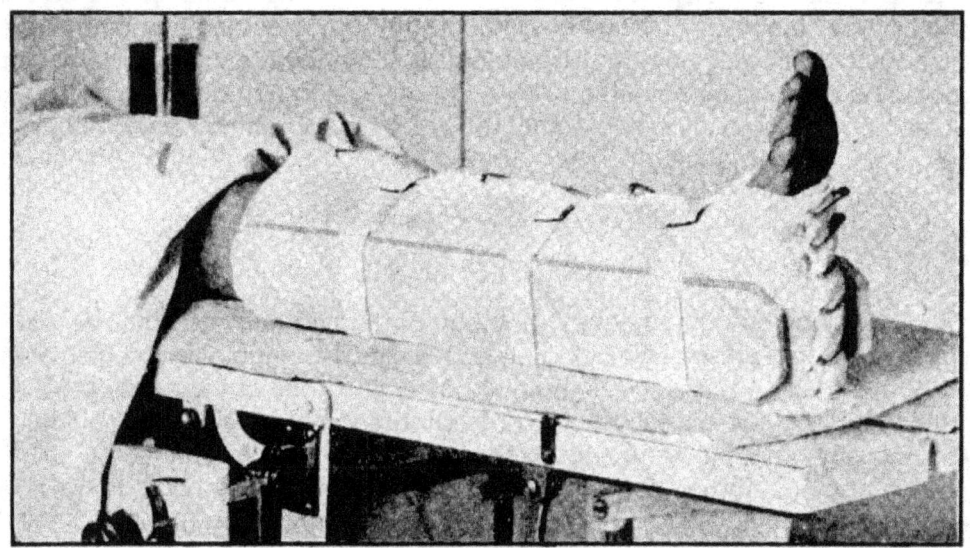

Pillow Splint.

FRACTURES.

Never allow a person with a broken bone to be moved until the part is properly splinted. Any firm object such as a lath, bed slat, stave, or cane will serve as a splint in case of emergency. Permanent splints should be made of soft pine, about four inches wide. The splints should be long enough to confine the joint above and below the seat of fracture and should be broader than the limb itself. Temporary splints may be applied over the clothing, but should always be well padded, as the hard board against the limb is very painful. A pillow strapped firmly about the fracture often makes a satisfactory support.

The fractured member should be dressed by holding the limb in as nearly normal position as possible while a second person applies the support, which may be bound in place by use of cord, rope, or piece of clothing or handkerchief. If the fracture is of the lower limbs, never allow the person to walk even after the dressing has been applied. After the physician or surgeon has properly "set" the fracture the patient usually requires six weeks or more before complete recovery is assured.

FREEZING.

Symptoms.—In those who are frozen the limbs become stiff and the skin white.

First Aid Treatment.

Never take a frozen person into a warm room or apply any warmth. The temperature must be raised gradually. Take patient into a cold room, remove clothing and rub the body carefully with snow or cold water. Later, when the limbs lose some of their rigidity, the hand or a piece of flannel may be used instead of the snow to produce friction. As soon as nourishment can be taken, give hot beef tea or milk. The body should then be protected from further cold but no heat applied. If parts become dark blue or mottled in color, circulation has not been completely restored and there is danger of development of gangrene. For more than a slight and localized frozen condition, a doctor's care and advice must be sought.

FROST BITES.—(See Freezing.)

GAS POISONING.

Great care should be taken in using gas stoves and gas lights—that the wind, or reduced pressure does not extinguish the flame unknown to the occupant of the room. Never sleep in a room with the gas stove or gas jet lighted. The gas may become low and the flame go out, later it may come on with full force and the occupant of the room become asphyxiated.

Symptoms.—When a person has been overcome by gas, the face is of a purplish color, and swollen. The breathing is very difficult and convulsive. Soon unconsciousness and death will follow.

First Aid Treatment.

Do not light a match in the room but throw open the windows. If in a well or any enclosure where gas has escaped, remove the patient immediately. If any hope of life still remains, use artificial respiration at once. The ambulance should be called and the patient removed to the hospital as soon as possible. Let the rescuer be cautious that he, too, does not remain too long in these same surroundings. (See Artificial Respiration.)

GUNSHOT WOUNDS.

Gunshot wounds include all wounds caused by explosion of gunpowder, by rifle and pistol balls, shot shells, etc. The danger resulting from such depends on the structure of the parts involved, the hemorrhages occurring, and the inflammation and infection which may result from parts of clothing being carried into the flesh. Wounds from small shots vary in degree of danger according to the range and velocity of the shot from the place of firing.

Wounds from large shot and shell are characterized by great tearing of the tissues which often proves very serious. Gunshot wounds are accompanied by the usual symptoms of other wounds, as pain, hemorrhage and shock.

First Aid Treatment.

Arrest the hemorrhage from the wound as quickly as possible, and carefully apply a temporary dressing but do not probe the wound. Place the patient in a hospital or under a surgeon's care.

In wounds from small shots simply imbedded in the skin, cleanse the skin and remove the shot with a knife point, which has been thoroughly cleansed by scrubbing or holding in alcohol.

Wounds from toy pistols should be cared for immediately, since in many cases they have proven very dangerous. when neglected, by causing lockjaw. (See Lockjaw or Tetanus.)

Remove all wadding or other foreign matter which might be carried into the tissues, wash thoroughly with peroxide of hydrogen and apply an antiseptic dressing.

HEAT EXHAUSTION.

This is due to excessive heat.

Symptoms.—The symptoms are the same as for shock. The skin is cold and clammy, pulse rapid and weak, breathing feeble. The blood leaves the brain and the surface of the body.

First Aid Treatment.

Remove to a cool place, lower the head, give hot bath or put blankets over the body. Apply heat to feet, rub limbs towards the heart. Give hot drinks.

HEMORRHAGE.

Hemorrhage is due to the escape of blood from its vessels. The hemorrhage is known by the name of the vessel from which it escapes, and can be recognized by the color of the blood and manner of its escape. Hemorrhage is usually caused by wounds or diseased condition of the blood vessels. Arterial hemorrhage is bright red, while hemorrhage from the veins, or venous hemorrhage is dark red, and apt to be less profuse. Hemorrhage from a large artery is one of the most troublesome forms of accident. Presence of mind and promptness are all important, since lack of these may be followed by fatal results. A loss of one-third the amount of blood in the body usually results fatally

Symptoms.—The principal symptoms are sighing, respiration, a growing pallor, cold skin, profuse perspiration, rapid but feeble pulse, darkness before the eyes, roaring in ears, restlessness, and falling temperature. Bleeding is evident except in internal hemorrhage. If hemorrhage is from one of the larger arteries, death may occur in a few minutes.

Nature's Treatment of Hemorrhage.

1. Because of the elastic nature of the walls of the blood vessels when they are cut, they contract and thus diminish the opening

2. Blood tends to coagulate as soon as it comes in contact with air.

3. Because of the weakened condition of the heart, caused by the hemorrhage, the blood is propelled through the vessels with less force.

Principal Points in Treatment.—Therefore the principal points in treatment of hemorrhage are—

1. Keep the patient as quiet as possible since excitement increases the rapidity of the heart's action.

2. Do not use stimulants as they increase the action of the heart.

3. Use pressure to hinder the escape of blood.

4. Elevate the wounded member or place it in some other position which will tend to cut off the blood supply.

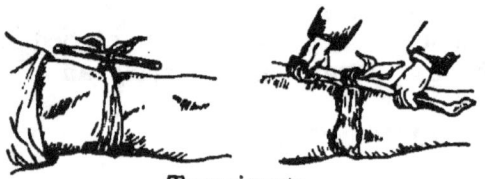 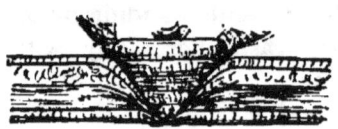

Tourniquets.   Graduated Compress.

5. Use hot or cold applications as they tend to contract the walls of the vessels and coagulate the blood. Styptics such as alum, alcohol and turpentine serve the same purpose, but should only be used when other treatments are impossible since they are apt to infect the wound.

6. Ligation, the tying of the severed parts of the vessels with silk or catgut is a sure and safe method of controlling hemorrhage, but generally the instruments are not at hand, and this should not be tried by an unskilled person.

First Aid Treatment.

Pressure should be applied at once to the wound to stop the hemorrhage.

If the hemorrhage is from an artery, the blood is of a bright red color and comes in spurts. For this kind of hemorrhage, pressure must be applied at some point between the wound and the heart. If the bleeding is from a vein, the blood is a dark red color and comes in a steady stream. For this kind of hemorrhage, pressure must be applied on the side farthest from the heart.

Arterial Hemorrhage.—Be quick. Grasp the limb with the thumbs pressing on the bleeding artery at some point between the wound and the heart, as indicated in the special cases given below. If the location of the artery is not known, tie a rope or handkerchief tightly around the limb above the wound, between the wound and the heart. Then, a clean compress or tourniquet may be made and applied to the wound.

Elevate the injured part.

Keep the patient quiet till the surgeon arrives.

Venous Hemorrhage.—In this form the pressure, by tourniquet or other means must be applied beyond the wound, on the side farthest from the heart because the blood is flowing to the heart. Remove any clothing which might constrict between the wound and heart.

Capillary Hemorrhage.—Apply an ice compress or cloth wrung out of very hot water. The water must be at a high temperature (about 125°), not warm, as warm water stimulates and thus increases the flow of blood.

Hemorrhage from the Scalp and Face may be controlled by pressing the bleeding vessel against the skull till assistance arrives. These are not so hard to control because they are not imbedded in much flesh and can easily be pressed against a bone.

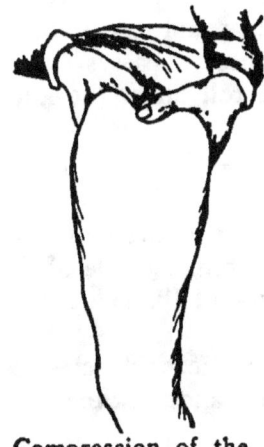
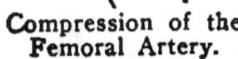

Compression of the Femoral Artery.

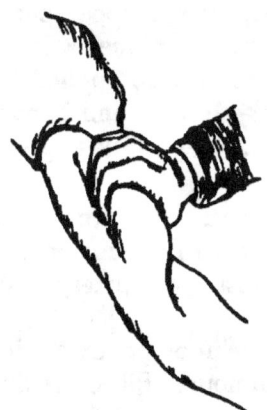

Compression of the Brachial Artery.

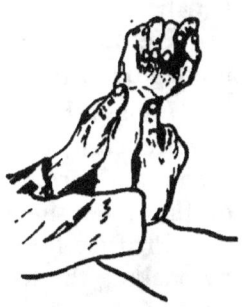

Compression of Arteries at the Wrist.

Hemorrhage from the Nose.—Bleeding of the nose is sometimes just nature's effort to relieve the head or it may be the result of accident. To check the bleeding, place cold applications on the forehead and back of the neck, and press the artery at the root of the nose. Press nostrils between thumb and forefinger.

If bleeding persists, pack the nose well with linen or cotton. If it still persists, call a physician.

Make pressure by placing the thumb in the little hollow of the jaw bone where the pulse can be felt. This affects the blood supply of the nose.

Hemorrhage of the Gum.—If caused by extraction of a tooth, pack the cavity with linen or cotton or apply ice to the cavity.

If this fails saturate a piece of cotton or linen in a solution of alum or strong tea, and pack the cavity.

Hemorrhage from the Neck.—The carotid arteries which supply the neck can readily be felt at either side of the throat. Do not apply a tourniquet to the neck, it will strangle the injured one.

Press the artery between the thumb and spinal column till efficient aid is procured.

Hemorrhage from the Arms.—The artery supplying the arms runs down on the inside of the arm to the center of the bend of the elbow, where it can be easily felt. Apply pressure here, either by fingers or tourniquet.

Hemorrhage from Forearm.—This can best be dealt with by using pressure on the artery of the upper arm, mentioned just above, or by placing a pad in the bend of the elbow and bending the forearm tight against the upper arm.

Hemorrhage from the Hand.—This can be controlled by pressure on the artery in the upper arm as mentioned above, or pressure at the middle of the bend of the elbow, or on both the arteries in the wrist. (See Page 181.)

For bleeding of the palm, place a large, hard compress in the hand and close fingers over it and bandage tightly.

Hemorrhage from the Thigh.—The artery supplying the thigh extends down the inner side of the leg in the upper part of its course and can be compressed either by the fingers or tourniquet. In its lower course it passes to the back of the thigh and pressure may be applied by placing a roll under the knee and bending the leg as far as possible and bandaging it so.

Hemorrhage from the Leg.—Apply a pressure to the artery high up in the leg or at the knee.

Hemorrhage from the Foot.—Bleeding of the upper part of the foot may be checked by pressing the artery of the instep, and bleeding from the sole of the foot may be controlled by pressing the artery just a little back of the ankle bone on the inner side of the limb.

Profuse bleeding from the foot or lower limb has been effectively checked by packing the foot or limb in flour. Place the limb in a vessel and pack the flour around it.

Hemorrhage from Varicose Veins.—Varicose veins may occur in any part of the body, but are usually in the legs. They are due to a weakened condition of the walls of the veins or to the circulation being interfered with.

Elevate the injured part and apply pressure to the wound.

Hemorrhage from the Lungs.—The symptoms of hemorrhage of the lungs are—fits of coughing, and spitting up of frothy bright red blood.

This cannot be controlled by first aid treatment. .All that can be done is to keep the patient in a reclining position and absolutely quiet. Keep ice in the mouth. An ice bag may also be applied to the chest. Do not use stimulants. Call a doctor.

Because blood is expectorated is not always a sign of hemorrhage of the lungs. It may have been swallowed, originally coming from the nose or mouth.

Put the patient to bed and keep him quiet. Give cracked ice, but do not give stimulants or food for some time after bleeding has ceased.

Hemorrhage of the Stomach.—The symptoms of hemorrhage of the stomach are—fullness in the stomach, pain and vomiting of dark clotted blood resembling coffee grounds.

HYSTERIA.

Hysteria is caused by condition of the mind and nervous system, usually affecting women. The attack usually begins with causeless sobbing, screaming or laughing and temporary lack of will power. It sometimes assumes a form similar to epilepsy or apoplexy for which it is sometimes mistaken. However, it can be easily distinguished from epilepsy as there is no grinding of the teeth and biting of the tongue; the patient is conscious, extremities and face are warm, and the patient will resist any attempt to raise the eyelids. All these symptoms being the opposite of epilepsy.

First Aid Treatment.

Sometimes the patient falls, however, usually in a comfortable position. Watch the patient closely, but as a rule, it is best to leave her alone. Do not sympathize with her, as this usually aggravates the case. Sometimes it is advisable, if there is much demonstration, to throw cold water in the face. It is rarely necessary to attempt much treatment. See that the patient is comfortable and leave her entirely alone. Frequent recurrence of attacks denotes need for proper medical care.

INSECT BITES OR STINGS.—(See Bites.)
LOCKJAW.—(See Tetanus—Medical Dept.)
MAD DOG OR CAT BITES.—(See Bites.)
NAIL IN FOOT.—(See Wounds.)
NOSE-BLEED.—(See Hemorrhage.)
POISONS.—(See Drugs and Poisons.)

SHOCK.

Shock is a great depression of the vital organs of the body, usually brought on by injury, surgical operation, or mental shock such as joy, grief, and fright.

Symptoms.—A weak, rapid fluttering pulse; sighing; feeble respiration; temperature normal or a little below; face pale with a pinched look; body cold and clammy; mind dull.

First Aid Treatment.

Remove clothing, keep the patient lying down, absolutely quiet with the head lowered so as to stimulate circulation in the brain. Rub the feet and hands and place hot water bags at sides and extremities. A mustard plaster or hot water bag may be applied over the heart. Rub the limbs upward toward the heart.

Hot tea, coffee or beef tea may be given if it can be retained, or give a stimulating enema of warm coffee or a salt solution.

Send for the doctor.

SNAKE BITES.

The most poisonous snakes in the United States are the rattlesnake, copper head, water moccasin, and the viper. There is also a certain kind of lizard called "Gila Monster" which is poisonous.

First Aid Treatment.

In case of a poisonous snake bite immediate and strenuous action is demanded by all present to save the patient's life. There is no time to wait for help.

The first thing is to extract the poison.

Tie a handkerchief, small piece of rope, or rubber tube above the bite or between the heart and the wound, fo keep the poison from being carried to the rest of the body, by means of the circulation.

Cut open the wound made by the serpent's fangs. Use knife, razor or whatever may be most handy. Cut considerably deeper than the bite so that the wound may bleed freely.

The wound may be cauterized with a hot iron, or with nitric or carbolic acid. Hunters may pour powder into this wound and apply a spark or lay a live coal upon it.

If the patient becomes weak, due to the poisoning, give some stimulant—strong coffee, aromatic spirits of ammonia or anything that will increase the action of the heart. Strychnine, ether and digitalis, hypodermically applied are valuable as stimulants.

Quick action is absolutely necessary in case of poisonous snake bites.

The after care for the wound is the same as for other surgical cases, a physician usually giving the directions.

SPLINTERS.

Seize splinter between the point of a penknife (inserted beneath splinter) and the thumb nail. It is well to apply tincture of iodine to the puncture after removal of splinter.

SPLINTS.—(Red Cross First Aid.)

Splints are used to prevent movement at the point where a bone is broken. They must, therefore, be made of a stiff and rigid material. For first-aid purposes splints must generally be improvised from something which may easily be procured on the spot. Such articles are pieces of wood, broom handles, laths, rules, squares, wire netting, heavy cardboard, umbrellas, canes, pick handles, spades, rolls made of blankets or cloths, pillows alone or with pieces of board outside, rifles, swords and bayonets. With a broken leg it is even possible to use the other leg as a splint.

In improvising splints a few precautions should be observed. Besides being rigid enough to prevent movement at the point where a bone is broken, they should be long enough to prevent movement at the nearest joints, as this will move the broken bone, and they should be as wide as the limb to which they are applied, as otherwise the bandages holding them will press on the limb as well as on the splint and thus cause pain and perhaps displace the ends of the broken bone. On account of the danger from swelling and in order to promote the comfort of the patient and not to rub the skin, splints should be well padded on the inner side with some soft material. The clothing sometimes answers this purpose fairly well when it is not removed. Substances generally used are cotton batting, waste, tow, flannel, pieces of cloth, grass, etc. If splints are not well padded, the limb to which they are applied must be watched with special care because the swelling is likely to make the splints too tight which will cut off the circulation and may cause mortification.

SPRAINS.

A sprain is the result of a severe strain of a joint, and is accompanied by intense pain and swelling. The tendons and ligaments are often badly torn by twisting or wrenching of the joint. A sprain is always troublesome and may result in stiffness of the joint. Proper medical care should be given immediately, as a sprain may prove more serious than a fracture. The wrist and ankle are the joints most often affected.

First Aid Treatment.

Elevate the part.

Ice Bag.—Prevent the further congestion of blood at the injured joint by applying an ice bag or cloths wrung out of cold water.

Hot Applications.—Very hot applications are good to stop the pain.

Alcohol or Salt Water.—After the pain and swelling have subsided, the cold applications may be discontinued, and the application of salt water or alcohol with gentle friction may be substituted.

Soap Liniment.—This will be found good to take out soreness and stiffness.

Massage.—Massage accompanied with slight exercise of the joint will prevent stiffness.

Arnica.—Bathe the parts freely with tincture of arnica.

If the sprain is severe, the parts should be kept quiet for several weeks and then exercise be begun gradually and continued under the direction of a physician.

STINGS.—(See Bites.)

SUFFOCATION.—(See Gas Poison.)

SUNSTROKE OR HEAT STROKE.

Sunstroke is due to long exposure to the direct rays of the sun. Those persons addicted to alcoholic habits are more susceptible than others. However, those in a weakened condition, from any cause, if exercising actively or doing hard, physical labor may be affected.

Symptoms.—At first there is a feeling of weakness, dizziness, and oppression followed by unconsciousness. Breathing is rapid and noisy, pulse weak and irregular; the skin is very hot and dry, the temperature at times reaching 110° or 112°. Death may occur instantly or in a very short time.

First Aid Treatment.

Reduce the temperature as rapidly as possible. Remove the patient to a shady place; remove clothing and rub the body with ice. If this is not to be had, put him in a tub of cold water, at the same time rubbing the body briskly to bring the heated blood to the surface. An enema of cold water may also be given. Continue this till the temperature falls, if there is depression give stimulants.

Heart failure may cause death at any moment, therefore careful watch should be kept over the pulse and if there is a marked drop of temperature, remove the patient from the cold bath and apply heat to the extremities.

TETANUS.—(See Medical Department.)

TOURNIQUETS.

Tourniquets are instruments used to stop bleeding from an artery. Each has a strap to go around the limb, a pad to place on the artery and some means by which the pad may be made to press on the artery and thus stop the flow of blood. In an improvised tourniquet, which is the type most commonly used, the strap may be made of a handkerchief, towel, bandage or cravat, and a smooth round stone, a cork or some object of similar shape and size may be used for the pad. The stone, etc., had best be wrapped in a small piece of cloth so that it will not bruise the skin too much. It is then placed over the artery above the wound and the strap is best passed twice around the limb and ties loosely at its outer side. A stick is introduced between the two layers thus formed and is twisted around until the bleeding is stopped. If desired, another bandage may be used to loop over and to hold the end of the stick from twisting back and so relieving the pressure of the pad on the artery. One layer of bandage may be used for the strap if more is not procurable. In order to avoid bruising in using this it is best after introducing the stick into the loop to twist away from the body. The inner tube of a bicycle tire makes an excellent tourniquet. Its end is used for the pad.

Besides the bruising of the muscles and skin which is certain to occur to some extent with any tourniquet, there is a much graver danger connected with their use. This is due to the fact that in consequence of cutting off the circulation, mortification and death of the part may follow. If a tourniquet has been in place for an hour, therefore, it is desirable to loosen it and to allow it to remain loose if no bleeding occurs. It should not be removed as it may be necessary to tighten it again quickly as possible, for if three or four hours pass with a tourniquet in place, mortification is very liable to follow.

Instead of tourniquets, appliances to make pressure on the whole circumference of a limb and thus to stop bleeding are sometimes employed. The strap which has just been described, without the pad, may be used for this purpose. A special elastic bandage and elastic suspenders have also been recommended. When possible, however, use the tourniquet, as cutting off the whole circulation by pressure on the entire circumference of a limb is much more likely to cause mortification than the tourniquet, which presses to the greatest extent on the artery alone. If circular constriction is used it should not be employed for over an hour.

WOUNDS.

A wound is the severing of the tissues of the body by violence. There are various kinds of wounds, usually named according to their causes, such as: incised wounds, punctured wounds, lacerated or contused wounds, gunshot wounds, etc.

Wounds heal by first intention or by second intention.

First Aid Treatment.

First Intention.—The edges of the wound are brought together and heal rapidly and naturally without granulation or suppuration.

Second Intention.—When the edges are ragged and cannot be brought together, granulations which are soft, bright red elevations, fill up the wound from the bottom and sides.

Proud Flesh.—The granulations which are growths, usually resembling bright red particles, appear in the wound and are called "proud flesh." These particles grow very rapidly and must be removed before the wound can heal naturally. This may be done by applying nitrate of silver, or burnt alum.

Great care must be taken to have everything about a wound thoroughly clean. All bandages and instruments used must be sterilized.

Incised Wounds.—The incised wound is one made with a knife or any sharp instrument which cuts the parts with an even edge. Hemorrhage is more likely to result from the incised wound. (See Hemorrhage.)

Lacerated or Contused Wounds.—These wounds are made by blunt or dull instruments such as stones, clubs, or any object that destroys the tissue. Local inflammation and constitutional trouble is likely to result from this kind of wound. (See Treatment for Lacerated Wound.)

Gunshot Wounds.—Gunshot wounds are made by bullets, cannon balls, pieces of stone, iron or wood which penetrate the body. Internal hemorrhage or blood poisoning frequently result from gunshot wound. (See Treatment for Gunshot Wounds).

Aseptic Wounds.—These are wounds which are free from bacteria, and are not liable to any poisonous infection.

Septic or Poisonous Wounds.—These are wounds which have been infected by bacteria. This may have gained entrance at the time of the injury or during the treatment.

PUNCTURED WOUNDS.—(See Tetanus.)

A punctured wound is one made by some sharp instrument such as, nails, pins, splinters, slivers, arrows, daggers, bullets and all similar objects or instruments. They are the most dangerous of wounds as they often penetrate the tissues deeply and carry poisonous matter with them which is often difficult to remove.

First Aid Treatment.

In case a wound is made by bullets or dagger, a surgeon should be summoned at once, or the patient taken to a hospital. The object or instrument may have penetrated a vital organ of the body or severed an artery in which case the wound may result fatally very soon.

In all cases of punctured wounds, regardless of how trivial, the first thing to be done in the way of treatment after the object causing the injury has been removed, is to remove all poisonous or foreign matter which may have been left in the wound. This may be largely accomplished by causing the wound to bleed freely.

Never probe a wound, if it has been caused by a bullet or an object which cannot easily be removed, a good surgeon should do the probing.

NAIL IN FOOT.

Allow to bleed freely but do not squeeze the part or walk unnecessarily as it may tend to hasten absorption of infected material, if present.

Apply tincture of iodine into the wound and bandage gauze in place.

INFECTION OF WOUNDS.

Germs are practically everywhere, on hands, chairs, tables, etc. However, the air is practically germ-free. Never touch a wound with your fingers. Do not touch any part of sterile gauze directly over the wound, even if the hands have been sterilized. Exposure to air is better than an unclean dressing.

Before dressing wounds, scrub the hands (particularly the nails) with soap and water for several minutes, using a hand brush, then soak the hands in 1 : 5000 solution of bichloride of mercury for a few minutes. If in a hurry, one can cleanse the hands and nails with cotton soaked in alcohol.

These precautions are, of course, impossible in severe hemorrhage.

NURSING AND FIRST AID TREATMENT OF SPECIAL DISEASES.

ABSCESS.

DESCRIPTION.—An abscess is a collection of pus in a cavity, the result of inflammation. External abscesses are noticed by swelling, throbbing and pain. When they occur internally they are not readily recognized except by a physician, and if there is any reason to believe an internal abscess exists a physician should be consulted at once.

NURSING.—When the pus has formed in the external abscess and it feels soft to touch, it should be opened. The surface should be washed with hot water and pure soap and then with an antiseptic solution, such as alcohol, listerine or boric acid solution.

The knife or instrument used should be sterilized and the hands perfectly clean. The pus should be removed by pressing gently on the sides but do not use much pressure. The opening should be dressed with sterilized gauze to keep the abscess open and to allow the pus to drain. The dressing should be changed twice a week and the opening kept clean with an antiseptic wash, such as one pint of boiled water to which one teaspoonful of carbolic acid, 5 percent solution, is added, this being applied with absorbent cotton. Severe cases must be attended by a physician.

Catarrh may lead to the formation of an abscess in a cavity of the mastoid process, which is a prominent bone just behind the middle ear. An abscess in this region of the head may become very serious, as it is so near the brain and should be cared for by a physician.

An abscess near the surface may be poulticed with flaxseed meal or bread and milk. Never poultice an abscess after it has been opened.

Take a good blood purifier and keep the bowels regular. Seek the cause of all abscess and take measures to remove.

ADENOIDS.

DESCRIPTION.—Adenoids are soft, glandular, whitish masses which grow in the back of the mouth, near the posterior opening of the nostrils, partially closing the air passages. Children having adenoids breathe almost entirely through the mouth, and breathe noisily when they eat and drink. They sleep with the mouth open, snore, have night terrors, toss about and moan. During the colder months of the year, they are troubled almost constantly with colds in the head, coughs and recurring attacks of bronchitis. When the adenoids are very large, the child breathes almost entirely through the mouth, the lower jaw drops and the mouth is open constantly. The face has a vacant and stupid expression, the nose is pinched and narrow, and when it occurs in young children the palate is often high-arched. If this state continues, the palate becomes more pointed at the top causing the upper jaw to elongate, the teeth to be crowded and the front teeth to project far beyond the lower jaw. The speech is also affected, the child not being able to articulate plainly, and often the Eustachian tube is closed causing inflammation of the ears and sometimes deafness. Adenoids predispose to diphtheria and tuberculosis and are the direct causes of the mouth-breathing habit, imperfect speech, nervousness, stunted growth and backwardness.

An operation is frequently advisable, the child usually convalescing rapidly. See that it gets plenty of good food and fresh air.

APPENDICITIS.

DESCRIPTION.—This is an inflammation of the vermiform appendix which is a small tube about 3½ inches in length, situated at the lower back part of that part of the large bowel called the caecum. The inflammation is liable to occur at any age, however, it is more common between the ages of twenty and thirty. Men are more liable to an attack than women. People who take violent exercise or lift heavy weights are also more subject to the disease. The tendency may also be inherited. Indiscretions in diet, constipation, inflammation of surrounding organs may bring it on. It is also due sometimes to the presence in the appendix of foreign bodies such as grape, orange, lemon, or melon seeds, or concretions of fecal matter from the intestines. It may also develop from typhoid fever or tuberculosis.

SYMPTOMS.—An attack of appendicitis generally commences with a sudden onset of pain in the abdomen which is often very severe. It comes on without previous warning and often appears to be all over the abdomen, however, it soon becomes localized to the region of the appendix, which is situated about half way between the navel and the point of the hip-bone on the right side of the body. In a short time the pain is followed by nausea and vomiting, rigidity of the muscles on the right side of the abdomen, rise in temperature and tenderness over the region of the appendix. The pain may be mistaken for colic, renal colic or the pain of indigestion. Where the vomiting continues and especially if the vomited matter looks like coffee grounds, the case is very unfavorable as this is evidence of general septic infection.

NURSING.—This might be divided into expectant and operative. The expectant treatment consists in keeping the patient in bed on a strictly liquid or milk diet and watching the course of events. To relieve the pain, apply hot fomentations to the abdomen such as turpentine or mustard fomentations or poultices. However, the application of an ice-bag to the affected part is preferable as it not only relieves the pain but leaves the skin and superficial parts in good condition, should an operation afterwards be necessary. Hot fomentations or poultices often blister the skin or make it raw and thus very hard to cleanse and prepare for the operation. Purgatives should not be given, as they cause much harm in the early stages of the disease. The bowels may be moved by means of a soapsuds or oil enema gently and carefully given. If the case does not improve by the end of 48 hours, that is, if the vomiting continues, the temperature remaining high or continuing to rise, the muscles becoming more rigid and the pulse rate 120 or over, the matter of an operation should be seriously considered. In case an operation is decided upon, it should be done by an experienced, reliable surgeon in a good hospital.

Persons having a tendency to appendicitis or who have had one attack can do much to prevent a recurrent attack by careful attention to diet, regular habits, personal hygiene, especially avoiding constipation, hearty meals at night, indigestible foods, over exertion, exposure to cold, etc. However, although the greatest care is taken, attacks will recur. In these cases nothing but an operation will bring relief. A person who has had several attacks better have the offending organ removed.

First Aid and Home Treatment.

If the pain is severe a physician should be sent for. In the meantime relieve the patient as much as possible.

The patient should be put to bed and kept quiet. The bowels should be moved by giving an injection of hot water and soapsuds.

Epsom Salts.—To move the bowels give a tablespoonful of Epsom Salts dissolved in hot water.

Cold Compress.—Cloths wrung out of cold water and applied to the painful part will give relief.

Ice Bag.—An ice bag may be used to reduce the pain but a piece of flannel should be placed next to the skin.

Hot Compress.—Wring a piece of flannel out of hot water and apply to the affected part.

ASTHMA.

DESCRIPTION.—This term is applied to recurrent paroxysms of difficult breathing accompanied by a sense of suffocation. It very often develops from what appears to be an ordinary catarrh, the paroxysm of difficult breathing usually coming on during the night and lasting a few or many hours. The first attack may come after a prolonged attack of bronchitis, or an after-effect of measles, whooping-cough or some other ailment. It also very often springs from the catarrhal condition connected with hay fever. It is generally chronic and not dangerous till other complications follow. It usually begins in the young and affects men more often than women.

SYMPTOMS.—The attack generally comes on suddenly at night. The patient may wake up and find himself wheezing and hardly able to get his breath. In severe cases there is an expression of terror on the face, the hands and feet are cold, pulse small and quick. This may last for a few hours or for days.

NURSING.—The main treatment for this disease lies in preventive measures. Remove the conditions which cause the attack. A person with this tendency should be free from excitement as this invariably makes the disease worse. Careful attention should be given to the mucous membranes of the nose and bronchial tubes, and any abnormal condition of these remedied. Conditions which may bring on colds, catarrh, bronchitis, or any affection of the air passages should be carefully avoided. Also avoid the inhalation of such irritating substances as dust, smoke, pollen of grass, etc. It is also made worse by the patient being around animals or certain plants.

The climate also has a great deal to do with the disease, however there is no especially suitable place. Each patient must select the best climate for his individual case by trial. Some like the sea air, some a high dry climate, etc.

The application of heat over the heart and lungs, hot footbaths, hot drinks, inhalations of steam, the inhalation of the fumes of the vapo-cresolene lamp, etc., will all give relief during an attack. The diet should also be carefully attended to, the bowels kept open and the general health built up.

First Aid and Home Treatment.

Saltpeter.—Saturate blotting paper with a strong solution of saltpeter, then dry this and burn, letting the patient inhale the smoke. This will relieve and shorten the attack.

Lobelia.—Make a tea out of the leaves, one ounce of leaves to one pint of water and give one teaspoonful every fifteen minutes until it causes free discharge of mucus.

Mineral Water and Lemon Juice.—Give a glassful of mineral water to which has been added one tablespoonful of lemon juice. This may be given three times a day.

BILIOUSNESS.

DESCRIPTION.—This is the common name for congestion of the liver. Too much bile is secreted by the liver and too little expelled from the bowels. One of the main causes is alcoholic excess. It is also due to indigestion and constipation, overeating, and may be caused by taking cold.

SYMPTOMS.—As a rule the liver is swollen and tender to the touch, there is pain in the right side, the skin and white of the eyes may have a yellowish appearance. The tongue is coated, there is a bitter taste in the mouth, headache, (nausea) accompanied by vomiting, highly colored urine, loss of appetite, etc.

NURSING.—The patient should be given a good cathartic and a dose of calomel given at night, followed in the morning by a saline purgative, such as rochelle salts. Drink a glass of hot water with a little lemon juice added before breakfast. The diet should be very light, in fact it is well to give the stomach a rest for at least a day. Take plenty of exercise in the open.

First Aid and Home Treatment.

Salts.—If there is a tendency to constipation, keep the bowels active by means of a good cathartic, such as Seidlitz powder or Epsom salts.

Dandelion.—A strong tea made from the roots of dandelion and taken several times a day is very good for biliousness. Hot fomentations over the liver are beneficial.

Lemon.—The juice of a lemon in hot or cold water is helpful.

Blue Flag, Golden Seal and Simple Elixir.—Fluid extract of blue flag one ounce, golden seal one ounce, and simple elixir two ounces. Take a dessert-spoonful in one-half glass of hot water before meals.

Camomile.—Make a tea of camomile one-half ounce to a pint of boiling water.

INFLAMMATION OF THE BLADDER.

Inflammation of the bladder or acute cystitis is accompanied by severe pain in the region of the bladder, frequent and painful urination with a feeling of scalding, urine is highly colored, hot, contains blood particles and looks ropy. Chronic inflammation of the bladder has practically the same symptoms as the acute, but is accompanied by less pain.

Tuberculosis is frequently a cause of cystitis. It may result from taking cold, from local irritation caused by the formation of gall stones or from the urine containing too much acid. It may also be caused by inflammation extending to the bladder from other diseased organs. Cancers and tumors are also causes.

NURSING.—The patient should be put to bed and hot applications applied over the bladder to ease the pain. Give plenty of mild drinks and water. The patient should also be given a good cathartic as this will not only open the bowels but act on the kidneys and bladder. Quiet and rest are very necessary. The bladder may also be washed out, however, this should be done by the physician.

Teas.—Make tea out of corn silks, pumpkin seeds, watermelon seeds, flax-seeds, etc., as these are very mild and have a soothing effect on the bladder. Hop tea is also very good.

Smartweed.—A hot fomentation of smartweed applied to the abdomen will be found very beneficial in allaying the pain and inflammation.

If the disease is chronic, alcoholic liquors and all vegetables such as asparagus and those containing salts, should be forbidden.

BOILS.

DESCRIPTION.—A boil is a painful inflammatory swelling which is imdiately under the skin. They were formally believed to be due to impurities in the blood. The system was thought to be throwing off poisons in this way. However, it is now known that they are due to infection from without, entering the skin through breaks such as scratches, slight wounds, etc. Therefore it will do little good to use blood purifier to treat the boil directly. As a rule a "run-down" or debilitated system is a predisposing cause and any general treatment which will build up the system will lessen the number of boils. They usually appear on the back of the neck, wrist or on the back of the hands, and are due to the parts being scratched with dirty finger nails or otherwise irritated. Irritation produced by worn collars often causes them on the neck.

NURSING.—Of course in this disease prevention is the thing and any break in the skin should be bathed with an antiseptic solution, such as witch hazel or alcohol, or dusted with antiseptic toilet powders. A good prevention is clean blood.

First Aid and Home Treatment.

Alcohol or Camphor.—Alcohol or camphor applied early will usually prevent them from developing.

Vinegar.—This is very good to use as a wash in the very beginning.

Hot Water.—Hot water will relieve suppuration. Some physicians do not advise the use of poultices at all, however if one desires to do so the following are good:

Mutton Tallow, Yoke of Egg and Salt.—Mix mutton tallow one tablespoonful, one yolk of egg and one teaspoonful of salt. Apply and repeat the second night if necessary.

Flaxseed.—Flaxseed meal makes a good poultice for boils. As a rule the boil finally ruptures without lancing. Pus will be discharged and a "core" of dead tissue will come away. When it breaks, or is opened, it must be thoroughly cleansed with antiseptics and dressing applied.

BRIGHT'S DISEASE.

Bright's disease is a term including many kinds of kidney trouble. It is an inflammation of the kidneys and is a very serious disease. However, it may not be fatal since there is no organ in the body more responsive to change from bad habits to good as the kidneys.

The young and men in the prime of life are more often afflicted with the disease.

Bright's disease is influenced more than any other disease by habits of eating and by life generally. Many men earn this disease by improper habits, some get it through poisoning by lead, alcohol or other poisons, some by infections with rheumatism or vernal disease. Overeating is a cause, eating too many eggs and especially too lean meat. The habit gradually wears out the kidneys. Scarlet fever, rheumatism, pregnancy, cold and diphtheria are also causes.

SYMPTOMS.—The most important symptoms are albumen and casts in the urine. The urine is passed frequently but the quantity diminishes. The complexion is waxy and yellow, the eyes and feet become swollen and puffed. Chills, headache, dizziness, light urination, stomach and bowel disturbance, rapid pulse, paleness and puffiness of the eyelids, and a peculiar acting heart, are important symptoms.

NURSING.—A great number of people who have this disease may live to an old age if they will follow proper eating and rest habits strictly, and live a quiet normal life. Milk, bread, vegetables and fruits should form the main part of the diet. A certain amount of protein is necessary, but it should be very small. Temperance in eating, drinking just water as a beverage, proper exercise and sleeping habits, care of the skin and bowels are all important in the disease.

Buttermilk or skimmed milk as a diet is often advised. One should begin the milk diet slowly and increase until nothing else is used. Hot air baths given under the bed covers have helped some people. Drugs are of little value, build up the patient in every way possible with good care, proper diet and rest. The patient should be under the care of a physician.

BRONCHITIS.

DESCRIPTION.—Bronchitis is an inflammation of the bronchial tubes or air passages, generally caused by taking cold. It may also develop as a complication of an infectious disease such as whooping cough, measles, grippe, etc. There are three forms of the disease, simple or acute, capillary and chronic.

SYMPTOMS.—Simple or acute bronchitis is practically the same as a cold in the chest. It affects the large and medium sized bronchial tubes and is characterized by hoarseness, cough, soreness and tightness about the chest. It is usually ushered in by chilliness, general discomfort and some fever. The cough is generally worse in the morning or after sleep and there is usually a great deal of expectoration. At first the cough is dry and the expectoration scanty and viscid, there being much pain and soreness beneath the breast-bone. Later the cough becomes looser, less painful and the expectoration more abundant.

(Capillary Bronchitis or Bronchial Pneumonia usually develops from the simple form and is an inflammation of the capillaries or small air passages. It is often difficult to tell just when it develops from the simple form, and is usually ushered in by a sharp chill.)

See Pneumonia, page 242.

Chronic Bronchitis is a chronic inflammation of the bronchial tubes generally brought on by repeated attacks of the acute form. It is more prevalent among old people and usually more severe in winter.

NURSING.—The care and treatment for this disease should be practically the same as that of a severe cold. The patient should be given a hot mustard foot-bath and put to bed. Hot water bottles or hot irons should be placed about him and he should be given a pint of hot lemonade or some ginger tea, causing him to perspire freely. The greatest of care should be taken to prevent him from taking additional cold. He must be protected from all draughts, although the room should be well ventilated as is the case in all diseases of the lungs. The pack should be given according to instructions given in the Nursing Department.

It is often well to apply poultices of onions to the back and chest, mustard plasters or paste may also be used. These aid in relieving the congestion. Steam inhalations are also good. Keep the bowels open and give light diet. The room should be well ventilated and the temperature kept at about 70 degrees. This disease may develop quickly into Broncho-Pneumonia which is very dangerous, so the patient should have the best of care and nursing.

First Aid and Home Treatment.

Lard, Camphor and Soda.—Cream together some lard and camphor gum, spread on a cloth and sprinkle with soda. Spread on the chest to relieve inflammation and tightness. Or rub the chest with camphorated oil.

Castor Oil or Onion Syrup.—When the phlegm becomes loose, give a dose of castor oil, onion syrup or some other good cathartic to carry off the phlegm, as children especially swallow some of it and it is poisonous to the system.

Codfish Oil.—One teaspoonful of codfish oil given three or four times a day with a small dose of glycerine will produce a good effect.

Hot Teas.—Give plenty of hot teas to drink.

Garlic or Mustard.—A garlic poultice or mustard plaster on the chest is good.

Hops and Vinegar.—Bathing the chest and throat with a solution made from hops and vinegar is effective.

Stramonium Leaves.—Inhale the steam from stramonium leaves steeped in hot water.

BUNIONS.

A bunion is an enlargement and inflammation of a small membraneous sac, usually occurring on the first joint of the great toe, caused generally by pressure, short, narrow-toed shoes, or sometimes by freezing. Bunions are generally incurable, but may be greatly relieved by treatment.

First Aid and Home Treatment.

Hot Water.—Let water as hot as you can stand, drop from as great a distance as possible, directly on the bunion for some time. This will greatly relieve the congested condition.

Salicylic Acid and Lard.—Mix one-half teaspoonful of salicylic acid to one tablespoonful of lard. Apply daily.

Smartweed.—Make a poultice of smartweed, and bandage the joint.

Iodine.—Paint the joint with tincture of iodine. Buy a properly fitted shoe.

CANCER.

DESCRIPTION.—Cancer is an animal spore or seed cell, capable of taking root and multiplying its kind in any favorable soil such as the epithelium of the secreting glands where cancer more often occurs. It is one of the most malignant forms of abnormal cell growths and usually occurs in the following parts of the body: the face, mouth, lips, nose, liver, stomach, uterus and ovaries.

Statistics prove that cancer is neither contagious nor hereditary, but that this very fatal disease is caused by irritation of some gland in a part of the body where resistance is not sufficient. The blood containing a great amount of impurity is congested in regions of the body of least resistance. It may be cured if taken in its first form.

SYMPTOMS.—An internal form of cancer may not be evident except by loss of appetite and weight. At first there are stinging, darting pains at intervals, then as the growth develops, the pain becomes more constant. In case of a surface cancer as on the face, a small hard lump is felt which bleeds easily and does not heal.

The first noticeable symptom of cancer of the breast is inflammation extending to the skin, giving it a puckered appearance. The skin appears dark and congested usually about the nipple.

Cancer of the stomach or any internal organ is very difficult to detect in its early stages. At the first appearance of continuous indigestion or food remaining in the stomach causing fermentation, consult a competent physician. Loss of weight and dull pain in the stomach are probably the first evident symptoms.

Cancer of the uterus often occurs at the change of life which comes about the age of forty or forty-four, though it may occur before that time. This change is seldom accompanied or preceded by excessive flow, discharge, or pain, but comes gradually. This is the period during which cancer is more apt to become evident. The first symptoms of cancer of the uterus are: profuse flowing, maybe only a few days more than usual, whites or leucorrhea at this time if not occurring before, spotting after bowel movement, pain in the region of the side, back or uterus. Loss of weight.

If any of these symptoms are noticed, a skilled physician should be consulted and a thorough examination made. Since cancer is a local disease, if taken in time, during its early stages, it can be cured.

CARBUNCLE.

DESCRIPTION.—A carbuncle is a severe inflammation of the skin and the adjoining tissues. It is larger than a boil and very painful, having several openings which are characteristic of it. These generally come together and a large core of dead tissue called a "slough" may come away.

Carbuncles more often appear on the back of the neck and on the back but may come on any part of the body. A large carbuncle is very painful and is often so exhaustive that the patient is frequently kept in bed several weeks.

First Aid and Home Treatment.

An incision should be made by a physician, and great care taken to keep the part clean by antiseptic washes. Particular attention must be paid to the diet, as carbuncles are a sign of a weakened constitution.

Flaxseed Meal or Linseed Meal.—Make a poultice of flaxseed meal or linseed meal and apply to the carbuncle.

Slippery Elm.—Poultice with slippery elm bark.

Bread and Milk.—Make a poultice of bread and milk and apply.

Lemons, Cream of Tartar and Sulphur.—Take the juice of two lemons, one-half ounce cream of tartar and one-half ounce pulverized sulphur. Mix and pour boiling water over mixture and stir thoroughly. Take a wineglassful every morning.

CATARRH.

Catarrh is an inflammation of the mucous membrane caused by irritation due to dust, acid vapors, hot or cold air, etc. Sometimes the secretions are thin and watery and sometimes thick and sticky. Secretions are often discharged into the throat and cause frequent expectoration.

First Aid and Home Treatment.

Camphor, Olive Oil and Ginger.—Dissolve as much camphor gum as possible in one-half ounce of olive oil and with this moisten a little ginger. Snuff this up the nostrils and into the head. Camphor contracts the swollen membrane and the oil is soothing.

Salt Water.—Make a solution of one teaspoonful of salt and a cupful of warm water and snuff up the nostrils every morning. It loosens the secretions and cleanses the nose.

Mullein Leaves.—Smoke dried mullein leaves. Spray the nose and throat. with salt water several times a day.

Borax.—Syringe the nose with two teaspoonfuls of powdered borax dissolved in one quart of warm water.

BRONCHIAL CATARRH.

This is inflammation affecting larynx, trachea, and larger bronchial tubes, sometimes commencing with nasal catarrh and working downward to the chest. The causes are: chilling a part of the skin, or a change of temperature caused by sitting in a draught with damp clothes on, or with wet feet, or while perspiring freely.

NURSING.—Prevent its occurrence if possible, but if you have already contracted a cough, bring on a good sweat by bathing the feet in a hot mustard bath before retiring. Wrap the throat in flannel and stay well covered at night.

GASTRIC CATARRH.

Catarrh of the stomach without fever is perhaps the commonest derangement among children. Bottle babies are often affected because undigested and fermenting milk, passing continually along the bowels, causes catarrh. This brings on repeated attacks of vomiting and diarrhea. The child is restless and uncomfortable. Change of food, less food, or greater care of food are necessary.

In childhood, a gastric or intestinal disorder is a familiar consequence of exposure to changes in temperature. The cause sometimes is damp feet or insufficient clothing. Flannel should be worn. Children suffering with rickets, or scrofulous children are especially susceptible to catarrh. As in an infant, so in older children, the kind of food is very important. Excess of rich sauces, starches, fruits or sweets should be avoided. Foods should consist of freshly made broths with dry toast. When milk is given it should be mixed with one fourth as much limewater.

CHAPPING.

Carelessness in rinsing and drying the hands and face is generally the cause of chapping, especially is this the case with tender skin. This may easily be prevented by thoroughly drying the hands and face each time after washing, especially during the cold weather and before going out in the wind. If the hands become chapped, the following simple treatments will be found to be all that is necessary in the way of treatment.

First Aid and Home Treatment.

Soak the hands in hot soapy water for ten or fifteen minutes, rinse well and rub with camphor ice, cold cream or vaseline.

Bay Rum, Glycerine, Pond's Extract.—After washing, rub with equal parts of bay rum, glycerine, and Pond's Extract.

Cold Cream.—Wash the face with hot water and castile soap, rinse, pat dry with a soft towel, and rub cold cream well into the pores.

For Lips.

Ointment.—Make an ointment of two ounces of fresh lard, the yolk of one egg, two teaspoonfuls of honey, rose water, and oat meal or almond flower.

Camphor or Cold Cream.—Apply camphor ice or cold cream night and morning.

Adhesive Tape.—After drying carefully, put a small piece of adhesive tape over the crack, drawing it well together. Leave on over night.

A Wash.—Soak one ounce of quince seeds in one quart of rain water over night, add two ounces of rose water, two ounces of glycerine, one ounce of alcohol, three drops of carbolic acid, the juice of three lemons from which the seeds have been removed. This solution will keep for a long time. Apply often.

Glycerine and Witch Hazel.—Equal parts of glycerine and witch hazel may be used.

Honey or Almond Oil.—Diluted honey or almond oil is good.

Carbolated Vaseline.—Use a good vaseline with a few drops of carbolic acid added.

CHICKEN POX.

DESCRIPTION.—Chicken-pox is a mild, contagious disease very common among children, especially very young children. It is generally contracted through direct exposure. However, it may be carried by means of a third person, and is contagious throughout its course. It occurs but once in the same individual. It is characterized by an eruption of vesicles.

INCUBATION.—As a rule from seven to fourteen days elapse after the exposure before the symptoms develop.

SYMPTOMS.—It usually comes on suddenly with slight fever and general illness the first day. The eruption appears the first or second day on the chest and back first, spreading rather slowly over the body. At first the spots are bright red, later they become vesicles filled with a clear liquid which soon turns to pus. By the end of a day or so they begin to dry, a crust forming over them which soon falls off. This eruption comes out in crops, new spots appearing as the first ones are drying up. Thus at the heighth of the disease, all stages of the eruption may be seen on the same part of the body. This eruption often causes a great deal of itching but should not be scratched, as the vesicles are liable to leave scars.

CHARACTERISTICS.—Certain characteristics distinguish it from other diseases. The disease is liable to be mistaken for small-pox, however, in small-pox eruption does not appear until the third or fourth day, and then appears on the face and forehead first. The vesicles do not form till about the fifth or sixth day, and do not come in crops as in chicken-pox. There is only one stage present at the same time. In small-pox there is often a rash resembling that of measles or scarlet fever at the beginning of the disease.

NURSING.—If there are very small, delicate children in the family, it is well to keep the child suffering with the disease isolated. The patient should not be allowed to return to school till the crusts have wholly disappeared and the skin is again smooth. If there is much fever, the child should be put to bed and kept on a liquid diet. Keep the bowels open with mild cathartics. Do not allow the child to scratch as this may cause scars, or serious infection.

First Aid and Home Treatment.

Very little treatment is needed.

Lard, Vaseline, Cocoa Butter.—To allay the irritation and stop the itching, apply fresh lard, carbolized vaseline or cocoa butter to the spots.

Flour, Corn Starch, Talcum Powder.—It is well to dust the itching parts with one of these.

Hot Teas.—Give hot teas such as saffron, pennyroyal, sage or catnip, to bring out the eruption.

Warm Sponge Baths.—Warm sponge baths may also be given. Give a daily bath with soda or boric acid in the water.

CHILBLAINS AND FROST BITE.

Chilblains and frost bite are inflammation of the tissues caused by cold. The parts at first become red and tingle, and if further exposed, they become white and dead looking.

First Aid and Home Treatment.

Ice Water.—A cloth wrung out of ice water should be applied or the feet immersed in snow or ice water, until congestion disappears. One troubled with chilblains should keep away from the fire and take hot drinks.

Bathing the feet in cold water in which has been put salt or a little ammonia is good. Dry thoroughly and rub vigorously then dust with talcum.

Oil of Sassafras.—After washing feet thoroughly, rub well with oil of sassafras.

White of Egg.—To the white of one egg add enough flour to make a paste; put this on a cloth and bind on the affected parts, leaving on till dry.

Lemon.—Cut a lemon in two and sprinkle with salt. Rub chilblains with this.

Cat-tails and Lard.—Take the fuzzy parts of cat-tails and mix with fresh lard and apply.

Brine.—Bathe in brine in which beef has been corned. Have the brine quite warm. You can get this at a meat market.

Iodine.—Paint with iodine. Put on one coat and after it drys apply another.

COLDS.

A cold is an inflamed condition of the air-passages due to infection received from without. It is an indication of improper living and of a weakened condition of the body. The strong, healthy, well kept body is practically immune to colds.

Study carefully and put into practice the simple suggestions on how to prevent colds as given in the "How To Keep Well" department.

First Aid and Home Treatment.

If a cold has been contracted, or if one has reason to believe he is taking cold, a good cathartic should be taken at once to clean out the system. This is best taken at night so as to act the first thing in the morning. Any simple cathartic may be used such as, calomel for adults or castor-oil for children. It should be followed in the morning by a Seidlitz powder or a mineral water to prevent the cathartic remaining in the system.

Sweating.—One of the best means of breaking up a cold right at the start, is to take a good sweat. Take a good hot mustard foot-bath, lasting one half hour, adding more hot water as it cools. Go to bed and cover up warm with hot water bottles, hot irons or bricks around the body and at the feet. When free perspiration has started, drink a pint of hot lemonade. This will cause profuse sweating, thus opening all the pores of the body and relieving congestion. The sweat should last an hour or an hour and a half, after which the irons and extra covers may be gradually removed. The patient should then be given a good rub-down under the covers and a dry gown put on, the greatest care being taken to prevent catching cold. This is very effective in breaking up a cold if taken in time and done carefully.

Camphorated Oil.—Neck, chest and nostrils may be rubbed with camphorated oil.

Camphor, Lard, Turpentine and Kerosene.—Saturate a piece of flannel with the mixture and apply to the chest and throat. Use one part each of spirits of camphor and turpentine and two parts of lard and kerosene.

Onion Poultice.—Onions fried in lard and applied to the chest, will draw congestion from the lungs.

Onion Syrup.—Slice an onion, cover with sugar and allow to stand until juice forms, or add a little water and simmer on the stove. Give freely.

Hot Roasted Onion.—Eat a hot roasted onion before going to bed.

Quinine.—Five or six grains of quinine taken before going to bed and again in the morning is very good in the beginning of cold.

Brisk Purge.—A brisk purge is advisable.

Hot Mustard Foot Bath.—Hot mustard foot bath one half hour will draw the fever down from the head and promote free perspiration. Also take hot lemonade or flaxseed tea; one-half ounce of whole flaxseed to one pint of boiling water. Flavor with lemon juice or licorice root. In the morning sponge the throat, chest and arms with cold water and take a glass of mineral water.

Oil of Tar.—Spread oil of tar on the throat well up under the ears and cover with a cloth. Lie down and cover up warm. You will be surprised when you get up. A sure relief.

Hoarhound.—Use one ounce of leaves and one pint of boiling water. Steep and strain. Take freely.

Hoarhound.—Dissolve hoarhound candy in a little boiling water and drink hot.

Marshmallow.—Use two ounces of roots and herbs and one pint water. Boil and strain.

Pennyroyal Tea.—Pennyroyal tea is very good for cold.

Lard, Mustard and Ammonia.—Mix one tablespoonful of lard and just enough dry mustard to make a light yellow salve, adding three drops of ammonia. Spread on the chest and cover with a flannel cloth.

Cold Water.—Drink a pint of cold water immediately before going to bed.

Sage Tea.—Drink hot sage tea. It cures a cold quickly.

Camphor.—A few drops of spirits of camphor on a lump of sugar or in a little water is very beneficial in the beginning.

Ground Mustard.—A small quantity of ground mustard placed in the bottom of the shoes will draw the inflammation away from the head thus relieving the congestion in the head. This will often cure a cold in the head in less than three days' time.

Camphor, Borax and Salt.—One ounce each of camphor, borax and fine salt mixed thoroughly and used as a snuff will greatly relieve a cold in the head. It should be used every three or four hours until the cold is cured.

Baking Soda and Salt.—Take a half teaspoonful each of baking soda and salt, stir well in a cup of lukewarm water. Snuff this through the nose daily to clear out the passages of the nose and head.

Salt and Albolene.—Make a douche of a warm salt solution, alternate this with warm liquid albolene. Snuff up and spray into the nose every three hours.

Restrict Diet.—In all colds the diet should be carefully guarded.

Cathartic.—A good cathartic is one of the first steps to take in the treatment of a cold.

Coal Oil and Gum Camphor.—Mix one pint of coal oil and 10 cents worth of gum camphor. Rub this ointment on chest. This is very good for cold on lungs.

Antiphlogistine.—This is one of the best ointments to apply to the chest and lungs. It is usually convenient to get and keep on hand.

COLIC.

DESCRIPTION.—This is simply pain in the abdomen due to the spasmodic contraction of the muscles of the digestive organs, caused by abnormal conditions. The trouble is generally due to indigestible matter in the intestines which not only excites pain, but through decomposition gives rise to gases which cause painful bloating of the bowels.

Flatulent, Wind Colic or Bilious Colic are practically the same, however, they must be distinguished from other forms of colic or inflammation of the digestive organs, such as inflammation of the bowels, appendicular colic, renal colic, etc. The main distinguishing symptoms are the absence of fever and the fact that pressure over the abdomen relieves the pain in flatulent or wind colic.

SYMPTOMS.—The onset is generally sudden and the pain is of a twisting or writhing nature, remittent or intermittent. That is, it may come on at regular intervals leaving the patient free from pain between these periods, or it may just subside but not entirely cease. It is generally relieved by pressure. The patient generally draws up the limbs and rolls about, the face is pale and drawn, skin cold and moist, the bowels may be felt or heard to be in an agitated state. The temperature is normal, pulse normal or slower, there may or may not be vomiting. Relief comes with the expulsion of the gaseous or other contents of the bowels.

NURSING.—In very severe cases the intense pain will soon cause serious collapse unless relieved. It may be necessary to call a physician in order that a hypodermic injection of morphia may be given, or whiffs of chloroform may quiet the patient. In less severe cases, a hot bath or hot fomentations or poultices applied to the abdomen will give relief. After the pain has been relieved and the patient becomes quiet, the cause of the trouble may be discovered and removed.

First Aid and Home Treatment.

Clear out the bowels by giving an enema. This usually entirely relieves the patient.

Massage.—Massage of the abdomen is good.

Castor Oil or Salts.—Give a dose of castor oil or salts.

Castor Oil, Baking Soda and Peppermint.—Give a dose of castor oil and in a short time ½ teaspoonful baking soda and ½ teaspoonful peppermint in one-half glass of hot water.

Hot Water.—Apply a hot water bottle to the painful part or use cloths wrung out of hot water.

Baking Soda.—Give one teaspoonful in a glass of water.

Olive Oil.—One half teacupful, taken frequently, is very good.

Ginger, Peppermint or Spearmint.—Hot drinks containing ½ teaspoonful of ginger, peppermint or spearmint are beneficial.

Hops and Vinegar.—Apply a poultice of hops and vinegar to the abdomen.

CONJUNCTIVITIS.

(Pink Eye).

DESCRIPTION.—This is an acute catarrhal inflammation of the conjunctiva, which is the mucous membrane covering the external surface of the ball of the eye and the inner surface of the lids. There is a discharge of mucus and pus. It is caused by germ infection and is very contagious.

NURSING.—Keep the eyes clean. Use a boric solution (one tablespoonful of boric acid powder to a pint of hot water) or salt water, and bathe the eyes freely.

Use absorbent cotton to wash the eyes and burn the cotton to prevent the infection spreading. Never use the same piece of cotton for both eyes.

CONSTIPATION.

"Mother of Disease."

DESCRIPTION.—A great many of the ills and troubles, the human body is heir to, may be directly attributed to constipation. The bowels are the main system of sewerage within the body and must be kept open and in good condition in order that the poisonous waste matter may be carried off. If it is not disposed of freely and regularly, it will be absorbed by the tissues and thus poison the system.

One of the main causes is carelessness in answering nature's call to the stool. This may be continued till the bowels become accustomed to the presence of the fecal matter and thus the main incentive to regular movement is lost. It may also be due to sedentary habits or occupations, sluggish circulation, feebleness of the abdominal muscles, etc.

Other causes are obstructions in the bowels themselves, defective nervous mechanism, food too soft and too easily digested, lack of the proper secretions in the lower bowel, the contents of the intestines being too dry, not enough water taken, etc.

NURSING.—Do not use drugs. The vigorous cathartic should only be used as a commencement of the thorough treatment. Of course, in constipation as in other diseases, the main thing is prevention which you will find thoroughly taken up in the "How to Keep Well" Department.

Habit.—Establish 'the habit of going to the stool regularly each day at the same hour. The best time as a rule is soon after a meal, however, the time must be chosen which will be the most convenient for every day. Be regular and punctual in the daily evacuation. This is one of the most important steps either in the prevention or treatment of this trouble. Answer nature's call at once, no difference how slight.

Diet.—Drink plenty of water at all times and especially just before going to bed and the first thing on arising in the morning. It may be taken hot or cold, however, it should be taken freely. A pint of water taken on going to bed and a half hour before breakfast will often be all that is necessary in the treatment of this trouble. Fruits either raw or cooked should be eaten freely. An orange, or grape-fruit eaten before breakfast is good. An apple before going to bed is also good. Figs, prunes, dates, and apricots, should be eaten freely. Vegetables of all kinds, especially those leaving a fibrous residue are good. Foods made of coarse grains, whole wheat, bread, whole meal porridge, well baked breads especially the crusts, oatmeal, graham bread and mush, corn bread, etc., are very healthful. Avoid rich pastries, cakes, new bread, fine meal porridges; also eat sparingly of sweets, nuts, cheese, milk, eggs, meats and such like. Do not drink spirituous liquors, strong coffee and tea, as they are all binding. Above all things suit the diet to the occupation.

A regular systematic massage of the abdomen is very good. Refer to the "How to Keep Well" Department for this and also for the special exercises to relieve and prevent constipation.

All exercises such as horseback riding, rapid walking, swimming, rowing, handball, golf and tennis, use the abdominal muscles and prevent constipation.

First Aid and Home Treatment.

Senna Leaves and Pumpkin Seed.—This is a safe and good purge. Two ounces of senna leaves, twelve pumpkin seeds, boil in two quarts of water one-half hour, strain and add a cup of sugar and boil down to a pint. Flavor with fifteen drops of wintergreen. Give one-half to one teaspoonful every night or as needed. This is recommended by a physician, as being cheap and very good.

Agar.—Some leading physicians advise the use of agar (a Japanese seaweed) which absorbs and holds water like a sponge. This goes through the intestines unused. It increases the residue and retains water in the intestinal tract. Eat a tablespoonful three or four times a day.

Extract of Cascara.—One teaspoonful of cascara in one-half glass of water. Take before going to bed.

Milk of Magnesia.—Take one teaspoonful every morning and evening.

Figs and Senna Leaves.—Take one pound of figs and five cents worth of senna leaves, grind together and take as needed.

Licorice Powder.—One teaspoonful dissolved in a glass of water is fine for constipation.

Senna Leaves.—Make an infusion of senna leaves and take a teacupful before going to bed. The same effect may be obtained by chewing the dry leaves.

COUGHS AND HOARSENESS.

First Aid and Home Treatment.

Lemon Juice and Sugar.—This is excellent for coughs and hoarseness. Cut the end off of a lemon and cover the cut end well with sugar. Suck the juice of this. Allow to remain in throat as long as possible.

Hoarhound.—Either the tea or candy is good for cough.

Marshmallow Tea.—Good for cough.

Oil of Sweet Almonds.—Good for hoarseness and cough.

White Pine Tar and Honey.—Taken every two hours will stop cough.

Licorice Root.—Is soothing to the throat and loosens a cough.

Flaxseed Tea.—A tea made out of flaxseed is very good to stop a cough.

Wild Cherry Bark.—This tea is good for cough.

Molasses and Vinegar for Cough.—Cook together until stringy one pint of molasses and one cup of vinegar. Add a generous pinch of red pepper and a piece of butter about the size of a small egg. This may be taken either hot or cold until the cough is cured.

Lemons.—Take three lemons, slice these and put to boil in one quart of water. Boil until tender, then strain. Put back on fire and add a large cupful of sugar. Boil down to a thick syrup. Dose: one tablespoonful every two or three hours.

Onions for Cough.—Take six medium sized onions, slice and put in a shallow baking dish. Cover with sugar and bake until the onions are done. Add one-fourth cup of water and let drain. Dose: One teaspoonful of juice every hour. This remedy is especially good for children.

Fresh Onions for Cough.—Cut a slice large enough to go into the mouth. Allow the onion to remain in the mouth. The juice going down the throat stops the irritation and thus will stop coughing when nothing else will have any effect.

Flaxseed and Honey.—Take two tablespoonfuls of flaxseed and one pint of water. Steep two hours; strain and add three tablespoonfuls of honey. Dose: a teaspoonful every time the coughing spell comes on.

Cold Baths.—Cold baths seldom fail to cure inveterate coughs.

Bran.—One-half pound of bran; one and one-half quarts of water; boil down to one quart, then add sugar. This makes a soothing and laxative drink for one suffering with sore throat or a cough.

Mullein Leaf Tea.—Two ounces of mullein leaves boiled in water. To this add sugar to suit the taste. This tea soothes and loosens the cough.

A physician should be called in any case of persistent cough, because of the danger of tuberculosis or consumption.

CORNS.

A corn is a thickening of the outer skin at some point, especially on the toes, caused by friction and pressure.

On retiring, wet a large cloth and wrap it around the feet, then wrap with flannel. In the morning scrape with a knife, but do not cut. Repeat for several nights.

Soft corns are relieved by rubbing with lemon and binding some lemon pulp on the corn with a piece of gauze. Soft corns are caused by improper drying and perspiration and are easily removed. After bathing well, in warm water and soap, apply turpentine to corn with a soft linen cloth.

Cover corns and callous places with finely shaven soap, every night for a week. Bandage with a clean cloth or carefully draw on clean white stockings. This will soon remove corns.

CROUP—SPASMODIC.

DESCRIPTION.—Croup consists in a spasm of the muscles of the glottis, or the top of the windpipe, following a catarrhal condition of the larynx. It usually affects small children from 6 months to 3 or 4 years of age, and is accompanied by a crowing or croupy cough and hard breathing. It is the result of irritation caused by teething, enlarged tonsils, adenoids, undue exposure to cold indigestion or constipation. A child often inherits a tendency to croup, and any one of the above causes is likely to bring it on. One attack makes a child more susceptible to another attack. Often a child has croup two or three nights in succession, then may not have another attack for a long time. Some children have attacks regularly every few weeks.

SYMPTOMS.—Although the real attack comes on suddenly and usually at night, it is often preceded during the day by a slight cold and hoarseness, becoming worse toward evening. Near midnight the child may wake up suddenly with a loud barking, metallic cough, anxious face, much difficulty in breathing, pulse rapid and with slight fever. If the attack is severe he will often sit up in his crib and struggle for breath till almost exhausted, the lips and tips of the fingers often becoming blue. Sometimes it is very alarming and the mother who has witnessed one attack will very readily recognize the symptoms the second time. Often the attack is not preceded by symptoms during the day, the child playing around apparently very well, the attack coming on suddenly late at night.

NURSING.—This form of croup very seldom proves fatal, therefore the mother should control herself or she may frighten the child and make him worse.

Produce vomiting by giving the child luke-warm water with a pinch of salt or mustard in it. This will throw off the mucus and make breathing easier.

The spasm of the larynx can often be relaxed by wringing flannels out of hot water and applying them to the throat as hot as can be borne without burning the skin. These should be changed just as soon as they begin to get cold. Many physicians apply the cold compress to the neck. This consists of a flannel wrung out of cold water and applied to the throat then covered with a dry flannel.

Give cathartic to keep the bowels active.

First Aid and Home Treatment.

Wine of Ipecac.—Give the child at once a teaspoonful of wine of ipecac or syrup of ipecac. Repeat dose every ten minutes until he vomits.

Powdered Alum and Honey.—Powdered alum one-half teaspoonful mixed with honey or molasses, given every one-half hour until vomiting occurs, is a good remedy.

Inhalations.—Inhalations from a croup kettle are very beneficial.

Hot and Cold Compresses.—Use hot compresses or flaxseed poultices alternating with ice cold compresses applied to the throat.

Slaking Lime.—Breathe vapor from slaking lime.

Oil.—Application of warm oil or lard over the neck and upper part of the chest is beneficial.

Turpentine and Oil.—Use spirits of turpentine combined with either sweet oil, goose oil, lard or cocoanut oil (two teaspoonfuls of turpentine to ten teaspoonfuls of whichever oil is used). A woolen cloth saturated with this and placed over the throat, with several layers of cloth dipped in hot water and wrung dry and placed over it, will be found very helpful.

Onion Poultice.—Apply onion poultice, consisting of onions fried in lard and applied to the throat as warm as possible.

Hops and Vinegar.—A poultice of hops and vinegar applied hot to the throat is very beneficial.

DIABETES.

DESCRIPTION.—Diabetes is a disturbance of the system of nutrition, by which glucose or grape sugar accumulates in the blood in excessive quantities, and must be thrown off in the urine, which often amounts to from six to forty pints per day.

There are two forms of diabetes, diabetes millitus and diabetes insipidus. It is a constitutional disease and is preceded by some disorders of the nervous system, promoted by sedentary habits, overindulgence in drinking and eating, chiefly that of sugar and starches, exposure to cold, wet and fatigue, or some injury to the nervous system. There are nervous complications of the disease.

The most serious form is that of diabetes millitus found more often among men than women, and more at middle age. Obesity is one of the first signs of diabetes, although lean persons develop the disease also. The most evident symptoms are great quantities of urine of high specific gravity, coated tongue, bad breath, craving for food, intense thirst, voracious appetite but continued loss of flesh, intestinal disorder, scanty saliva, great exhaustion. The disease comes on, stealthily by degrees, and proves fatal in most true cases.

NURSING.—The important and almost entire treatment is through the diet. A physician should be consulted concerning the specified diet which should be strictly followed. In general, avoid all sugars and starches. When able, take a moderate amount of exercise in the fresh air. Drink as little of fluids as possible, common tea being quite effective in quenching the thirst. Keep the skin perfectly clean, by frequent bathing. A warm alkaline or spirituous bath is good before retiring and a cold sponge bath in the morning.

Diabetes insipidis is known by the passing of a great amount of urine and intense thirst. This disease may be present in infants and may be caused by injury or fright or may follow some other disease. Urine should be examined at frequent intervals. The physician will attend to this.

DIARRHEA.

DESCRIPTION.—This is not a disease in itself, strictly speaking, but a symptom. However, there are cases where it is of sole importance and may be considered as a disease. It is due to numerous causes, such as local irritation, caused by the eating of improper food, exposure to cold, nervous agitation, microbes as those in connection with various diseases, or it may follow as a result of inflammation of the intestines. It is common to all ages, however, is most common and most serious in the very young and very old. In children under two years of age, 80 percent of the cases prove fatal.

SYMPTOMS.—There is usually gastric disturbance, a bloated feeling, pain, numerous evacuations, varying in number from two or three times a day to four or five every hour. There may be constant desire for passage. The stools are usually a light or dark brown or clay colored. However, in children they are often of a green color. If the diarrhea is the result of some disease, the stools often vary a great deal in appearance. There is often much irritation of the rectum and passage is often attended by severe pain and distress.

NURSING.—In slight cases there is little treatment needed except rest and abstaining from solid foods. However, it is well to give a good cathartic as soon as possible, such as ½ ounce of castor oil or a dose of rhubarb. If there are many and small movements, the rectum becoming much irritated, give an enema of one or two ounces of starch with fifteen to twenty drops of laudanum in it. The patient should be put to bed, kept quiet and warm. The diet should consist of milk and cereal foods which have been cooked for some hours.

First Aid and Home Treatment.

Milk.—Drink a glass of hot scalded milk.

Blackberry Root.—Make a tea of ¼ ounce blackberry root and ½ pint water. Boil 15 minutes, then strain. Take one teaspoonful every hour or two.

Milk and Limewater.—It is well to stop food and give milk or milk and limewater equal parts.

Castor Oil.—Take a dose of castor oil and stop solid food for a day or two. Avoid fruits and vegetables for a few days.

Blackberries.—Blackberries one quart, white sugar ½ pound, cloves ¼ pound and allspice ¼ pound. Boil and strain. Take one teaspoonful every two hours.

DIPHTHERIA.

DESCRIPTION.—Diphtheria is an extremely infectious disease, characterized by the formation of a false membrane on the tonsils and mucous membranes of the throat, which often extends to the larynx and nose. The disease may be mild in its form of attack, or alarmingly severe from the onset. The different epidemics exhibit different degrees of severity and it seems that the first cases of the epidemic are the most severe. It usually affects children from two to fifteen years of age, although it often affects adults also. Defective sanitary conditions and weak or inflamed conditions of the throat, tonsils and nose predispose one to its attack and favor its development. It may be communicated from one person to another in a great many ways, such as, coming in contact with the poison of the disease through infected bedding, clothing, coming in contact with the person infected, by excretions, secretions or portions of the membrane thrown off in coughing, etc. Once having it, does not make one immune to another attack.

INCUBATION.—It is usually from two to seven days after exposure to the disease, that the symptoms are noticed.

SYMPTOMS.—As a rule the first symptoms are much like those attending a slight cold; chilliness, some fever, fullness and irritation of the throat, uneasiness in swallowing, general lassitude. In a day or so, and sometimes in an hour or two, if the throat is carefully examined there will be found whitish-grey patches of false membrane forming on the tonsils and tissues of the throat which often spread rapidly even to the pharynx and air passages in the nose. The color of this membrane soon becomes a dirty grey or yellowish. If removed it leaves a raw bleeding surface on the tonsils over which another membrane will quickly form. This is a characteristic of Diphtheria which distinguishes it from other infections of the throat. When the membrane extends to the nose and larynx, this condition will be manifested by an offensive discharge from the nose, a gradual loss of the voice and difficult breathing, which are grave symptoms. As the disease progresses, the constitutional symptoms become more marked. The glands in the neck swell, delirium and stupor may occur, the heart becoming very weak.

LARYNGEAL DIPHTHERIA or MEMBRANEOUS CROUP.—In this form of the disease a membrane forms in the larynx or upper part of the windpipe. Hoarseness will first be noticed, coughing, difficult breathing, rough, croupy-like cough. After these symptoms have lasted for a day or so the child suddenly becomes worse, breathing more difficult, coming in paroxysms, at first and then the difficulty more continuous, the voice husky and reduced to a whisper, there is a bluish look in the face, the child becomes restless often grasping the throat with its hands vainly trying to get breath. If not quickly relieved the struggle for air will become less and less the child sinking into a sleep, death following quickly from suffocation.

COMPLICATIONS.—Paralysis of the muscles of the throat is not uncommon. There may also be temporary paralysis of the eyes and of the limbs. Inflammation of the kidneys very often occurs even early in the disease and in severe cases there may be complete suppression of the urine. Skin rashes often occur and in severe ulcerative cases there may be dangerous hemorrhages of the throat and nose.

SEQUELAE.—The paralysis caused by Diphtheria is usually recovered from, however, paralysis of the heart may occur when least expected, therefore the patient should be kept quiet while convalescing. Children have dropped over dead from heart paralysis caused by too severe exercise while recovering from an attack of diphtheria. Follow the instructions of the physician carefully and be sure not to allow the patient to take cold.

NURSING.—Diphtheria as a rule is confined to childhood. If a child complains of sore throat, its throat should be examined at once. If there are white spots found on the tonsils it should be isolated, placed in a room by itself, from which all unnecessary furniture and draperies have been removed. Of course it may only be a sore throat, however, as diphtheria starts that way it is wise to use every precaution. Begin at once using some of the first aid treatments given below. Ventilate the room properly. Temperature of the room should be about 65 degrees F. Watch the patient closely and if the throat becomes worse, other symptoms as given above developing, send for the doctor at once. Moist air is often desired in the room which can be obtained by boiling water in the room. Antitoxin should be given just as soon as the disease is known, however, this must be done by a doctor. The patient must be properly nourished as a rule with such liquid foods as milk, eggs, broth, etc. Also ice cream and chipped ice is very nourishing and gratifying to the patient. Very often there is danger of paralysis of the muscles of the throat, therefore no solid foods should be given without permission from the doctor. Watch the urine of the patient which is, as a rule, scanty, high colored and may be suppressed on account of paralysis of the bladder. Do not allow the patient to sit up unless instructed to do so by the doctor as the depression is very great and heart failure is liable to occur suddenly. As to the general care of the patient, follow the instructions as given in the Nursing Department and especially heed the instructions of the doctor.

The mother or nurse who cares for the patient should guard her own health, by eating plenty of good nourishing food, by getting rest and sleep, and exercise in the open air, faithful use of disinfectants. She should be careful that there are no wounds or sores on her hands as the germs of the disease may get into them and cause blood poison. After the case is ended, disinfection should be carried out as instructed under that subject.

First Aid and Home Treatment.

Peroxide of Hydrogen.—Swab out the throat with peroxide of hydrogen full strength if the throat is not too sensitive. It may also be sprayed with one part peroxide of hydrogen to four parts water.

Sulphur.—Blow sulphur onto the tonsils by means of a goosequill, straw or paper tube. Sulphur may also be given mixed with molasses.

Lemon and Sulphur.—Rub lemon juice and sulphur together till thick and smooth. Put a little at a time in the patient's mouth and allow him to swallow it.

Kerosene.—Swab the mouth and throat carefully with kerosene (coal oil). It may also be taken inwardly several times a day. The dose should be one teaspoonful for an adult and about one-third as much for a child.

Tannin.—Gargle with one-half teaspoonful of tannin to a cup of water several times a day.

Salt and Fat Bacon.—Rub a good amount of salt into a piece of fat bacon and tie about the throat.

Onion Poultice.—Apply an onion poultice to the throat.

Camphorated Oil.—Rub the throat well with camphorated oil. Also wet a soft cloth with the oil and bandage the throat with it.

Mountain Sage.—Take one teaspoonful of the fluid extract of mountain sage in a cup of hot lemonade.

Turpentine and Liquid Tar.—Burn equal parts of turpentine and liquid tar and have the patient inhale the fumes.

Hops.—Put some hops in a flannel bag, pour boiling water over them and apply to the throat. When the bag gets cool replace it with another one.

Gargle.—Gargle the throat with lemon juice and water equal parts, to which has been added a little sulphur.

Tannin and Glycerine.—Mix one dram of tannin and one ounce of glycerine. Heat and stir till tannin is well dissolved. Make a swab and apply the mixture to the sore spots on the throat.

Petroleum.—Rub petroleum well into the skin of the throat.

DYSENTERY.

DESCRIPTION.—Dysentery is an infectious disease occurring more in hot weather and more prevalent in tropical climates. It is practically the same as a severe case of diarrhea and is some times called "Bloody-Flux." It is an inflammation of the mucous membrane of the large colon and sometimes extends to the small bowel. Hot weather, unsanitary conditions, bad hygienic surroundings, unsuitable food and bad water are predisposing causes. The form found in the tropical sections is largely due to a little animal parasite.

SYMPTOMS.—The disease is characterized by severe colicky pains in the abdomen and frequent desire for movement of the bowels which is the most striking feature of the disease. The stools are small, containing blood, mucus and pus, but very little natural excrement. The symptoms are more severe during the night and early morning and there is always the distressing sensation that there is something in the bowels yet to be discharged. In very severe cases, the disease is not unlike typhoid fever in character, there being great prostration, temperature high and often vomiting. The toxema or poisoning is often so great that it proves fatal. However, in most cases where it results thus it is due simply to the patient becoming worn out. Convalescence may begin at the end of the first week, however, it is usually long drawn out and often the patient continues to suffer many months, the disease often resulting in extreme emaciation, anemia and other complications. It may also continue for some time in a less severe chronic form.

NURSING.—Absolute rest in bed, fresh air and cleanliness are very important. Be sure to remove the causes of the disease, if known. Give a cathartic such as castor oil, Epsom salts or Rochelle salts. Castor oil is preferable and the dose should be two tablespoonfuls for an adult and a teaspoonful for a baby. The laxative is given to dispose of any poisonous matter in the digestive tract. All discharges from the body should be immediately disinfected as in cases of typhoid fever. In case of infants, paper napkins should be used inside the diaper and should be burned.

The diet should consist only of liquids and foods most easily digested. In severe cases during the acute stage the patient is usually put on a pasteurized milk diet. Milk and limewater is good, also albumin water, made by mixing the unbeaten white of an egg in water. Raw eggs beaten up in milk, rice water, oatmeal water, barley water are good. The food should consist only of the blandest and most non-irritating substances.

First Aid and Home Treatments.

Make a thick syrup from blackberry roots and take three tablespoonfuls three times a day.

Raw Eggs.—Raw eggs eaten freely are excellent.

Dewberry.—Boil two ounces of dewberry roots in two quarts of water till the amount is one quart. Give one-half glassful every three hours.

Oak Bark.—Steep one ounce of oak bark in one pint of water and give one half teaspoonful every three hours.

Cream.—Two teaspoonfuls of thick cream given every hour is said to be good.

Salt and Lemon Juice.—Make a solution of salt and lemon juice, dilute and give every two or three hours.

EARACHE.

Earache is often caused by colds, scarlet fever, grippe, measles or adenoids. This should not be neglected as it may lead to something more serious. Do not allow pus to remain in the middle ear, as it causes inflammation and the hearing may be affected. Untreated discharges from the ears of infants or children are the chief cause of injured and lost hearing in later years.

First Aid and Home Treatment.

Hops or Salt.—Make a little bag out of soft cotton or woolen cloth, in the shape of a half moon, and fill with hops or salt. Heat until very hot and place around the ear, not directly over it, as this might cause the walls of the canal to swell.

Salt or Bran.—Fill a finger of a glove with hot salt or dry bran and insert in the ear a little way.

Heat.—Several magazines heated until very hot will hold the heat for several hours and will not blister.

Salt.—Make a salt solution of one-half teaspoonful of salt to one-half pint of boiling water. Cool until just warm, then wash the ear out carefully and thoroughly, using pledgets of cotton—burning the same after using. After drying well with a piece of medicated cotton, place dry cotton in the ear.

Boracic Acid.—Wash the ear with a warm solution of boracic acid, one half teaspoonful to half pint of water, using a syringe a little distance from ear.

Carbolic Acid.—Wash with a solution of carbolic acid two or three times a day.

Oil.—One is justified in putting oil in the ear only when the ear has been invaded by an insect. Oils are always injurious, although they give temporary relief.

Sometimes earache is caused by water or pus forming back of the ear drum. This should be opened by a physician. It should not be neglected, for if opened early, the discharge may last a week or so, while if allowed to burst, the discharging may continue for a much longer period.

All discharging ears should be examined by the doctor.

ECZEMA, TETTER, SALT RHEUM.

DESCRIPTION.—This is an inflammatory disease of the skin affecting all ages and classes. It appears in several different forms, the most common of which are the dry and weeping eczema. It is most likely to appear on the face, scalp, hands, and in the hollows of the elbows and knees. It is characterized in the beginning by redness, intense itching and burning, little pimples, vesicles or postules forming under the skin. If this is scratched or irritated the vesicles break, discharging a watery pus-like fluid. The skin of the affected part becomes thick, often breaks away leaving a raw surface of a deep red color.

This disease does not yield readily to treatment and therefore it takes a long time to cure it. The patient must be patient and persistent in trying to overcome it. As this disease is largely due to the system being "out of order," it manifesting itself in this way, one should look to the general health and diet. The person afflicted should eat very little rich, greasy or salty foods such as pork, salt fish, corned beef, rich pasteries, etc. The digestive organs should be kept in the best of condition, the bowels and kidneys active, in order that the poisonous waste matter may be carried from the system. The patient should take plenty of exercise in the open air and build up the general health.

Avoid scratching or irritating the affected parts. In children it often becomes necessary to tie the hands down, put little mittens on them, or fasten little splints on the arms to prevent bending at the elbows. The parts should not be washed with soap and water but may be cleansed with sweet oil or olive oil. If the hands are affected, rubber gloves should be used when they must be put into water.

First Aid and Home Treatment.

Scraped Potato and Camphor.—Scrape or grate a medium sized potato and add a tablespoonful of spirits of camphor. Mix well and apply as a poultice, binding on to keep in place.

"D. D. D." Remedy.—The "D. D. D." remedy for eczema, which may be obtained at any drug store, has been a great help to many people suffering with this disease.

Sulphur and Lard.—Sulphur and lard mixed and applied twice a day is very good in mild cases of eczema.

ERYSIPELAS.

DESCRIPTION.—This is an acute, infectious, inflammation of the skin, caused by a little germ which usually enters the system through a wound or break in the skin. It is accompanied by pain, heat, redness and general inflammation. Although it usually develops through a wound, it occasionally seems to arise spontaneously and in such cases affects the head and face more frequently than other parts of the body. It may be conveyed by a third person, or by the poison, which attaches itself to clothing, furniture, etc., coming in contact with an open wound.

INCUBATION.—Varies from one to eight days.

SYMPTOMS.—The disease comes on with a chill followed by a rise in temperature, other signs of fever, and the parts affected become red and swollen. When it affects the face and head, the first redness appears on the bridge of the nose and spreads over the cheeks and other parts. The eyes, ears, lips, etc., become very much swollen. The eyes frequently are swollen shut. There is a distinct line of demarcation between the diseased part and the healthy skin.

NURSING.—The patient should be isolated and it is well to disinfect all articles used in the sick room. The bowels should be kept open and strength sustained with good nourishing foods. Wash the parts with a solution of boric acid water and then apply a poultice of crushed cranberries.

First Aid and Home Treatment.

Take iron for the blood. Make a slippery elm poultice and apply to affected parts. Slippery elm is good for any skin disease. It may also be taken internally.

Cranberries.—Crush fresh cranberries and spread on a soft cloth and apply to sores.

Lard or Tallow.—Apply lard or tallow gently to relieve irritation.

Soda.—Bathe well with a soda solution, one teaspoonful of soda to one-half pint of water.

Witch Hazel.—Witch hazel is good for bathing the affected parts.

Bellwort.—Bellwort root boiled in water and applied is said to be good.

EYES—WEAK OR DISEASED.

No organ of the body is so easily affected by diseases as the eye. Many different kinds of diseases of the eye result from serious diseases of the constitution, such as, fevers, diabetes, syphilis, nephritis, etc. In case of an infected system causing the weakened condition of the eyes, treatment by a physician should not be delayed.

Often weak eyes are only a condition of the eye, corresponding to a weakened, starved or overworked system. Therefore build up the system with nutritious food and sufficient rest. Bathe the eyes as directed.

Everything connected with the treatment of the eye should be absolutely sterile and the hands must be clean.

If only one eye is infected, do not allow a drop of the discharge or fluid used in bathing, or any part of the apparatus, to come in contact with the sound eye, but discard every piece of cotton after each using.

First Aid and Home Treatment.

Boracic Acid.—Bathe the eyes several times a day, in warm water, in which has been dissolved several grains of boracic acid.

Salt.—Common salt water, used as a wash several times a day, is one of the best remedies for weak eyes.

Sweet Elder.—A wash made of the tea from the flowers of sweet elder has been proven very good for weak eyes.

Ice Compress.—If very painful, take a piece of cotton just large enough to cover the eye and saturate with ice cold boracic acid water (using one tablespoonful of boracic acid to one pint of water). Change every minute or half minute.

Sweet Oil.—When the eye surface is irritated wash the eye carefully and drop one drop of warm sweet oil into it.

Consult a good physician regarding the abnormal conditions.

FEET.

Perspiring Feet.—Bathe the feet in hot water and good soap, then dash some cold water over them. After bathing the feet thoroughly, apply often a mixture of one-half pint of alcohol and one dram of salicylic acid. This is a splendid deodorizer.

A twenty-five percent solution of ammonium chloride in distilled water will relieve perspiration if rubbed in well, about twice a week.

When the feet ache or burn make a thick lather of a brown laundry soap, rub on and soak well. This will remove soreness remarkably well.

Rawness Between Toes.—Do not wear patent leather shoes, since they do not allow the air to get at the feet. Wear sandals while in the house. After bathing, dust with a solution of salicylic acid one teaspoonful, starch four teaspoonfuls. Massage with olive oil or cocoa butter.

To Keep Feet from Tiring Quickly.—Massage in the morning, then bathe them in tepid alum water (one tablespoonful of powdered alum to one quart of water). At night, bathe again in warm water and soap. After drying, rub with alcohol and talcum. Do not wear pointed toed shoes or Louis XIV heels. Change shoes every day if possible.

FELONS.

DESCRIPTION.—A felon is a painful inflammation of the periosteum or covering of the bone of the finger. The last joint is the part more often affected. It is caused by the accumulation of pus germs underneath the bone covering.

SYMPTOMS.—The symptoms are throbbing pain, great tenderness and dark red colored condition of the affected part. The intense pain and fever often extend far up the arm, and if neglected, may infect the bone or joint to such an extent that the hand may be crippled.

When a felon is developed, it should be lanced as soon as possible, if it does not open of itself after several applications have been used. If a physician does not lance the felon, great care should be taken to have the instruments thoroughly sterilized. The incision must be deep enough to reach the pus formation underneath the periosteum or bone covering. The operation should always be done by a physician.

The superficial kind may be cured readily if taken in time.

First Aid and Home Treatment.

Bread and Milk or Flaxseed Poultice.—Poultice of bread and milk or of flaxseed is good.

Salt and Egg.—Salt and yolk of an egg mixed and applied as a salve is effective.

Indian Turnip and Blue Flag.—Stew roots of Indian turnip and blue flag in lard until well done. Strain, add four tablespoonfuls of castile soap, heat together and apply to the felon until it breaks.

Lye.—Hold the finger in hot weak lye, made from wood ashes, as long as possible, then repeat after a short time.

Alcohol.—As soon as a felon is detected, soak the finger in a solution of equal parts of alcohol and hot water.

Smartweed.—The bruised leaves of smartweed bound tightly on the finger is a good poultice.

Soap and Cornmeal.—As soon as a felon is noticed, bind in a poultice of soap and cornmeal.

Rock Salt and Turpentine.—Bind the affected finger in a poultice of pulverized rock salt and turpentine. Keep the poultice moist.

GALLSTONES.

DESCRIPTION.—Gallstones are hard concretions which form in the gall bladder, caused by the crystallization of certain properties of the bile. This may be due to a catarrhal condition of the mucous membrane caused by the presence of bacteria. They may occur at any age, however, are much more common in people of middle age, or later life, and in women than in men. They may be very small, so small that they will not be noticed, and again they may attain the size of a walnut or hen egg.

SYMPTOMS.—These stones may exist in the gall bladder for some time without the patient being aware of their presence, there being no marked symptoms. However, when they attempt to pass out through the gall duct or bile duct, which is very small, there is very severe pain of a griping, tearing nature called gallstone colic. The onset is sudden and may be marked by a chill and fever. It may last but a few minutes or it may last several days and may be so severe as to cause collapse. It often ends with the onset of vomiting. It is chiefly in the upper part of the abdomen and on the right side. There is often local peritonitis in greater or less degree, giving rise to rigidity of the muscles and tenderness over the gall bladder. These attacks may come every few days, or months may intervene.

NURSING.—It is very hard to dissolve these gallstones after they have once formed. It is said, however, that large doses of olive oil, as much as a half pint per day, will do much good. It will do much good if enough of it can be gotten to the stones. If the stones are large and give much trouble, it may be necessary to remove them by having an operation performed.

In very bad attacks when the pain is very severe it may be necessary to give a sedative such as morphine. This must be done by the physician. However, in less severe attacks the taking of a glass of hot water as hot as can be taken, will often give much relief. Also the application of hot fomentations over the gall bladder or the taking of hot baths will give much relief. The patient should be made as comfortable as possible during an attack.

It has been found that alcoholic excess, sedentary habits, insufficient exercise, poor digestion, etc., are predisposing causes. The diet is very important.

First Aid and Home Treatment.

Sweet Oil.—Sweet oil, one-half teacupful taken at bedtime and in the morning is very good.

Salts.—Take Rochelle salts or Seidlitz powder to keep the bowels active.

Hot Compress.—A piece of flannel wrung out of hot water and applied to the painful part will relieve pain.

Olive Oil.—Olive oil is a fine remedy. Take a tablespoonful every three hours.

GANGRENE.

DESCRIPTION.—Gangrene is the death of a part or parts of the body. It results from the blood supply being cut off, and most frequently affects the hands or feet.

CAUSES.—Causes are injuries, freezing, burning, diabetes, strangulated hernia, erysipelas, a heart too feeble to send blood to all parts of the body, hardened blood vessels, or old age. The cutting of a corn may cause it.

SYMPTOMS.—In dry gangrene there may be a sensation of coldness or numbness—sensation of heat and pain, or a dark spot or blister which discharges a little bloody fluid at times. In moist gangrene there are dark spots greatly swollen and gases which are very odious. This is the most dangerous kind, as it spreads very rapidly and quickly leads to death. A physician should be summoned at once.

Keep the part warm, quiet and level. Do not apply bandages tightly as they may interfere with the circulation. Do everything possible to improve the general health of the patient.

First Aid and Home Treatment.

Listerine or Iodoform.—For the dry form, keep very clean, apply listerine or iodoform.

Cabbage Leaves.—Put wilted cabbage leaves on the sore part, till they do not become colored any more. This treatment draws out the poison. Bathe with a weak solution of saleratus then cover with black pepper and bandage. Do this two or three times a day.

GOITRE.

DESCRIPTION.—This is an enlargement of the thyroid gland in front of the neck. The cause is not definitely known, however, it is thought by some to come from the drinking water. It is much more common in some districts than others and is hereditary in some families. It is also much more prevalent in certain sections of Europe than it is in this country. It is much more frequent in women than in men and although it may occur at any time in life, it is often first noticed about puberty.

NURSING.—If the patient is in a district in which goitre seems to be very common, removal from this district, or the boiling of all drinking water may be all that is necessary. Good results have also been obtained in the treating of young adults by giving thyroid extract. From one to three grains of the dry powder may be given twice or three times daily. In some instances this does good and in others it does not, so if the goitre does not diminish in size after six or eight weeks, stop the treatment. If it does, it may be continued for eight or ten weeks longer.

Wash the part externally with a solution of tincture of iodine diluted with half the amount of alcohol, or paint the neck with tincture of iodine every other day.

The only treatment which is sure of success is to remove the whole thyroid gland as early as possible.

GOUT.

DESCRIPTION.—This is a painful affection of the fibrous tissues of the small joints usually occurring first in the joint of the great toe. It is somewhat like rheumatism, although more severe in the pain it causes. It is thought by some to be caused by excess of uric acid in the blood, however, the direct cause is not fully known. The tendency is generally inherited, but it usually comes from high living, excess in wines and malt liquors, rich food with indolent habits, lack of exercise, etc. If the tendency is inherited it may show up early in life, however, if brought on by the mode of living it usually does not appear till later in life. It is more common in men than in women.

SYMPTOMS.—The disease usually comes on suddenly, the patient going to bed feeling fine and being wakened about midnight or a little after by a very severe pain in the joint of the great toe. Or the attack may be preceded by indigestion, loss of appetite, sour stomach, nausea and vomiting. The body may have a swollen, heavy feeling and there may be a sense of bloat in the legs and thighs. However, the gouty pain comes on suddenly accompanied by chills and a little fever, the chills dying out as the pain becomes more intense. The affected part becomes swollen, red and hot, very sensitive to the touch. The patient usually suffers intensely until near morning when the symptoms usually subside to reappear the next night. This may continue for several days, the attacks becoming less severe till they gradually die out. Another attack may not come on for three or four years. Although the inflammation is severe, there is no formation of pus, however, there may be a chalk-like deposit thrown out about the joints affected.

NURSING.—The affected limb should be raised so as to be level with the body. Apply hot fomentations, such as a flannel dipped in hot water, or the application of wet cloths soaked in laudanum and lead water. It is also well to bathe the parts with vinegar to which has been added all the salt it will dissolve. Drink freely of a tea made of wintergreen leaves. Hot baths followed by massage is also good.

Diet.—Regulation of the diet is of great importance in the treatment of gout. The patient should eat no more than is necessary to satisfy the hunger, and keep up the strength. It should be of the simplest foods, avoiding all sweets, fats, rich foods and alcoholic liquors. Drink plenty of water and take lots of exercise in the fresh air. Keep the bowels open and observe the laws of hygiene.

GRANULAR EYELIDS.

DESCRIPTION.—This is a form of conjunctivitis characterized by the formation of little granules on the conjunctiva. The secretion is contagious and the disease is very hard to get rid of.

NURSING.—Use boric acid as a wash, in an eye glass, several times a day. Do not strain the eyes by reading or sewing in a poor light. Have the eyes treated by an oculist.

GRIPPE—INFLUENZA.

DESCRIPTION.—It is an acute infectious disease caused by a germ taken into the system, by coming in contact with one who has the disease or from the air. It is often epidemic, attacking large numbers of people at the same time. It is no respecter of persons, attacking the young and old with equal severity. It occurs at any season, although the more severe epidemics have been in the colder seasons of the year. One attack does not protect one from another attack.

INCUBATION.—It is generally from two to four days after exposure that the first symptoms develop.

SYMPTOMS.—As a rule the onset is sudden, however, sometimes one may show lassitude and irritability for several days before the acute symptoms begin. There is fever, catarrhal conditions of the nose, throat and bronchial tubes, accompanied by a cough, running at the nose and eyes, sneezing, headache, pains in the joints, aching of the muscles of the back and legs. There is no appetite and great prostration. It often affects the stomach and bowels causing coated tongue, vomiting, diarrhea.

COMPLICATIONS.—The prostration is generally so great that many and often serious complications develop. The most serious and common of these are bronchitis and pneumonia.

SEQUELAE.—The disease often leaves the system in such a weakened condition that such serious after-effects develop as pneumonia, tuberculosis, heart trouble, kidney trouble, etc.

NURSING.—Great care should be taken that very young children and old people are not exposed to it. For this reason it is best to isolate the patient as much as practical. He should be put to bed at once and kept there till the attack is over. The room should be well ventilated, bowels should be kept open, diet light and easy to digest, but of good nourishing foods. The depression or prostration is generally so great both physically and mentally that everything should be done that is possible to nourish and keep the spirits up. If there is high fever it should be controlled by frequent sponge baths of alcohol and water. The patient should be kept in bed as long as there is any fever and several days after, if there is much prostration. The best of care should be given and the serious complications and after-effects well guarded against.

First Aid and Home Treatments.

The treatment varies with the different forms of the disease and the complications that arise. As a rule it is unnecessary to call a doctor if the patient is well taken care of and the following home treatments given.

Sweat.—Just as soon as one feels the attack coming on, he should take a good cathartic, a hot mustard foot-bath, go to bed and cover up warm. Put hot water-bottles, irons or bricks around him, and as soon as he begins to sweat, he should be given a pint of good hot lemonade or ginger tea, thus causing him to sweat profusely. After the sweat, the night clothes and bedding should be changed, the patient being very careful not to get chilled.

Poultices.—If the cough is severe or there is much bronchitis or soreness of the lungs, it is well to apply a mustard paste or an onion poultice to the chest and back. Refer to the Nursing Department for instructions as to how to make these. This poulticing relieves the inflammation and often prevents the development of serious lung troubles such as pneumonia.

If the patient is very weak, it may be necessary to give stimulants, however, this should be left to a physician.

For the sore throat, use some good gargle such as a solution of boric acid, listerine, peroxide of hydrogen, lemon juice, etc. Baking soda is also fine for any kind of sore throat.

Catnip or Pennyroyal.—Give plenty of hot catnip or pennyroyal tea to sweat the patient.

Peppermint.—Rub forehead, ears and neck with oil of peppermint.

Quinine.—Give quinine, about four grains every four hours.

For headache, bathe the face, temples and neck well with hot water.

Give a mild cathartic to keep the system clean.

HAY FEVER.

DESCRIPTION.—This is a catarrhal condition of the nose, throat and upper air passages. There is sneezing, burning sensation of the eyes and nose, followed by an increase in the secretions of all the air passages of the head. Sometimes in a severe form it is very much like asthma. It generally develops about the middle of August or during the haying season, from which it gets its name, and continues until there is a hard frost in the fall. It is caused by the pollen of ragweed, hay or golden rod.

First Aid and Home Treatment.

There is no known cure for the disease, however, relief may be obtained by change in climate. The patient often gets relief by going to the seaside or to some high, dry climate. Build up the nervous system.

Calcium Chloride.—Dissolve two ounces of calcium chloride crystals in one pint of distilled water. Give one teaspoonful after each meal. Give fifteen grains of calcium chloride three times a day. Many claim this to be a very effective cure.

Salt and Alcohol.—Heat salt and alcohol together till very hot and breathe the vapor for five or ten minutes several times a day.

Camphor.—The inhaling of camphor also gives relief.

Chlorate of Potash.—To relieve the tickling sensation, gargle with chlorate of potash several times daily.

Ground Coffee.—It is said that sprinkling ground coffee over the coals and inhaling the smoke will give relief.

Quinine.—Use powdered quinine as a snuff to give relief from tightness in the head.

Preventive Measures.—Keep the eyes and nose in a healthy condition. The nose may be sprayed with alkaline or oily sprays.

If possible, sleep in a tent all summer. Keep away from cultivated lands, and do not live in thick woods or close to them.

Travel by water whenever you can, and not by rail. Do not travel in dusty weather.

Keep away from vacant lots in the city. There is sure to be ragweed.

HEADACHES.

This is one of the most common ailments the human body is heir to and appears in many different forms and with practically all diseases. The most common forms are the sick headache, nervous headache, neuralgic headache and catarrhal headache. This is not a disease in itself but a symptom of a disease or deranged part of the body. The most common causes are: poor digestion, diseases of the kidneys, liver and nerves; catarrh, weak eyes, anaemic conditions and disorders of the generative organs. In order to treat it successfully, the cause must be discovered and removed and not the symptom treated as is often done.

HEADACHE—CATARRHAL.

This form of headache is usually due to a catarrhal condition of the air passages of the head resulting from a heavy cold or exposure. There are dull aching pains in the fore part of the head over the eyes.

NURSING.—As this is due to a severe cold, treat the same as a cold. Take a hot foot-bath, go to bed and sweat. This will open up the pores of the body and relieve the congestion. Take a good cathartic and clean out the system.

HEADACHE—NERVOUS.

This form of headache denotes a weak, impaired condition of the nervous system, brought on by over work, illness, excitement, worry, weak eyes, ill-fitting glasses, lack of sleep and rest, etc. In fact anything which affects the nerves seriously is likely to cause this form of headache.

SYMPTOMS.—As this is an affection of the nerves, the headache usually starts at the back of the neck or the base of the skull. The patient has a general nervous "unstrung" feeling. The head feels big and heavy, the eyesight is often affected, the patient may be sleepless, yet tired and weary.

NURSING.—Anything that will quiet or build up the nervous system will not only relieve the attack but prevent its recurrence. A good, sound, restful sleep will often be all that is necessary. Do not take a lot of drugs in the form of patent headache remedies, as these simply deaden the nerves by means of the narcotics which they contain and have no lasting beneficial effects.

Take lots of exercise in the open air, sleep with the bedroom windows wide open and keep the mind free from worry.

Cold Cloths.—The application of cold packs or cloths wrung out of cold water to the back of the neck and base of the skull will often give much relief.

Hot Foot Bath.—This will draw the blood from the head and thus relieve congestion.

HEADACHE—NEURALGIC.

This is a form of headache in which neuralgic symptoms are combined with ordinary headache. It is usually limited to one side of the head or face and comes in paroxysms. Women are more subject to it than men and it often comes from bad teeth.

SYMPTOMS.—This form generally comes on in the morning soon after waking, the face is hot and throbbing, eyes red and inflamed. The symptoms usually develop rapidly until there is an almost unbearable headache. The location of the pain varies according to the nerve affected and is of a stabbing nature.

NURSING.—Build up the nervous system with plenty of sleep and rest, good nutritious foods, outdoor exercise, etc. As long as the nerves are in bad condition one is subject to neuralgic headache. Have the teeth examined and keep them healthy.

HEADACHE—SICK.

This form of headache is due largely to a derangement of the digestive tract, or act of digestion, unhealthy condition of the kidneys, liver, womb and ovaries. There is no trouble in the head and, in treating the disease, the remedy must be applied to the cause of the headache.

SYMPTOMS.—The headache due to gastric disturbances is generally located in the forehead. It begins as a rule in the morning and continues throughout the day. There is nausea, vomiting, and the patient is very sick. The symptoms are too well known to need further description.

NURSING.—The first thing to do in the treatment of the trouble is to discover the cause. If it is due to digestive disorder, limit the diet to the simplest, easily digested foods. Take much exercise in the open, keep the bowels regular and the kidneys active. Drink lots of water and get plenty of sleep and rest. Don't take drugs or headache medicines, but build up the general health through proper diet, exercise, rest and recreation.

HERNIA (Rupture).

DESCRIPTION.—Hernia or rupture is the protrusion of a part of the intestine of any internal organ through the abdominal wall. It is more common in case of the bowels and occurs generally at the navel or in the groin. That occurring at the navel is known as umbilical hernia, while that in the groin is called inguinal hernia. It generally occurs at these places as these are natural openings in the abdominal wall. In the early stages of life the testicles are in the abdominal cavity and descend into the scrotum before birth through a natural passage-way. The opening at the navel was the natural passage-way for the umbilical cord while attached to the foetus. During severe strain or exertion the peritoneum or lining of the abdominal cavity is not strong enough to prevent intestines from protruding through these openings.

Hernia which can be returned into the abdominal cavity is called reducible hernia. That which cannot be returned is known as irreducible hernia. When the protrusion is so great and the opening so tightly constricted that the hernia cannot be returned, the circulation being interfered with, it is called strangulated hernia. This is the most serious form of the trouble.

SYMPTOMS.—There is a protrusion of the bowels at the navel or in the groin, or at the point of the hernia, great pain, and in case of strangulation the bowel becomes hard and dark looking. Often in the case of children the pain is so severe that there will be vomiting and convulsions.

NURSING.—The only sure cure for hernia is an operation which should be performed by a skilled surgeon as early as possible. At the time of the protrusion, the patient should be put to bed and the muscles allowed to relax. Give no food and very little to drink. Avoid a cathartic.

Ice Bag.—Place an ice bag or cold pack over the swelling to reduce the inflammation.

Hot Fomentations.—Apply hot fomentations or place the patient in a hot bath. This will help to relax the muscles and allow the protrusion to return.

A physician should be consulted as soon as the rupture is discovered.

Truss.—A truss will often effect a cure if used in time.

HIVES.

DESCRIPTION.—This is a circular eruption of the skin due to indigestion, or eating of certain foods, or constipation. In curing hives the greatest care should be taken in choosing food, because there are many kinds of food which cause hives. Some of these are: strawberries, pickles, cheese and certain kinds of shell fish. Insect bites may also cause hives.

First Aid and Home Treatment.

Rye Flour and Water.—Mix fresh rye flour with water and drink as much of this as possible. Dust with starch, buckwheat or rye flour. This is very effective.

Salt.—Put a handful of salt in the bath water. Salt relieves the itching and strengthens and beautifies the body.

Slippery Elm.—Use slippery elm both internally and externally. It throws off impurities, and is very good for any skin irritation.

Limewater and Zinc.—Make a solution of limewater and zinc and apply to the hives with a soft cloth.

Hot Bath.—A hot bath will relieve the irritation.

Baking Soda.—Make a strong solution of soda water and bathe hives or apply soda directly to hives.·

Buttermilk.—To bathe in buttermilk is good.

Catnip or Sassafras.—Drink catnip or sassafras tea.

Bran.—Bran baths are helpful.

Vinegar.—Bathe with a weak solution of vinegar.

Carbolated Vaseline.—Carbolated vaseline will relieve the itching and burning.

Take a good cathartic.

HYDROPHOBIA (Rabies).

DESCRIPTION.—Hydrophobia is an acute infectious disease transmitted to man by the bite of an animal suffering with the disease. The specific virus which causes the disease is conveyed through the saliva of the animal and affects the nervous system of man. A very large percent of the cases is due to the bites of rabid dogs, however, it is also caused by the bites of cats, horses, foxes, etc.

Incubation.—The incubation period of this disease is from six weeks to six months. It very seldom develops six months after the wound is received. As the disease is transmitted by the saliva of the animal it may even be contracted from a dog, suffering with the disease, licking an open wound. However, deep wounds are more dangerous than one made through the clothing as the saliva of the animal is not so likely to reach the broken skin in the latter case.

Whether the wound is severe or not it should be taken care of at once if there is any chance whatever that the animal is suffering with rabies. A good physician should be called, the wound should be opened up well and cauterized or burned with crude carbolic acid, caustic soda, nitric acid or a red-hot iron. If the bite is on a limb, apply a tight bandage between the wound and the body, however, this should not be kept on longer than 30 to 45 minutes. After this has been done, the patient should be taken if possible to an institute where the Pasteur Treatment can be given. These Pasteur Institutes are located in the following towns: Chicago, Illinois; Minneapolis, Minnesota; New York City; Baltimore, Maryland; Austin, Texas; Ann Arbor, Michigan; Toronto, Ontario. At the present time the Health Department of any large city can handle these cases.

The treatment given above is preventative and is practically the only successful treatment, as the patient very seldom recovers after the disease has once developed. In case the preventative treatment is unsuccessful, the first symptoms that the disease is developing may be slight. There is usually pain and swelling at the point of the wound, although it may have previously healed. There is chilliness, headache, anxiety, uneasiness, the patient being very excitable, sometimes thrown into convulsions by a sudden noise, draught of air or by attempting to swallow. There is foaming at the mouth, due to the excessive flow of saliva caused by the constant spasm of the jaws. This is followed by paralysis and death in a short time.

INDIGESTION OR DYSPEPSIA.

DESCRIPTION.—The term covers a number of digestive troubles. It is an interruption or disturbance of the act of digestion. It is the symptom of digestive unrest and not a disease in itself. It appears in different forms and develops from various causes.

Improper diet is the chief cause of indigestion or dyspepsia. Insufficient mastication of food, bolting of meals, ice-cold drinks, over-hot drinks, alcoholic stimulants taken to excess, overloading the stomach too often, etc., etc., are causes. These errors, persisted in, will result in chronic dyspepsia, as well as attacks of indigestion. Irregular and unsuitable meals, insufficient and badly prepared foods, often initiate chronic indigestion or dyspepsia. The diet must also be suited to the habits. A very common starting point for indigestion is shown by a person accustomed previously to an outdoor life or much in the open air, to take up a sedentary position or occupation.

SYMPTOMS.—There is a local sensation of discomfort, as of a ball or weight pressing down in the stomach. There may be a gnawing pain definitely located or diffused through the entire organ. There is likely to be a bloated feeling due to the collection of gas in the stomach, coated tongue, loss of appetite, bad taste in the mouth, foul breath, and a raw or burning feeling right back of the breast bone, commonly called heartburn. This may be accompanied by belching of gas, sour food and sometimes vomiting.

NURSING.—In slight cases of indigestion due to errors in diet, the symptoms will readily subside if a light diet be taken and the bowels kept open. The idea is to remove the cause. In acute cases of much severity, it is well to give an emetic and thus empty the stomach of the irritating material. The local distress may be relieved by the application of a mustard plaster or external heat. The diet should consist of milk and broths taken every two or three hours during the day. No coffee, tea, alcohol, fruits or vegetables, cooked or raw, should be eaten. Hot water, water containing soda or milk, milk and lime water, etc., may be taken as desired.

Many remedies have been suggested and much doctoring done for this trouble, however, the less medicine used the better. Most all mild cases will yield to regulation of diet and habit and by giving the stomach periods of comparative rest. The cure is largely in the hands of the patient himself.

First Aid and Home Treatment.

Give a good cathartic and keep bowels regular.

Restrict the diet or abstain entirely from food for a day or two.

Extract of Cascara.—A teaspoonful of cascara in one-half glass of water will relieve indigestion and constipation.

Eat regularly and slowly. Do not eat between meals. Rest immediately after eating and never eat when tired, excited or angry.

Take regular systematic exercise several times a day or a cold bath and a good rub with a coarse towel, two or three hours after meals. Avoid sweets, pastries and foods hard to digest.

All defective teeth should be attended to.

Baking Soda.—One-half teaspoonful of baking soda dissolved in one-half glass of cold water is very good.

Milk of Magnesia.—Take one teaspoonful of milk of magnesia every two or three hours.

Charcoal.—Take charcoal tablets before and after meals and before going to bed.

Figs and Senna Leaves.—A lady from Cambridge, Wisconsin, says: "Take one pound of figs, five cents worth of senna leaves and grind thoroughly. Take dry as needed."

Salt.—One teaspoonful of salt in a glass of hot water is good for indigestion.

Fruit Diet.—Exclusive fruit diet for a few days is good.

Peppermint.—Add ten drops of essence of peppermint and one-half teaspoonful of baking soda to one-half glass of water. Take all at once. Repeat in one-half hour if necessary.

Creosote and Tolu.—Mix twenty-four drops of creosote and three ounces of syrup of tolu. Take one teaspoonful stirred up well in one-half glass of water, after meals.

Drink a pint of hot water before going to bed and again the first thing in the morning. To add lemon juice to the water is good.

Soda Mint.—Use one teaspoonful of spirits of hartshorn, one and one-half teaspoonsful of baking soda, one and one-half teaspoonsful of mint water and six ounces of soft water. Heat a part of the water and pour on the soda, when dissolved, add the remainder of water, cold, and other ingredients. Take one dessertspoonful after each meal.

INFANTILE PARALYSIS.

This is a disease peculiar to childhood, usually affecting children under three or four years of age and those of weakly constitution. It is an inflammation of the spinal cord caused by germs entering the system through the nose and throat.

SYMPTOMS.—As a rule the child first appears dull, tired and irritable, there is a flushed appearance, temperature rising to about 102 degrees F., eyes become bright and glassy and the child often has convulsions. These symptoms are followed by paralysis in one or more of the extremities, usually the legs.

PREVENTION.—As this disease is peculiar to small children and to warm weather, children should be kept in the best of condition, especially during an epidemic of the disease. It seldom affects those of robust constitution. Keep them away from public gatherings where they may be exposed to germ carriers, also beware of people coughing and sneezing. Watch for signs of running nose or sniffles. There should be no operation on the nose or throat during an epidemic of the disease, and in case the nose, lips or mouth are sore, the sores should be washed with boric acid solution or touched with the dry powder every few hours. The nose should also be irrigated with a five or ten percent solution of boric acid. Keep the child well nourished with the best of foods. Be very careful of its diet. Never use raw milk. Prevention is very important as a child seldom fully recovers from the disease.

NURSING.—In case the symptoms as enumerated above develop, a physician should be consulted at once and the child placed under his care. An operation is often necessary. The child should be well nourished during the disease. Exercising and massaging the affected limb often gives very satisfactory results.

INFLAMMATION OF LARGE INTESTINES.

This is a simple catarrhal inflammation of the colon or large intestines, similar to bronchitis or inflammation of the air passages. It may be caused by large doses of purgatives, poisoning, or it may come from inflammation of the other organs extending to the large intestines.

SYMPTOMS.—The main symptom is diarrhea, which may come on suddenly. There is much mucus and often blood in the stools. The bowels may move many times a day and there may be difficulty and pain at stool. Pain in the stomach is a common symptom and is of a griping nature, often very severe. The patient is usually at ease between attacks. There is tenderness over the abdomen, the tongue is furred with a very white coat, there is loss of appetite, nausea and vomiting. The patient is often very much depressed mentally.

NURSING.—Keep the patient absolutely quiet and in bed until the diarrhea has stopped, until the passages are normal or well formed, there being no more blood in them and until the temperature is normal. The application of heat in the form of hot fomentations, poultices, etc., to the abdomen will often give much relief. The patient should have nothing but a milk diet and only about two fluid ounces of that at a time, the total amount per day depending on the severity of the attack and the general condition of the patient. The diarrhea may be checked or relieved by a rectal injection of six or eight ounces of warm olive oil or a drachm of glycerine. A good long rest among new surroundings will greatly aid convalescence.

First Aid and Home Treatment.

Hot Water.—Apply to the stomach a piece of flannel wrung out of hot water.

Cold Water.—Cloths wrung out of cold water are good, cover with dry cloth.

Flaxseed.—Flaxseed poultice, applied hot, is very beneficial. Change as soon as cool.

Salt.—Hot salt bag placed on affected part gives relief.

INFLAMMATION OF SMALL INTESTINE.

This is a catarrhal condition of the small intestine caused by an irritant coming in contact with the intestinal walls or by the inflammation being extended from other neighboring organs. Children are more subject to it than older people, however, debility either in old or young is a predisposing cause. Common causes are indigestible or undigested foods, such as form coagulated milk, especially in young children, the eating of too much unripe food, intestinal worms, poisons and violent purgatives. It may also be caused by bacteria. The disease occurs most frequently during the months of July, August and September.

SYMPTOMS.—The symptoms vary greatly in severity according to the cause. There is chilliness, a feeling of uneasiness in the abdomen, colicky pains, loss of appetite and nausea. The tongue is dry and coated, there is an anxious expression, the face having a pinched appearance. The diarrhea soon commences. The stools are at first semi-solid but soon become watery, acid, scalding and containing more or less mucus. They may have a greenish color, however, they are usually clear and watery. The abdomen may be bloated and there may be palpitation of the heart. The urine is scanty and highly colored. The patient quickly loses his strength, especially if the diarrhea is profuse.

NURSING.—The first thing to do is to ascertain and remove the cause. Slight cases generally cure themselves, nature removing the irritating cause or substance by the diarrhea. If the cause is undigested food, give a dose of castor oil. In case the colicky pains are severe, the application of hot fomentations to the abdomen, or hot poultices will often give much relief. These should be changed frequently and kept warm. If the case is one of eating spoiled food and the irritating matter remains in the stomach, an emetic should be given followed by a dose of castor oil.

In all cases the digestive organs should be given a rest and then the diet should be of the simplest, easily digested food until the recovery is complete.

INFLAMMATION OF STOMACH (Acute Gastritis).

This is a catarrhal condition of the stomach much like that met within the throat and air passages. It is characterized by congestion and excessive secretion and excessive secretion of mucus. It is generally caused by overloading the stomach, eating too much indigestible food, too many sweets, drinking ice water and other cold drinks when patient is warm, etc. It is also caused by taking irritant poisons into the stomach, by alcoholic excess and may occur as a symptom of some of the eruptive fevers.

SYMPTOMS.—The symptoms are too well known to really need description. There are pains and tenderness over the pit of the stomach, which are increased by taking food and may be relieved by vomiting. There is nausea, vomiting, tongue is coated, bowels inactive, urine scanty and highly colored, there is also likely to be headache and other fever symptoms.

NURSING.—If the trouble is caused by some poison or irritating substance in the stomach, the patient should be given an emetic causing him to vomit. This should be followed by a good cathartic in order that the offending substance may be removed as quickly as possible. Poultices of flaxseed meal or mustard applied over the stomach will often give much relief. Hot fomentations or hot flannels are also good. As the membranes of the stomach are usually very sore and irritated, the patient should eat very little and that of the most easily digested foods taken in small quantities at a time. In fact it is better to give the stomach a complete rest for a day or so. One afflicted in this way should be very careful of the diet even for some time after the attack is past. Drink plenty of hot water and let the diet consist of milk, broth, etc.

INGROWN TOENAILS.

Wear broad-toed shoes and do not cut the corners of toenails. Let them grow square.

Cotton.—Put a small piece of cotton under the corner of nail to lift the nail. Change this daily. Increase the size of piece till the nail is raised.

Adhesive Tape.—Draw a piece of adhesive tape tightly around the toe so as to pull back the flesh from the edge of the nail. This will give great relief.

Mutton Tallow.—Pour in at the corner of nail, some very hot mutton tallow. A couple of these applications will curl the nail and the ingrown nail will be cured.

Cut a "U" in the top of the nail. As this grows together it will tend to draw the nail away from the flesh at the sides.

INSOMNIA.

Insomnia is a term used to signify sleeplessness. Do not use drugs for this, as they are often very harmful and powerful. Moderate stimulation with some hot drink will help if weariness is the cause. A warm bath or some quieting occupation before retiring will often help.

First Aid and Home Treatment.

Hot Tea.—A cup of hot tea before retiring and the use of a pillow made of hops has a soothing effect.

Ginger Tea.—If the stomach is out of order, a cup of ginger tea will stimulate it and draw the blood from the head.

Hot Milk.—A cup of hot milk is quieting.

Cold Water.—Dip a cloth, folded several times, into cold water and apply to the forehead.

Heat.—Applications of heat to the abdomen and feet may give relief.

Vigorous Stretching.—Vigorous stretching until tired, will draw the blood from the head, and sleep will follow.

Exercise in a bathtub containing about a foot of cold water until feet are red, then wrap them in towels or blankets without drying, and go to bed.

Bathing the spine and abdomen with cold water and retiring without drying is soothing, but be sure to keep well covered.

The following method is a good one: Fill a large hot-water bottle with cold water and put it at the back of the head and neck against the pillow. It will give relief, then remove pillow and go to sleep. The room should be kept dark and a cloth folded and laid over the eyes.

Do not allow yourself to become excited just before going to bed.

Do not eat later than two hours before retiring. Be in the sunlight as much as possible.

Insomnia often brings on grayness, baldness, wrinkles, furrows, crow's feet and lines. If the patient awakens during the early morning hours, a light meal such as a cup of hot cocoa and a cracker, or cup of hot milk will induce sleep by drawing blood from the head to the stomach.

ITCH.

Itch is due to the presence of animal parasite and is contagious. This disease is accompanied by intense itching, generally between the fingers and on other tender parts of the body.

First Aid and Home Treatment.

Sulphur Bath.—A sulphur bath from 20 minutes to a half hour is generally advised. This is prepared by adding 4 ounces of potassium sulphide to about 35 gallons of tepid water.

Fresh Lard and Dry Mustard.—Cream together a cupful of fresh lard and a tablespoonful of dry mustard. Apply to the affected parts.

Synol Soap.—This is especially good. It can be bought at the drug store.

Sulphur Ointment.—Take a warm bath and scrub well with soft soap for twenty minutes, then lie in bath for half an hour, after being thoroughly rubbed dry, rub with a compound of sulphur ointment.

Baking Soda.—Plenty of baking soda in the bath water and an occasional dose of castor oil is very good.

Vaseline.—Vaseline is very effective.

Balm of Pine Balsam.—Six to ten drops taken with a little sugar is very effective.

Naphthol, Lanolin, Powdered Sulphur and Lard.—Take ½ dram of naphthol, ½ ounce of lanolin, 1 ounce of powdered sulphur and 4 ounces of lard.

IVY POISON.

DESCRIPTION.—This is an inflammation of the skin characterized by pronounced redness, pimples or blisters containing serum or pus and accompanied by swelling, severe burning and itching. It occurs more often on the face and hands, but after contact other parts of the body are also frequently affected.

First Aid and Home Treatment.

Bathe the poisoned parts with hot water and dry with care.

Ichthyol.—Spread ichthyol ointment on a cloth and bandage loosely or fasten securely with adhesive plaster. In case the face is poisoned, cut holes in the cloth for eyes, nose and mouth, and wear as a mask. This may be changed twice a day, using clean cloth and fresh ointment each time.

Carbolic Acid.—Use water to which a little carbolic acid is added to bathe the affected parts.

Boric Acid or Baking Soda.—One tablespoonful of boric acid dissolved in one pint of water or a teaspoonful of baking soda added to a tumblerful of water is a soothing lotion for bathing poisoned parts.

Bismuth Subnitrate or Lead Acetate.—Use dusting powders such as bismuth subnitrate or lead acetate.

Borax.—Wash affected parts with a solution of borax water using one teaspoonful of borax to one pint of warm water. Apply cold cream after using this solution.

Lye.—Bathe the poisoned parts in lye made of wood ashes and you will be relieved immediately.

Wood Ashes.—Dry wood ashes rubbed over affected parts will give relief.

Sugar of Lead.—Make a wash by mixing one-half ounce of sugar of lead in one pint of water. Dip a piece of cotton in the solution and apply.

JAUNDICE.

DESCRIPTION.—This is caused by the stopping-up of the gallduct, thus throwing bile into the blood which is carried throughout the circulation. It gives the whole body a yellow appearance. The bile passes into the circulation instead of into the intestines. This is due to several different causes, the principal of which are: congestion of the bile ducts, gallstones, overeating and drinking, anger, malaria or simply taking cold.

SYMPTOMS.—Temperature is usually low, pulse slow, with general debility. The skin becomes yellow and in bad cases takes on even an olive-green color. The whites of the eyes and all the mucous membranes take on the yellow appearance. The urine is of a saffron color, however, the discharge from the bowels is a pale, putty appearance, devoid of the natural brownish-yellow tint.

NURSING.—The patient should have rest, be kept on a milk diet, encouraged to drink plenty of water. The bowels should be kept open by means of small doses of calomel for a few days. As soon as action is obtained from the calomel the patient should be given some kind of mineral water or salts, such as seidlitz powder, phosphate of soda or rochelle salts to prevent the calomel from remaining in the system. A glass of water with a half a teaspoonful of common baking soda added is good taken before meals. It is well to consult a physician.

First Aid and Home Treatment.

Dandelion Greens.—Dandelion greens are good. A strong tea made from the roots and taken several times every day. This is very good for liver and bowels.

Boneset Tea.—Boneset tea is an excellent remedy for liver trouble. It should be taken three or four times during the day.

CONGESTION OF THE KIDNEYS.

There are two kinds of congestion of the kidneys—the acute and the chronic. The kidneys become distended and dark red. The urine is scanty and highly colored.

CAUSES.—The acute form is caused by injuries to the back, chilling of the skin, medicines such as turpentine, carbolic acid, alcohol, ether and other anesthetics. The chronic form comes from diseases of the liver, lungs, heart and from the acute. This is the more common form.

SYMPTOMS.—A slight fever, a tired feeling in the back or sometimes an ache in the back, urine scanty, highly colored, and has albumin in it.

NURSING.—One suffering with this disease should take absolute rest in bed, on a fluid diet, such as milk, broths, etc. Drink watermelon seed tea, pumpkin or flaxseed tea are also good. One may use injections of warm normal salt solutions into the bowels every day or so. It is also well to take a good sweat.

Make a tea from four ounces of roots and seeds of burdock to a quart of water. This may be taken internally.

Carrots are good for kidney trouble and should be eaten freely.

LICE.

DESCRIPTION.—There are several kinds of lice which infest the head and body of man, usually due to filth. They can be destroyed by thorough cleanliness, frequent bathing and by the following treatments:

First Aid and Home Treatment.

Louse-wort Seeds.—Crushed louse-wort seeds, made into a paste and rubbed on the head is effective.

Mercurial Ointment.—After bathing carefully with warm water and soap, rub mercurial ointment diluted with five times its bulk of lard, on the scalp or affected parts. It is better to leave some time intervene between bathing the head and applying this ointment, and do not apply too strongly or leave it on too long.

Kerosene and Lard.—Kerosene and lard rubbed well into the scalp is a good old remedy.

Sassafras Oil.—Sassafras oil rubbed on at night and washed off in the morning is good.

Larkspur.—Put on tincture of larkspur and tie the hair up in a large cloth for several hours. This is a harmless remedy. Shampoo thoroughly. Larkspur should not be taken internally or be left where children are likely to get it as it is poison.

Kerosene and Olive Oil.—Rub on equal parts of kerosene and olive oil or sweet oil. Saturate the hair and scalp thoroughly, tie up and leave for about twelve hours. Keep away from the fire. Wash well, dip comb in vinegar when hair is ready to comb.

MALARIA FEVER.

DESCRIPTION.—This is an infectious disease characterized by paroxysms of chills, fever and sweating. It is caused by the entrance into the system of an animal parasite which is transmitted from the sick to the well by the bite of a certain kind of mosquito. It occurs more often in low lands and swampy places and in the warmer sections of the country. There are three varieties: intermittent, remittent and chronic.

SYMPTOMS.—The symptoms of **Intermittent Fever** are paroxysms of chills, fever and sweating. These paroxysms recur at regular intervals but the length of time between attacks may vary in different cases. Usually at the same hour every day or every other day. During these intervals the patient's temperature is almost normal. This is the commonest form and is sometimes called ague.

Remittent Fever is more severe than intermittent fever. The attacks of chills, fever and sweating occur in regular order but there is very little or no recession of fever. The intervals are sometimes irregular and the paroxysms last longer. Sometimes the chills do not take place and after the "hot stage" the temperature falls gradually.

Pernicious Malaria Fever is practically the same as ordinary ague and remittent fever except that it is much more severe in every respect. The patient may lose consciousness very soon, perhaps due to the great amount of poison and its effect on the brain. The fever is very high, the skin hot and dry. Vomiting and purging are also marked symptoms. The disease may prove fatal in a short time.

NURSING.—The patient should be screened from mosquitoes to prevent spreading of the disease. He should be put to bed and when the chill comes on be well covered and hot-water bottles, irons, etc., be put to his feet and armpits. When the hot stage comes on the fever may be reduced by applying cold compresses to the head and by sponge baths or alcohol rubs. Give a cathartic to keep the bowels open. Give plenty of pure water and keep kidneys active. If there is danger of congestion apply hot poultices across the back. Bathe the patient frequently to cleanse the body of waste matter thrown off through the pores. Give nourishing food, when there is much fever give liquid diet.

First Aid and Home Treatment.

Quinine.—Quinine is probably the best treatment. Take five grains four or five times a day on days the chills and fever occur. In milder form, a smaller dose may be taken.

Lemons.—Make an infusion of two sliced lemons, four tablespoonfuls of sugar and one quart of boiling water; cool and drink often.

Salt.—Common salt, one dessertspoonful in a glass of water.

Boneset, Pennyroyal, Catnip or Ginger.—During chills give hot boneset, pennyroyal, catnip or ginger tea.

Dogwood.—Use one-half ounce of dogwood root and one pint water, boiled down to one-half pint. Give two tablespoonfuls every two hours.

MEASLES.

DESCRIPTION.—Measles is a highly infectious and contagious disease, sparing practically no exposed person who has not had it. It is especially common among children, and one attack usually protects them from a second attack, however, persons sometimes have a second and even a third attack. It occurs more often and more severely in cold weather, as people are more closely crowded together and conditions are more unsanitary. The infection is spread by the secretions of the nose, mouth, throat and by one coming in direct contact with one coming down with the disease. It may also be spread by a third person. It is well to keep a child who is known to have the disease well isolated till he has entirely recovered.

INCUBATION.—The period of incubation as a rule is from 10 to 20 days.

SYMPTOMS.—In the average case of measles the symptoms very much resemble those of a common cold. The child feels drowsy, irritable and complains of chilly sensations, headache and there is some fever. The eyes become red and watery, nose runs, the throat feels parched and dry and an irritating cough increases the discomfort. If the throat is examined the hard palate will be found to be a dull red color, little red spots may be found on it. If closely examined there will be found little white-tipped red spots on the lining membrane of the cheeks. At night the irritation increases, the child is feverish, tosses about a great deal and asks for water often. This continues for three or four days as a rule. About the fourth day the eruption appears first on the forehead, face and neck and in 24 hours extends all over the surface of the body. At first it appears as small red spots but soon enlarges into blotches leaving distinct white portions of skin between, later these blotches assume a crescent shape. This eruption remains at its height about two days and then begins to fade, in the order of its appearance. In two or three days the eruption will have disappeared and the skin will then begin to peel off in bran-like scales which lasts from a week to ten days.

COMPLICATIONS.—The most common and most fatal of all complications is broncho-pneumonia. This usually follows taking of cold from being exposed to draughts. Bronchitis and diarrhea are also frequent complications.

SEQUELAE.—Weak eyes is often a result of inflammation of the eyes caused by allowing the patient to read while suffering with the disease or by exposing the eyes to too bright a light. This is often very serious sometimes resulting in total loss of sight. Impaired hearing and chronic catarrh also very often follow an attack of measles.

NURSING.—A child with measles should be put to bed and kept there, in a room by itself and other children kept away. This should be done early as soon as he shows any symptoms of the disease as measles are particularly infectious during the incubation period. The room should be kept slightly darkened and the eyes well shaded as long as they show any signs of weakness. The child should be kept warm, however, the covers should not be too heavy as he may become too warm throwing the bedding off, thus taking cold. The room should be well ventilated. Do not allow the child to read, and the eyes should be bathed with warm water containing boric acid. If the eruption appears delayed or for any reason is driven in, which may be caused by chilling, give the patient hot drinks such as lemonade, saffron tea, etc., causing him to sweat. When this is done, great care should be taken that he does not cool off too rapidly. The food should be light, consisting chiefly of nutritious broths, milk, soft-boiled eggs, etc. Allow the patient to have all the cool water he wants to drink. Lemonade is very beneficial and relieves the inflammation of the throat; however, too much should not be taken at once as it may cause the patient to chill. When the fever and cough are gone, the child may be allowed to get up and be about the room but should not exercise too violently as the heart muscle is often weakened. The diet may be increased when the fever is gone, to good, plain strong food. The nurse should be particularly careful to guard against the complications and after-effects of this disease, as measles is not so dangerous in itself   It is the complications such as broncho-pneumonia that are dangerous. It is unnecessary to have a doctor for this disease unless complications develop. Take good care of the patient and use the simple first aid and home treatments given on page 237.

First Aid and Home Treatment.

Hot Teas.—To aid in bringing out the rash, drink plenty of hot lemonade, saffron tea, etc.

Flaxseed Tea.—To relieve the cough, drink freely of flaxseed tea with a little sugar and lemon juice. Or just sugar and lemon juice.

Baking Soda.—To relieve the irritation of the skin, sponge the patient with warm water containing baking soda.

Alcohol.—If the fever is very high and the patient restless, sponge him off with tepid water containing alcohol or soda.

Boric Acid.—For inflammation of the eyes, drop a little luke warm boric acid water into the eyes several times a day.

Castor Oil.—In case of diarrhea give castor oil or blackberry root tea.

In case of broncho-pneumonia, or other complications develop, use the treatments given for those diseases. Call a physician.

Hoarhound.—For cough after measles, steep hoarhound, make a syrup and give freely.

Talcum Powder or Corn Starch.—To relieve the itching dust with talcum powder or corn starch.

Elder Blossoms.—Make a strong tea of elder blossoms, sweeten and give warm; one teaspoonful every hour.

Mustard.—If the rash recedes, give a warm mustard bath. Rub hands and feet gently with fat to remove heat and tightness caused by the rash.

MEASLES—GERMAN.

DESCRIPTION.—This is a mild but infectious, contagious disease, resembling measles in many points, but quite distinct from them. Children of any age may have it, but it is not likely to be contracted by infants under six months. Very seldom do complications arise, or after-effects of any serious nature follow.

INCUBATION.—It generally develops in from eight to sixteen days after exposure.

SYMPTOMS.—Very often the first symptom to appear is the rash, much like that in true measles, which comes on the face first and then spreads rapidly over the entire body. At the end of the first day the body is generally covered by the rash. In the course of two or three days it fades away and is followed by a slight scaling of bran-like scales. This is accompanied by slight fever, mild catarrhal symptoms and often by swelling of the glands of the neck.

CHARACTERISTICS.—The most distinguishing characteristic of this disease, and one which serves to tell it from true measles or scarlet fever, when the rash somewhat resembles these diseases, is the swelling of the glands at the sides and back of the neck.

NURSING.—Until the disease is really known and one is sure that it is nothing more serious, the child should be kept in a room by itself, apart from the rest of the family. After the disease is definitely known there is very little need of special diet or nursing. Keep the bowels open with mild cathartics, and be sure to keep the child from taking cold. As long as there is any fever the diet should be light, consisting principally of milk and broths.

First Aid and Home Treatment.

Hot Teas.—Give hot teas, such as sage, pennyroyal, saffron, etc., to bring out the rash.

Hot Lemonade.—This is good to bring out the rash and is also refreshing to the child.

Cocoa Butter or Olive Oil.—The body may be rubbed gently with either of these to allay itching.

Caution.—Don't let the child go out too soon, even though it is not very sick, as serious results have often followed, especially if the child takes cold.

MUMPS.

DESCRIPTION.—Mumps are an acute, infectious and contagious disease of children, usually affecting those of from two to fourteen years of age, although children of all ages, and sometimes adults, may have them. They are characterized by the swelling of the glands at the sides of the face and neck which are called parotid glands. Other glands of the body are also affected. They are generally contracted by direct exposure, although they may be carried by clothing, or by a third party. It is not as contagious a disease as some others, and, although a child may be exposed to it, it is not at all certain that he will contract the disease. They are contagious from the very beginning to the end of the attack. One attack gives immunity.

INCUBATION.—The average time for the disease to develop after exposure is from seven to fourteen days.

SYMPTOMS.—In most cases swelling of the glands is the first symptom, however, there may be pains in the back and legs and considerable fever, also pain on moving the jaws before the swelling is noticed. The disease may just affect one side; both sides may be affected at once, or one side several days after the other side. The pain is generally most severe at the lower back part of the jaw and just below the ear. The swelling extends upwards back of the ear and forward in front of the ear and onto the face. The most prominent part of the swelling being as a rule about the lobe of the ear, causing it to stand out from the side of the head. The pain is often very severe on trying to eat, and especially on taking acids such as vinegar or lemon juice into the mouth. The temperature is generally from 100 to 102° F. The mouth, as a rule, is dry, can be opened but very little making the child very uncomfortable.

COMPLICATIONS.—Complications are very infrequent with this disease. Sometimes the swelling extends to other glandular organs of the body, such as the generative organs, and in boys and men this is often very severe. Kidney disease may follow a case of the mumps, but is very rare. One should be very careful not to take cold.

NURSING.—As the disease is contagious, the child should be put in bed in a room by himself, kept there while there is any fever, and confined to one room while the swelling lasts. The bowels must be kept open by some simple laxative, such as magnesia. The diet should be simple, consisting of milk, broths, gruels, etc., while the fever lasts. No solid foods or acid fruits, or other sour things, should be given as they increase the pain. The nose, mouth and throat should be kept clean with some mild antiseptic wash. The patient should also be given frequent drinks of cool water to relieve the dry condition of the mouth and throat.

First Aid and Home Treatment.

Very little treatment is necessary in this disease. Local treatment, such as the application of hot packs to the swollen glands, will often give much relief.

Camphorated Oil.—Camphorated oil on a piece of flannel is a good application.

Herb Teas.—If the pain is severe, drink freely of herb teas and cause sweating. Keep the feet warm.

Hops.—Hops applied to the parts in the form of a poultice will often give much relief.

NEURALGIA.

DESCRIPTION.—Neuralgia is a painful nerve affection due to a condition of debility following disease, worry, lead poisoning, overwork, lack of sleep and rest. Such diseases as diabetes, nephritis, syphilis, and uterine diseases are especially predisposing causes. Different names are given to the disease according to its location in the body, such as facial, hemicrania, or that affecting the side of the head, sciatic or that of the hip, angina pectoris, chiefly a neuralgic affection of the heart. Probably the most common form is that of facial neuralgia resulting from decayed teeth.

NURSING.—The main thing in treating this disease is to remove the causes. Keep up the general health. Get out in the fresh air and breathe deeply. Do not bundle up and sit by the fire. If the teeth are decayed or are giving any trouble, they should be taken care of at once. Anything that tends to build up the general health, and free the system of poison, will help cure neuralgia and prevent its recurrence. There are many simple treatments which may be applied locally and which will give much relief. The pain is often very severe and everything possible should be done to lessen it. It is well to have a thorough examination by a physician to locate the cause.

First Aid and Home Treatment.

Hot Flannel.—A piece of flannel wrung out of hot water and applied to the affected part will give relief.

Cold Cloths or Ice Bag.—Cloths wrung out of cold water or an ice bag are also good.

Black Pepper and Yoke of Egg.—A plaster made of one teaspoonful of black pepper and the yoke of an egg, mixed, makes a good application.

Cayenne Pepper and Vinegar.—Mix cayenne pepper and vinegar to a paste and spread on a piece of cloth and apply to the affected part.

Effervescing Salts.—Take a large dose of effervescing salts.

Horse Radish Leaves.—Neuralgia of the head or body is effectively relieved by a poultice made of wilted horse radish leaves tied to the bottom of the foot, outside of the stocking, as the leaves next to the skin will blister. The leaf is prepared by placing it in a hot frying pan over the fire and turning occasionally till well wilted. Apply as directed.

Ground Mustard and Lard.—Ground mustard mixed with lard is a good substitute for horse radish.

Lemon Juice.—Cut a lemon in two, squeeze the juice on the affected parts and rub in, after which place hot cloths over the place.

Hot Salt or Vinegar.—A small sack of hot salt applied to the place of pain, or to steam the place with vinegar is effective.

Quinine.—Two grains of quinine several times a day for two days followed by a cathartic is good. The cathartic is to remove the quinine from the system. This remedy is especially good when neuralgia is due to malarial conditions.

Vinegar, Mustard, Peppermint and Egg.—The following is a good simple remedy: One pint of vinegar, one-fourth ounce oil of mustard, one ounce oil of peppermint and the white of one egg. Beat the egg and stir all together.

PERITONITIS—ACUTE.

DESCRIPTION.—This is an acute inflammation of the peritoneum which is the membrane that lines the walls of the abdominal cavity and surrounds the intestines. One of the most common causes in both sexes is appendicitis. However, it may develop from any one of the following causes: hernia, external or internal, a blow on the abdomen, perforation of the abdomen by a foreign body, operation upon the abdomen, by the inflammation of other organs of the abdominal cavity extending to the peritoneum, typhoid fever in case the bowels are perforated, erysipelas, etc.

SYMPTOMS.—The acute form generally begins with a sudden chill, severe pain in the abdomen which at first seems general, however, soon becomes localized to the region of the navel. The abdomen is rigid, bloated and very tender. In order to diminish the tension, the patient generally lies on the back with the knees drawn up. The pulse is small, rapid, wiry. Temperature at first runs as high as 103 or 104 degrees F. and then later drops to about 101 degrees F. There is vomiting which generally sets in early in the disease. The ordinary contents of the stomach are first thrown up, then later the vomit becomes a characteristic green and still later a brownish black with a very offensive odor. Thirst is intense, mouth and tongue dry and parched. When these symptoms become fully developed the face has a characteristic appearance, the eyes are sunken, temples hollow, ears cold, forehead rough and dry, the face is tinged with a dark blue color. This disease generally runs its course in a very short time, often terminating fatally in from three to five days and sometimes sooner.

NURSING.—The weight of the bed clothes should be relieved by means of a cradle or support over the abdomen. Pillows may be placed under the knees to hold the legs up and thus relieve the strain. Hot fomentations or poultices may be applied to the abdomen to relieve the inflammation. The thirst may be relieved by allowing the patient to hold little pieces of ice in his mouth or by rinsing the mouth with water to which has been added a little lemon juice. Keep the patient quiet and relieve the suffering as much as possible.

It is very often necessary to have an operation performed for when the disease is left to run its course it almost always results fatally.

First Aid and Home Treatment.

Give enema of hot water and soap suds to empty the bowels. Bathe the feet in hot water.

Hot Compress.—Apply a piece of flannel wrung out of hot water to the abdomen.

Cold Compress.—Wring a piece of flannel out of cold water and apply to the affected part.

Alcohol.—Keep the patient quiet by rubbing and sponging often with alcohol.

PILES.

DESCRIPTION.—These are varicose veins or tumors about the anus. There are two kinds, the external or the "blind piles" and the internal or "bleeding piles." The external are the less important. There are a great variety of causes which bring about these formations and no class of persons are exempt. The main causes are constipation and pregnancy, however, they may be brought on by excessive smoking, rich diet, sedentary occupation, violent, prolonged, exercise, etc.

SYMPTOMS.—There is a sensation of fullness and pulsation in the anus, itching of a very annoying nature, and the anus is a little swollen and tender. In case of internal piles there is generally bleeding from the anus which is increased by movement of the bowels. Sometimes these protrude and in these cases are very painful.

NURSING.—As a rule, these will disappear with very simple treatment, however, if neglected may become very severe. In the first place secure proper and regular action of the bowels as constipation is one of the main causes. This should be done by means of a mild laxative. There should be rest, light diet, reduction of smoking and the application of a sedative and astringent ointment or lotion to the affected parts.

First Aid and Home Treatment.

Mentholatum.—Mentholatum applied to parts affected is very good.

Flowers of Sulphur and Vaseline.—Take one dram of flowers of sulphur and one tablespoonful of vaseline. Mix and apply several times a day.

Crushed Cranberries.—Crushed Cranberries are beneficial.

Lard and Smart Weed.—Take one ounce of lard and one-fourth ounce of smart weed and boil. Apply several times a day.

Witch-Hazel.—Witch-hazel applied externally is good. Use as an injection for bleeding piles.

Salt.—Use injections of salt water.

Keep the bowels open with mild laxatives such as compound licorice powder, cascara, etc.

PIMPLES AND BLACKHEADS.

To get rid of pimples regulate the bowels, take laxative if necessary. Wash the face with hot water and pure soap three times a day for several days, then once a day, being careful to use a clean wash cloth each time, and rinse the face thoroughly, changing the water several times. After removing all traces of soap, rinse in cold water to close the pores, and dry gently but thoroughly.

When the pimple comes to a head, pick it with a needle which has been dipped in boiling water or an antiseptic solution, and gently force out the pus using a piece of cotton or clean cloth. Sponge off with hydrogen peroxide, salt water or other antiseptic solution. Cold cream may be used occasionally and wiped off with a soft cloth.

Eat simple foods avoiding those which are rich and greasy; do not overeat, drink water freely, take plenty of outdoor exercise and breathe fresh air.

Blood Purifier.—One cupful of molasses, one teaspoonful of cream of tartar and enough sulphur to make as thick as cake batter. Take one-half tablespoonful each day for three days, skip three days and resume.

Lemons, Cream of Tartar and Sulphur.—Take the juice of two lemons, one-half ounce cream of tartar and one-half ounce pulverized sulphur. Mix and pour boiling water over the mixture and stir thoroughly. Take a wineglassful every morning.

A little cream of tartar in a glass of water, taken each morning is beneficial.

Use one-half teaspoonful powdered alum in one pint of water and sponge the face. Sponge the face in hot water in which two teaspoonsful of borax is dissolved.

In case of blackheads, steam the face to soften the skin and gently press out the large blackheads. Rinse in cold water to close the pores.

PLEURISY.

DESCRIPTION.—This is an inflammation of the pleura, which is the delicate membrane surrounding the lungs. It often presents two forms, the chronic and the acute, and is caused by exposure to cold or by wounds which have injured the pleura. It may also follow infectious diseases, inflammatory rheumatism, pneumonia, etc. It is very likely to be confused with bronchitis or pneumonia. However, it may be distinguished from bronchitis, since there is very little coughing in pleurisy, and also on account of the peculiar, sharp, piercing pain. It can be distinguished from pneumonia as there is very little fever, little difficulty in breathing and no rusty expectoration, which symptoms are all prominent in pneumonia.

SYMPTOMS.—When the disease results from exposure to severe cold, which is the commonest cause, the onset is usually sudden. There is a sense of chilliness, sharp pain at or near the nipple of the affected side, little fever, no expectoration, cough short and dry, the patient coughing as little as possible, as coughing increases the suffering. The tongue is sometimes slightly coated, appetite impaired and bowels inactive.

NURSING.—The patient should be put into a warm bed and given a good sweat in order to relieve the congestion and equalize the circulation. The sweat should be given as described in the chapter on nursing. Great care should be used that the patient does not take cold. Keep the bowels open and the kidneys active by a good cathartic. A counter-irritant, such as a mustard poultice, may be applied to the affected side. A hot fomentation of hops, catnip or oats will often give much relief. These must be applied hot and kept hot, great care being taken not to get the night gown or the bedding wet so that the patient might be chilled. He should be made comfortable and kept quiet, given good nourishing food and plenty of fresh air. The room should be well ventilated. In order to lessen the movement of the pleura, in breathing, and thus lessen the pain, it is well to use a tight binder around the body. This is placed around the chest, just under the arms, extending down as low as the lower border of the ribs. Adhesive plaster may be used instead of a binder.

First Aid and Home Treatment.

Flaxseed Meal and Hops.—Poultices of flaxseed meal and hops, applied hot and kept hot, will give much relief.

Salt.—Hot salt bags applied will do good.

Prickly Ash Bark.—Boil two ounces of prickly ash bark in two pints of water, strain, cool and give one tablespoonful four or five times a day.

PNEUMONIA.

This term may be applied to any inflammatory process affecting the lung tissues. However, it is usually applied to a specific general infection of the air passages or vesicles of the lungs of bacterial origin. It is communicated from one to another through the spray blown from the mouth while coughing and through the dried expectoration. Men are more subject to it than women, and it is more prevalent among children under 4 years of age and adults between the ages of 45 and 65 years. It is not a disease of winter, but rather of spring and that of late spring more especially. There are two main forms as given below.

Broncho-Pneumonia or Catarrhal Pneumonia are names applied to that form of disease affecting especially the smaller bronchi and their distribution. This is the kind that usually affects children.

Acute-Lobar, Fibrinous, or Croupous-Pneumonia are terms applied to that form of the disease which affects and involves large continuous tracts of lung tissue, such as an entire lobe or the greater part of a lobe.

INCUBATION.—This is from a few hours to a few days. Often there is really no incubation period, the patient becoming sick soon after exposure.

SYMPTOMS.—In general the symptoms are much like those of a continued fever setting in after an incubation period of short duration. There are chills, headache, pain in the affected side, usually near the nipple, loss of appetite, constipation, high temperature, rapid pulse, difficult breathing, shallow, and irregular, a cough and finally expectoration of a peculiar kind. However, these symptoms, may be preceded by hours and sometimes days of general prostration, loss of appetite, constipation, languor, headache, dull pains in various parts of the body, chills and flashes of heat alternating.

The onset may be sudden, accompanied by a violent chill, racking headache, thick coated tongue, foul breath, nausea and vomiting, and delirium. Very soon after these symptoms set in, there will be signs of consolidation of the lung.

The more typical cases begin with sharp chest pains, quick shallow breathing, the nostrils expanding with the inhalation, hard dry cough, usually suppressed on account of the pain it causes, the skin is dry and hot, temperature often runs to 104 or 105 degrees, a deep hectic flush settling on one or the other cheek. Soon there will be a marked difference between the affected side and the sound side.

There is little or no expectoration when the cough first begins, however, it soon begins to come up and is generally attended with much pain and suffering. At first it is usually of a frothy, colorless bronchitic character. It may also be rust colored, semi-clear and very viscid as in acute-lobar-pneumonia. The color is due to the presence of blood corpuscles in it. It may also be dark, watery and offensive, resembling prune juice. This is often so in unfavorable cases. In the final stages the sputum becomes mere frothy mucus.

The nervous system may also be affected, the patient showing signs of restlessness, sleeplessness, wandering of the mind or delirium.

In children, the symptoms may differ to quite an extent from those in adults. There may be convulsions at the onset of the disease, the temperature running very high. There may also be a slight rash or blush like scarlatina over the body, vomiting, diarrhea, abdominal pain and tenderness. In the aged it is very fatal, the heart often being unable to stand the strain of the disease, death coming from heart failure.

COMPLICATIONS.—A number of serious complications are likely to develop with this disease, the most important of which are:

Pleuritis—in which the inflammation extends to the pleura. When the pleura is much affected in this way, the disease is often called pleuro-pneumonia.

Chronic congestion of the kidneys may develop or follow as an after-effect.

Bronchitis is very common in the young and the aged.

Pericarditis and Endocarditis, diseases of the heart, are very rare, yet very serious complications.

Spinal Meningitis, in the epidemic form, very often follows the disease, especially croupous-pneumonia.

Pulmonary Consumption frequently follows an attack of catarrhal pneumonia.

NURSING.—This is a constitutional disease, self-limited in duration and should be treated in general as other infectious fevers. As the disease is contagious, the patient should be isolated. He should be put to bed as early as possible in a large, airy, warm, well lighted room. Pure air, sunlight and warmth are the most powerful remedies which can be applied.

The nursing is also of the greatest importance. As the disease is self-limited the nurse must do all within her power to sustain life till it has run its course. Economize the patient's strength as much as possible. Do not lift him up or turn him from side to side any more than is absolutely necessary. Raising him up may cause heart failure. He must refrain from talking as this is hard on the respiration or breathing and may cause fits of coughing. He must have absolute quiet and rest.

A cold bath which not only reduces the fever, but quiets the respirations and soothes the patient is often ordered by the physician. As the cold bath is often hard to give and inconvenient, the patient may be given a sponge bath of vinegar and tepid water, one part in four, which is a useful modification of the cold bath.

At the very beginning of the disease, great good may be done by giving the patient a good sweat. Place hot water bottles at the feet and around the body or hot irons may be used, then give the patient all the hot lemonade he can drink until he sweats freely. Hot fomentations of hops, corn meal and vinegar or hot linseed meal poultices may also be applied to the chest and back. These should be changed often so as to keep them hot. A little mustard may be added to these poultices which will cause a more decided counter-irritation. The corn-sweat may be given, which is done by packing around the patient ears of corn which have been placed in boiling water till they are steaming hot. The ears should be wrapped in cloths and packed around the body from the waist up, and also at the feet. In any case where the sweating treatment is used, great care must be taken that the patient does not catch cold. Onion poultices may also be applied to the chest. Rub the chest with turpentine and lard or apply turpentine stupes. Camphorated oil is also good.

The cough may be relieved by allowing the patient to sip cold water or half ounce each of glycerine and lemon juice mixed with an ounce of water. A teaspoonful sipped occasionally will relieve the cough.

The diet is of great importance. The food should be given in liquid form, very nourishing, easily digested, given in moderate quantities and at rather short intervals. The total amount per day should not exceed 3½ pints of liquid. If the stomach is very weak and irritated, equal parts of whey and egg water can be borne better than anything else. The egg water is made by stirring the whites of two or four eggs in a pint of cold water. The solution should then be strained. Milk and soda water, carbonized water, peptonized milk, strained mutton broth are nourishing and make good beverages. Egg-flip is a good food and stimulant combined. However, raw meat juice is not only very nourishing, but, mixed with a little port wine, makes a powerful restorative.

Tea with milk or cream and a little toast may also be given. As the patient's strength increases, he may be given custards, puddings, cream toast, eggs, etc. Cold water may be given in addition freely. The patient should not be allowed to suffer from thirst.

The vital points in the nursing and treatment are to conserve the patient's strength, relieve the congestion and keep the heart going, till the disease has run its course.

First Aid and Home Treatment.

Hot Foot Bath and Hot Lemonade.—On the first sign of pneumonia, which starts with a cold, break it up by taking a hot foot bath for half an hour and drink hot lemonade or flaxseed tea flavored with lemon or licorice root. Go to bed and keep warm.

Purge.—A brisk purge is very beneficial.

Camphorated Oil.—Rub the chest and nostrils with camphorated oil.

Peroxide of Hydrogen.—If the throat is sore, gargle or spray with peroxide of hydrogen, one part to three parts of water. Use often.

Cold Compress.—Apply cold compresses or cloths, saturated with equal parts of water and alcohol, to the throat. Cover with dry cloths.

PTOMAINE POISONING.

This is a form of inflammation of the small intestine which requires special mention. It comes from eating poisoned food such as tinned, preserved and potted meats, putrifying meat, over-ripe fruit, etc. An hour or two maybe twenty-four hours after the food has been taken into the stomach, the patient will become restless, complaining of nausea and sickness. This will soon be followed by vomiting and abdominal pain which often becomes very agonizing. There may be cramps of the muscles especially in the legs. Soon there is intense prostration, cold sweats, nervous depression and heart failure. Diarrhea develops early and is very profuse, watery and sometimes bloody. The temperature is high, pulse quick, urine scanty. If the dose of poison has been large and has not been quickly removed by vomiting and diarrhea, the patient may soon lapse into a state of unconsciousness and coma. The severity of the symptoms varies not only with the amount of the poison taken but may also vary with the individual. A number of people partaking of the same meal may have symptoms varying in severity. It does not affect all the same. The symptoms may begin to abate in an hour or so, however, convalescence is usually very slow.

NURSING.—This must be treated as a case of poisoning. The offending substance should be removed from the stomach at once by means of an emetic or the stomach pump. Give the patient a glass of warm water (lukewarm) to which a teaspoonful of common table salt has been added, causing him to vomit. As soon as this one has been thrown up, another glassful should be given at once and when that has been thrown up, he should be given another, and this time a mustard poultice should be put on the abdomen at once in order to keep the salt water down and quiet the stomach. He should then be given a good dose of Rochelle or Epsom salts, put to bed and kept warm. It may be necessary to apply hot bricks or irons to the feet. Of course, in all cases of this kind a physician should be called as quickly as possible, as the trouble may terminate seriously in a very short time.

RHEUMATISM (Muscular, Chronic and Sciatic).

As rheumatism is due to the presence of bacteria in the system and as the presence of these bacteria is due to infection of the mouth, throat, tonsils, etc., the first thing to do is to do away with the conditions which promote the development of these bacteria. See that the mouth, throat and tonsils are kept in a good healthy condition and that the resistance of the body be kept at its highest point. There is no specific cure for rheumatism; however, good nursing and the application of simple remedies will give much relief.

Very beneficial effects have been obtained by some from baths taken at the various places indicated below: Hot Springs, Arkansas; Mt. Clemens and Battle Creek, Michigan; Waukesha, Wisconsin; Virginia and Banff, Canada. There are other places, however these are the most noted.

RHEUMATISM—MUSCULAR.

DESCRIPTION.—Muscular rheumatism is an affection of one or a group of muscles. It may occur in any muscle, but it usually affects those used most. When it affects the large muscles in the "small of the back," those constantly used in supporting the body, it is known as lumbago. It sometimes affects the large muscles at side of the head, behind the ear, and is then commonly called "stiff neck." The disease often affects the large muscles of the chest used in breathing and the pain caused resembles that of pleurisy and is often mistaken for that disease.

SYMPTOMS.—When the form of the disease is very mild there may be soreness and stiffness, which, if the body be kept in one position for some time, may cause pain in certain muscles when changing the position. This is relieved by using or exercising the muscles affected. In more severe cases, the pain comes on suddenly. When the muscles of the back are affected, it is much as though one had sprained his back. Sometimes it is almost impossible to move for a time. When the muscles of the neck are affected, it causes the head to lean toward the affected side as this lessens the pain by relaxing the tension.

NURSING.—Make the affected parts as comfortable as possible by complete relaxation and by assuming a restful position. The application of hot and cold packs to the affected parts will often give much relief. Also a good sweat may give much relief.

Those with a tendency to rheumatism should always keep the feet warm and dry and avoid damp clothing. If warm or sweaty, do not cool off too quickly. Never sleep in a bed that is damp or one that has not been aired for some time. One troubled much with rheumatism should live in a warm dry climate, keep the bowels and kidneys in good condition and avoid colds.

RHEUMATISM—CHRONIC.

DESCRIPTION.—This is a disease of the joints and the tissues or membranes connecting, lining and surrounding them. It comes on slowly, insidiously and persistently. Inherited constitutional conditions often predispose one to its attacks. It is also common to persons who have suffered from exposure and hard labor.

SYMPTOMS.—The disease is characterized in the beginning by slight stiffness of the joints, usually more noticeable after a rest. There is also pain and soreness which is more severe in damp weather. These symptoms increase as the disease advances, the joints becoming stiff, and in time may become deformed. As a rule there is no fever or discoloration. The appetite is good and the digestion normal.

NURSING.—The pouring of hot water continuously over the affected parts for some time will give much relief. Hot water baths, vapor baths, hot dry air baths and mineral baths will all give relief.

There are numerous liniments and local treatments which will often give much relief. It is not necessary to name all of these here. However, such liniments as contain oil of wintergreen, oil of turpentine, oil of sassafras, ammonia and laudanum diluted with soap are beneficial. Where there is considerable pain, chloroform or aconite liniment may be applied.

RHEUMATISM—SCIATIC

DESCRIPTION.—This is an inflammation of the sciatic nerve which extends from the hip down the back part of the leg branching into the foot. This nerve is the largest nerve in the body, supplying the entire lower limb. The disease is often very severe and persistent. It may be brought on by any of the numerous conditions which cause other forms of rheumatism or neuralgia. The main and most immediate causes are, getting overheated and cooling off too rapidly, undue exposure to wet and cold, etc.

SYMPTOMS.—Pain in the hip, back part of the knee, the heel, in fact the entire course of the sciatic nerve may be affected. It may be more severe in one of these points at the beginning, then suddenly attack another point or the whole limb may be affected. The pain is very severe and persistent.

NURSING.—Absolute rest in bed. As the cause of the disease is inflammation of the sciatic nerve or surrounding tissues, the simplest treatment and one which often gives much relief, is the application of counter-irritants to the parts affected. A mustard plaster may be used for this purpose. Fly blisters are also used. Application of hot fomentations of hops and vinegar, hot and cold packs (alternate application) will all give relief.

First Aid and Home Treatment.

Porous Plaster.—Use porous plaster or rubber tissue about nine inches wide and long enough to go across the back and around the side. Put over painful part and cover with a hot water bottle or hot applications. Keep on a couple of days.

Hot Applications.—If severe, cover with flannel and apply a hot water bottle or other hot applications.

Baking Soda.—A teaspoonful of baking soda dissolved in a glass of cold water taken several times a day is very good.

Salt Water.—Warm salt water baths are good.

Salicylate of Soda.—Salicylate of soda, three drams; simple elixir, three ounces. Take one teaspoonful after each meal, dissolved in one-half tumblerful of water. This aids in eliminating uric acid.

Coal Oil and Gum Camphor.—One pint of coal oil and ten cents worth of gum camphor. When mixed the oil will dissolve the camphor. This is good and inexpensive.

Oil of Wintergreen and Olive Oil.—Oil of wintergreen, two ounces, and olive oil, two ounces, used externally is beneficial, and is especially good in such forms as stiff neck and lumbago.

Sun Baths.—Sun baths are very good for rheumatism.

Alcohol.—When the muscles are stiff take a hot bath and rub vigorously with alcohol.

Vapor Bath.—Much relief is obtained by vapor baths and by sweating.

Hot Fomentations.—The applications of hot fomentations such as hops and vinegar, heavy towels wrung out of hot water (about a gallon) to which a cupful of vinegar has been added, or use the hot water alone.

Turpentine.—Hot turpentine stupes applied will give much relief.

Liniments.—Liniments such as chloroform liniment, camphor liniment or those containing oil of turpentine, oil of sassafras, etc., are all beneficial.

RHEUMATISM.

(Rheumatic Fever, Acute Articular and Inflammatory Rheumatism.)

DESCRIPTION.—Rheumatic fever, acute rheumatism and inflammatory rheumatism are practically the same. They are an inflammation of the fibrous membrane of the joints and are characterized by pain, redness and swelling of the joints affected and general fever. There has been a great deal of difference of opinion as to the cause or origin of the disease. The conditions of the system which are predisposing causes of the disease are often hereditary. It is also particularly prevalent in cold damp seasons and climate. At least one form of the disease is thought to be caused by an excess of a substance called fibrin in the blood. It is also generally believed that the attack is often caused by diseased tonsils, tonsilitis being a predisposing cause. All ages are subject to the disease, however, it is more common among adults and rarely affects children under five years of age.

SYMPTOMS.—The disease comes on suddenly, however, it may be preceded by sore throat, fever, and pain in the joints. The joints rapidly become red, swollen and painful. It may not affect all of them at one time, but as it leaves one joint it quickly appears in another. Sometimes only one joint is affected. Although there is often much fever, the temperature ranging from 102 to 104 degrees F. There is often profuse sweating, the perspiration having an acid odor. The urine is generally scanty, highly colored and strongly acid.

As a rule it affects the larger joints: the knees, elbows, ankles, wrists and hips. The pain is often little noticed when the patient is perfectly quiet, however, it is very severe on the slightest movement rendering the patient almost helpless. The disease often affects the heart, especially in the young, this being indicated by difficulty of breathing, feeble though rapid and jerky pulse and violent, panicky heart action.

NURSING.—The patient should be put to bed in a warm, sunny room, upstairs room preferable, as dampness and darkness aid the disease. The room should be kept at an even temperature, about 68 degrees F and the patient guarded well against draughts. Soft pillows should be arranged about and under the affected parts so as to make the patient as comfortable as possible. The joints affected may be wrapped in cotton batting. They may also be protected from the weight of the bed clothes by the use of "cradles" or supports. It is well to use blankets on the bed and for the patient to wear a flannel night-gown as muslin becomes very wet and cold with the perspiration. The nurse must be very careful not to move the patient unnecessarily or jar the bed in any way as often the slightest movement causes much pain to the patient. Even one walking across the floor affects the patient. Also one should exercise the greatest patience and gentleness with one affected with this disease. The heart action must be watched carefully as it is often seriously affected, especially in the young, and in most cases where the disease results fatally, it is due to heart failure. If the disease affects the heart, the attending physician must be notified at once. The patient should not be allowed to eat more than just enough to satisfy the hunger. The food should be very simple and such as will easily digest, milk, soups, egg-nog, etc. The patient should be encouraged to drink as much water as possible.

First Aid and Home Treatment.

Cathartic.—Give a cathartic to keep the bowels open and the kidneys active.

Cold Baths.—The fever may be controlled by cold baths or by bathing with tepid water.

Vapor Baths.—Hot vapor baths are very beneficial.

Salicylate of Soda.—Salicylate of soda three drams, simple elixir three ounces. Take one teaspoonful after each meal, dissolved in one tumblerful of water. This aids in eliminating uric acid.

RINGWORM.

DESCRIPTION.—Ringworm is a severe circular irritation of the skin caused by a vegetable parasite, burrowing into and under the skin. The female leaves its track strewn with eggs which later hatch out and cause much trouble. The ring generally starts with a little pimple, increasing in a circle till about the size of a dollar or larger. The spot seems to heal in the center making it look like a healthy spot of flesh surrounded by a ring of very irritated skin about one-fourth of an inch wide. This shows that the germs have exhausted the material there, necessary for development.

First Aid and Home Treatment.

Tobacco.—Apply a strong solution of tobacco leaves till cured.

Limewater.—If the irritation is on the head, it is difficult to cure. The head should be shaved and a cap of oil silk should be worn. Wash with lime-water.

Gunpowder and Vinegar.—Apply a paste of gunpowder and vinegar.

Kerosene.—Kerosene applied several times daily is good.

Burdock and Vinegar.—Make a tea of burdock roots, to which add as much vinegar as tea.

Alum and White of Egg.—Mix alum with the white of an egg and heat thoroughly, then apply the paste.

Iodine.—Painting with tincture of iodine has often cured ringworm.

Ringworm is easily cured if taken in time, but becomes very serious if allowed to spread. It is contagious.

SCARLET FEVER.

DESCRIPTION.—Scarlet fever is one of the most serious, infectious and contagious of the diseases of childhood. It is characterized by fever, sore throat and a bright red flush or rash which covers more or less of the whole body. The rash is followed by a desquamation or peeling off the outer skin and it seems that the contagion or infection is contained in this as well as all the secretions, especially those of the nose and the throat. These scales retain the power to convey the disease for long periods of time. One attack generally protects from another.

INCUBATION.—It is generally from one to ten or twelve days after exposure that the first symptoms of the disease develop.

SYMPTOMS.—The onset of the disease is generally very sudden. There are chills, high fever, the temperature ranging from 103 to 105 degrees, face flushed, inflammation of the throat, headache, vomiting, tongue coated with red points extending above the surrounding surface much like the surface of a strawberry, hence often called the "strawberry tongue." Within eighteen to thirty-six hours the rash appears, first on the neck, chest and abdomen extending quickly over the entire body. It is most noticed in the flexures of the joints and where the surface of the body is particularly subjected to pressure or heat. It is bright red in character and in fine red dots which are so close together that at a distance it appears as a red blush over the body. This rash causes a burning, itchy sensation over all or parts of the body, and there is swelling of the skin. This generally lasts from two to five days and then the rash will gradually fade and the outer skin begin to peel off in scales of variable sizes. This scaling may continue for two or three weeks and sometimes much longer. The palms of the hands and the soles of the feet are usually the last to undergo this process, however, as a rule the peeling is very extensive on these parts. By means of these scales which lodge in books, upholstered furniture, clothing, etc., the disease is transmitted to others often years after. The source of contagion lies largely, though not exclusively, in these scales. In very mild cases of the disease scaling is often not perceptible. Other children should not be allowed to go near the patient during this period of scaling, neither should they be allowed to play with cats or dogs which have been around the sick, as the scales are often carrried in the hair or fur of these animals and may transmit the disease to others.

CHARACTERISTICS which distinguish it from other diseases: In measles the rash does not appear quite so early and has a blotchy appearance instead of the uniformity found in scarlet fever. Catarrhal symptoms of the nose and throat are prominent in measles while in scarlet fever the sore throat and "strawberry tongue" are prominent features. The onset of the disease is sudden instead of a gradual development as in measles.

In diphtheria the false membrane appears in the throat at the very beginning of the disease, while in scarlet fever not for a number of days after the beginning of illness. The characteristic rash showing up early in scarlet fever also serves to distinguish it from diphtheria.

COMPLICATIONS.—The most dreaded complications are acute inflammation of the kidneys—of greater or less intensity. Inflammation of the middle ear often resulting in perforation of the ear-drum and deafness. There is often swelling of the glands of the neck and also swelling of the joints. With small children there may also be convulsions.

SEQUELAE.—Chronic endocarditis or inflammation of the membranes lining the inside of the heart, chronic kidney trouble or Bright's disease, dropsy, inflammation of the middle ear often resulting in deafness, weak eyes, chronic tonsilitis and often paralysis. The most common of these are inflammation of the ears and kidney trouble, which should be particularly guarded against.

NURSING.—If the disease is prevalent, or if one has been exposed to it, as soon as he begins to show symptoms of illness he should be put to bed in a room apart from the rest of the family and watched closely. The room should be kept well ventilated, but free from draughts and at a temperature of about 68 degrees F. It is well to begin giving warm drinks so as to bring the rash out as quickly as possible. Herb teas are the best. If the onset is very severe, the child having convulsions, the doctor should be called immediately. As soon as the rash appears it is well to grease the body all over as suggested below under the home treatments. Cover the patient lightly in bed, give plenty of good pure water to drink. Lemonade may be given which is not only greatly desired by most children, but has a beneficial effect on the inflammation of the throat and digestive tract. A warm bath at the beginning of the disease will aid in bringing out the rash, and frequent bathing with lukewarm water throughout the attack will help to control the fever and allay the itching, burning sensation. Two tablespoonfuls of alcohol may be added to a basin of water for the bath. The body should be greased right after the bath.

The nurse or mother should be especially careful not to allow the child to take cold during the attack or while getting well, as some of the serious after-effects or complications are liable to develop. The urine should be watched and if there are symptoms of inflammation of the kidneys, this should be attended to at once by the doctor. Also in the case of inflammation of the ear, the doctor should take care of this at once as deafness may result. For the sore throat use the gargles or sprays suggested below. The bowels should be kept open daily by the use of the milk or citrate of magnesia. If the fever runs from 103 to 105 degrees, and remains that way for any length of time, the patient may become delirious and cold water or the ice cap may be applied to the head. This should be done under the supervision of the physician.

Until all fever has left, the patient should be kept on a milk diet. They may also be given instead of milk and for the sake of variety, orange juice several times a day. When the fever is gone, the patient may have broths, cereals, milk toast, junket, also a little ice cream may be given, but nothing more substantial for three or four weeks.

In order to prevent the spreading of the disease to other members of the family, the nurse should be very careful not to carry any of the scales on her clothing or in any other way to others. The greasing of the patient will prevent the flying of these scales and there should also be sheets spread on the floor around the bed to catch the scales which should immediately be burned. After the disease is over everything should be thoroughly disinfected according to directions given in a former chapter on that subject.

For the general care of the patient, follow the instructions on nursing as given in a previous chapter and be careful to follow the instructions of the doctor fully.

First Aid and Home Treatment.

Lemon Juice and Water.—Gargle the throat with equal parts of lemon juice and water.

Soda.—Take one teaspoonful baking soda to a glass of water. Use frequently as a gargle.

Listerine or Salt.—A teaspoonful of listerine or of table salt to a glass of water is very good as a gargle.

Peroxide of Hydrogen.—Gargle or spray the throat with peroxide of hydrogen one part to four parts water.

Vinegar and Water.—Take one-half glass each of vinegar and water to which add one-half teaspoonful salt and use as a gargle.

Pineapple.—Gargle with the juice of pineapple.

Hot Salt Water, Coal oil and Turpentine.—Hot salt water, coal oil and turpentine, mix and apply to the throat.

Vinegar.—Saturate a flannel cloth with vinegar and place around the throat; cover with a dry cloth.

Cold Pack.—Wring a piece of flannel out of cold water and put around the neck. Cover well with dry cloths.

Saffron and Pennyroyal.—Drink hot teas such as saffron and pennyroyal to bring out the rash.

Catnip and Sage.—Catnip and sage teas also, are good to bring out the rash.

Bathing.—Bathing with warm water helps to keep out the eruption and removes poisons from the body.

Mountain Sage.—A teaspoonful of the fluid extract of mountain sage added to a glass of hot lemonade and given every half hour, is very good to allay fever.

Unsalted Lard or Unsalted Butter.—To allay itching and to prevent the scales flying about use unsalted lard or unsalted butter. Fat bacon is also very good.

Sweet Oil or Olive Oil.—It is well to use sweet oil or olive oil for rubbing the patient.

Carbolated Vaseline.—Carbolated vaseline is also very good to use for this purpose.

Cocoa Butter.—Cocoa butter is very highly recommended for rubbing the patient.

SEPTICEMIA (Blood Poison).

DESCRIPTIVE.—It is a poisonous condition of the blood caused by the entrance into the system of bacteria or germs through a wound of some kind, such as running a nail into the foot, splinter into the finger, or any slight wound. It may also follow severe wounds, operations and also cases of confinement. However, whether it results from a wound, operation or confinement, it is almost always due to the unsanitary handling of the case.

SYMPTOMS.—The first symptoms generally appear in about twenty-four hours, however, they may appear in from two to three hours to three or four days. In confinement cases, the symptoms usually develop four or five days after labor. The first symptom is a chill varying in severity. This is usually followed by high fever (the temperature reaching 103 to 104 degrees F.) and profuse sweating. These symptoms reappear daily or at regular intervals. The patient loses his appetite, there is nausea, vomiting and general emaciation.

NURSING.—Especially when these symptoms develop after a case of confinement, send for the physician at once. Move the bowels thoroughly once or twice a day by means of a cathartic or an enema. The room should be well ventilated, the patient given plenty of pure water and the most nourishing food. The skin should be kept active by bath and brisk rubbing. In case the poisoning results from a wound, thoroughly cleanse with a strong antiseptic solution. Then dress it carefully with antiseptic cloths and bandages so that no further poison may develop. The dressing of the wound should be changed once or twice per day as the case demands, antiseptics being freely used. In case the wound is on the hand, foot or leg, and the member becomes badly swollen, the inflammation extending toward the body, which is noticed by red lines running from the wound toward the body, a physician should be sent for at once. Every wound whether slight or serious should be cleansed and taken care of at once in order to prevent the development of this disease. Often the blood is in bad condition and the slightest wounds result seriously if not taken care of.

First Aid and Home Treatment.

Preventive.—Every wound, no difference how small, should be thoroughly cleansed at once with some good antiseptic solution, bandaged and kept clean.

Poultices.—In case a wound becomes infected and swollen the inflammation extending toward the body, it should be poulticed with some good drawing poultice, such as flaxseed poultice, so as to draw the poison out ond keep it from spreading through the body.

Massage or Rub.—To keep the poison from spreading through the system, rub or massage the limb, always rubbing away from the body and toward the wound.

Antiseptics.—Keep the wound open well and wash often with some good antiseptic such as one part carbolic acid to 100 parts water, or hydrogen peroxide full strength.

Blood Purifiers.—Take some good blood purifier to rid the system of the poison. An infusion of red clover blossoms or elder flowers is good.

SMALLPOX.

DESCRIPTION.—Smallpox is a highly communicable, infectious disease, characterized by a high fever and a typical eruption which occurs in five stages. One attack protects a person from the second attack, also vaccination, which is described later, makes a person immune. The disease is very fatal to small children.

INCUBATION.—The attack comes on in from one to three weeks after exposure, the usual period being 12 days.

SYMPTOMS.—The onset of the disease is sudden with high fever ranging from 102 to 104 degrees F. and sometimes higher. This is often preceded by chills, however, not always. In children there may be convulsions. There is a very severe headache which is characteristic of the disease, also often intense pains in the back and extremities, vomiting and sometimes delirium.

The fever which is peculiar to this disease comes on suddenly at the onset, as a rule, is very high, often reaching 104 or 105 degrees F. as stated above. It then disappears when the eruption takes place, the temperature dropping to about normal. There is very little fever then till the pus forms in the eruption when it again rises to the same height as before. This is known as the secondary fever which reaches its highest point about the ninth day.

The peculiar eruption which is a characteristic of this disease, passes through five distinct stages. First there is noticed a little lump or macule under the skin. This continues for about three days when the lump develops into a pimple or vesicle above the skin containing a clear fluid. This continues about the same length of time, then the clear fluid in the pimple turns to pus and looks "mattery." The length of this period depends on the severity of the attack. The pus then begins to dry, forming a crust over the top which in mild cases is little more than scales of skin. In severe cases they are thick and crusty and when these drop off at the end of the third or fourth week they often leave a deep pit called the "pox-mark."

VARIOLOID.—This is smallpox in a mild form. It usually occurs in people who have been vaccinated or who have once had smallpox. It has all the symptoms of a severe case but in a much milder form.

VACCINATION.—It is agreed by the best authorities that vaccination does prevent smallpox and that it is one of the best means to prevent the spread of the dread disease. The best time to vaccinate a healthy child is at the age of three or four months. If the vaccination takes well, it makes the child immune to the disease for about seven years when he should be vaccinated again. Especially should the child be vaccinated if there is an epidemic prevailing.

The operation of vaccination is simple, but important and should be done by a physician. The usual place for the vaccination is on the outer fleshy part of either the arm or leg about midway between the joints. It should never be done near a joint. In infants not old enough to walk or creep, it is best to select the leg for the seat of vaccination, and the right side is preferable to the left.

The operation, which should be performed by a physician as stated above, consists in scraping or scratching the skin with a sterile needle or instrument until it appears raw or a little blood is seen, however, it should not be cut or scratched so deep that it bleeds much, as the blood will wash the virus out. The spot does not need to be large, about one-fourth inch across in each direction. The virus is then well rubbed into the spot and left dry before the part is covered. In order to keep the place clean and protect it from the stocking or shirt sleeve, it is well to bandage it loosely or at least baste a soft piece of linen inside the clothing over the spot.

The fourth or fifth day after the operation has been performed, the vaccination will begin "to take." An area of redness will appear around the spot and a vesicle form. This becomes fully developed about the ninth or tenth day, the redness around it being quite extended and there being some swelling and soreness. The vesicle then discharges or dries up and forms a crust which later falls off leaving a scar. If the vesicle discharges it may be dusted over with boric acid powder several times a day. If the vaccinated spot is well taken care of there is very little trouble experienced. Often young infants feel no general symptoms while others may have a little fever for a day or so and loss of appetite.

NURSING.—As smallpox is one of the most infectious diseases, the patient should be immediately isolated on development of any of the symptoms characteristic of the disease. The strictest quarantine should be observed from the onset to the disappearance of the last vestige of the disease, and the complete recovery of the patient. The nurse or mother should follow strictly the directions given on caring for patients suffering from contagious diseases as given in the chapter on Nursing. It is well for the nurse to wear a large cover-all apron and cap which should be removed on leaving the sick room.

On account of the danger of pneumonia or pleurisy developing, much care must be taken to keep the patient from taking cold, although the room should be well ventilated and the patient should have plenty of fresh air. In case the patient becomes delirious, which may occur in severe cases, he should be carefully watched to prevent him from injuring himself or others.

To relieve the itching, frequent sponge baths may be given or the crusts soaked with oil or vaseline. The application of equal parts of limewater and sweet oil mixed, is good for this. The patient should never be allowed to scratch himself especially on the face as this will leave scars. It may be necessary to wear gloves on his hands and tie them down, or instead of this, splints may be fastened to the arms to prevent bending the elbows, so he cannot reach his face. It is often well to wear the "mask" over the face, however, this should be prepared and used under directions from the doctor.

The eyes should be cleansed often with a mild antiseptic solution, such as boric acid water, made by dissolving one teaspoonful of boric acid in a tumbler full of warm water. The mouth may also be cleansed with boric acid water, which should be done before each feeding.

As in all diseases where there is much fever, the diet should be light, consisting principally of such foods as milk, rice, corn-starch, junket, etc. Oranges and lemonade may also be given. However, as the successful combating of the disease depends largely on keeping up the strength of the patient, in case his strength begins to fail, the pulse becoming very weak, good nourishing foods should be given, such as nutritious broths, milk-punch, egg-nog, etc., which are stimulating.

First Aid and Home Treatment

As stated above, the main thing in taking care of a patient suffering with this disease consists in proper nursing and good nourishing food. This can be administered by the nurse or mother, however, on first indication that the disease is smallpox, a good reliable physician should be called at once and his instructions followed carefully.

Boric Acid.—Rinse the mouth often with a solution of boric acid and water.

Vaseline or Sweet Oil.—To relieve the itching, soak the crusts with vaseline or sweet oil. Also sponge the patient often with tepid water.

Peroxide of Hydrogen.—Spray the mouth, throat and nose with peroxide of hydrogen and water equal parts, several times a day.

SORE MOUTH.
(Cold Sores and Cankers.)

Proper diet and a clean system will prevent cold sores and cankers since they are the result of a disordered stomach usually.

First Aid and Home Treatment.

Camphor.—Wet a small piece of cotton with a few drops of spirits of camphor and touch the sores several times a day with it. They will soon disappear.

Aromatic Sulphuric Acid.—Touch canker sores every few minutes for a while with a bit of aromatic sulphuric acid on the end of a little stick.

Burnt Alum.—Put one teaspoonful of burnt alum in a glass of warm water and use for a mouth wash.

Carbolic Acid.—Wrap a little piece of cotton around a toothpick and wet in 75 percent solution carbolic acid and touch to the sores. Immediately after, touch the sores with alcohol 95 percent.

Alum.—Touch the cankers with a lump of alum.

Hedge Mustard, Honey and Sugar.—Mix and make a syrup of the juice of hedge mustard, honey and sugar. Use as a gargle.

Green, Golden Seal and Sage Leaves.—Mix the tea made from green tea leaves, golden seal leaves and sage leaves. Use as a gargle.

SORE THROAT.

First Aid and Home Treatment.

Lemon Juice and Salt.—Lemon juice and salt used as a gargle will cure ordinary sore throat in a very short time.

Listerine.—Makes a good gargle for the throat.

Vinegar, Sugar, and Butter.—Make a gargle by boiling together, one-half cup of vinegar, enough sugar to make a syrup. To this add two tablespoonfuls of butter. This makes a splendid gargle for sore throats or hoarseness.

Sage Tea, Lemon Juice, Alum, and Borax.—Make a sage tea, add enough sugar to tea to make a syrup, then add the juice of one lemon, a little alum, and borax. Give a teaspoonful at a time and give often.

Sage Tea, Vinegar, Black Pepper.—Take a handful of green or dried sage leaves, boil down until you have a pint of the liquid. Strain, then add one tablespoonful of vinegar, one teaspoonful of black pepper, one teaspoonful of salt, alum the size of a lima bean. Mix well in the tea. Gargle the throat every half hour. Use the tea hot. After gargling, blow some sulphur into the throat.

Baking Soda and Salt Gargle.—To one cup of lukewarm water add a half teaspoonful of baking soda and a half teaspoonful of salt. Use warm.

Cold Water.—Take a pint of cold water, drink while lying down in bed. Allow to remain in throat as long as possible.

Pineapples.—Fresh, cooked, or canned pineapples are good for sore throat.

Hot or Cold Application.—Place a hot or a cold pack about the neck to relieve inflammation. Gargle frequently with one of the above mentioned gargles. Keep the patient on a liquid diet. Give a good laxative.

In severe cases call a physician as it may be more serious than should be treated at home, etc.

Steam from Vinegar.—Wring a cloth out of vinegar and place over a hot iron. Inhale the steam through the mouth. If the vinegar is very strong it may be diluted a little with water.

Kerosene.—Saturate a piece of flannel cloth with kerosene (coal oil) and place about the throat. Care should be taken as this may blister the skin.

Menthol Oil.—A mild menthol oil used occasionally is good to spray the nose and throat.

Peroxide of Hydrogen.—Makes a good gargle for sore throat. To one part of the peroxide add four parts water. This may be used frequently.

STYE.

DESCRIPTION.—A stye is an acute inflammation of the hair follicles and surrounding tissues. It appears as a little boil on the edge of the eyelid.

Eye strain is thought to be the most important cause of sties. It was formerly thought that they came from stomach trouble or a run-down condition of the body.

A severe itching and burning followed by a red swollen spot at the edge of the lid are the symptoms.

First Aid and Home Treatment.

Boracic Acid.—Every hour apply a hot boracic acid solution compress. Use a boracic acid eye-wash.

If the stye does not yield to this treatment, it is well to see a physician as it may result seriously.

SUPPRESSION OF THE URINE.

The bladder is the organ or receptacle of the body which holds the urine, and when distended contains about one pint, but may contain more. It should be entirely emptied several times a day.

When the work of the kidneys is defective, there is little or no secretion of urine; the system is affected very quickly as shown by pain in the back, irritation of the bladder, the patient becomes restless and anxious, dull and drowsy, and in severe cases may die after seven or eight days. . In cases where no urine has been passed for ten days hysteria, may and often does result. When children are teething, many times little or no urine is passed for several days. Other diseases may also cause suppression of the urine in children.

First Aid and Home Treatment.

Pumpkin Seeds.—No better or simpler remedy can be used than a tea made of pumpkin seeds and given freely to the child. Cut the seeds and steep for two hours, and give two teaspoonfuls several times a day.

Baths.—Frequent baths, hot or cold are good.

Peppermint.—Peppermint tea given frequently is very effective in the relief of suppression of the urine.

Pennyroyal.—A strong tea made from this plant and taken freely and often is very good. The pennyroyal plant is found in almost every part of the United States. It is very good for relief from the suppression of the urine or menses.

Partridge Berry.—The partridge berry infusion or taken freely in syrup is good to relieve suppression of the urine.

Buchu.—Make a tea of buchu leaves by adding one ounce of the leaves to a pint of boiling water. Take 3 or 4 tablespoonfuls three times a day. The leaves may be purchased at any drug store.

TETANUS OR LOCK JAW.

DESCRIPTION.—This is an infective disease of the voluntary muscles caused by a germ which usually enters the body through a wound. These germs exist in great numbers in the soil and usually enter the wound at the time of injury or a few days later. The disease as a rule results from a wound of the foot or hand, made by a blunt object such as a rusty nail.

SYMPTOMS.—The first symptoms noticed are pain and stiffness of the muscles of the neck and jaws. They soon become rigid so that the patient cannot open his mouth. This condition is called lockjaw from which the disease receives its common name. The stiffness or rigidity soon extends to the other muscles of the body. The large muscles of the back are sometimes so contracted that the body is drawn out of shape. The muscles of the face are also often so drawn as to produce a peculiar grinning expression. The muscles of the upper extremities are not much affected in mild cases.

NURSING.—The patient should be put to bed in a darkened room and kept perfectly quiet, much care being taken to disturb him as little as possible. The strength should be kept up by good nourishing liquid foods such as milk, beef teas, broths, etc. These must be carefully poured into the mouth between the teeth and cheeks. Sometimes it may be necessary to give nourishment and stimulants by the rectum. The bowels must be kept open and the kidneys active. Keep the patient as quiet as possible, free from all excitement and well nourished, as this is far more important than any medicine which can be given in this disease.

First Aid and Home Treatment.

Just as soon as it is suspected that the disease is developing, call the physician at once.

Antitoxin or serum treatment is often used with much success, however, this must be administered by a skilled physician.

Preventive.—Attend to every wound at once regardless of how slight. Cleanse with some good antiseptic. Apply equal parts of tincture iodine and alcohol to the wound and keep it clean.

Tobacco.—Moistened tobacco laid on the stomach has been known to relax the muscles. It must not be kept on too long as it is liable to make patient sick.

TONSILS—ENLARGED.

Enlarged tonsils may often accompany adenoids but sometimes are found without them. They cause inflammation of the throat, tonsilitis, bronchitis, and the child is more susceptible to rheumatism and heart disease, caused by rheumatism, diphtheria, tuberculosis and scarlet fever.

If the patient has repeated attacks of sore throat and tonsilitis, and the doctor advises an operation, the tonsils should be removed.

TONSILITIS—QUINSY.

DESCRIPTION.—This is an acute inflammation of the tonsils. It affects children more often than adults and often appears in epidemic form during the spring and fall of the year. It has been found in recent years that a rheumatic tendency is one of the most important results. Colds, enlarged tonsils, poison matter from decayed teeth, etc., are predisposing causes.

SYMPTOMS.—There is a general aching of the entire body, chilliness, sore throat, fever, coated foul tongue, scanty highly colored urine, constipation and general prostration. The tonsils become so sore and swollen that the patient can hardly swallow, the voice is thick, the surrounding tissues may become so inflamed that opening the mouth or turning the head causes much pain. Only one tonsil may be swollen and inflamed at first, however, as the inflammation subsides in one it develops in the other. These symptoms are accompanied by the formation of whitish or light yellow cheesy masses on the tonsils, or by abscess formations, which may easily be removed, leaving a smooth glossy surface. The suppuration or formation of pus usually takes place in four or five days after the onset of the disease. This may be distinguished from diphtheria by the fact that in diphtheria a false membrane of a dark grey or leathery appearance develops on the tonsils which, on being removed, leaves a raw, bleeding surface.

NURSING.—As this disease may be confused or mistaken for diphtheria or scarlet fever, the patient should be isolated till the disease is fully determined. Also some forms of this disease are contagious and for this reason isolation is best. Give a good cathartic and keep the bowels open. Give hot lemonade or teas to keep up a free perspiration. Surround the neck with hot packs by taking a long heavy towel, wringing one end out of hot water as hot as can be borne and applying this to the neck from the ears to the shoulders, with the wet end next to the skin.

First Aid and Home Treatment.

Steam.—The inhalation of steam from water to which has been added a little vinegar or turpentine is very beneficial. This may be done by placing a large funnel, made of paper, over a vessel containing the water and holding the small end of the funnel in the mouth. This is also good for hoarseness.

Baking Soda.—The application of baking soda to the tonsils by means of a swab or the moistened finger is also good.

Alkaline Solution.—Spray the throat with a hot alkaline solution to which has been added a small amount of listerine.

Peroxide of Hydrogen.—Wash the mouth and throat with an antiseptic solution such as peroxide of hydrogen and water, equal parts, or hot water to which has been added common baking soda. Alum water is also good.

Ice Pack.—In severe cases the application of an ice pack to the throat will bring great relief by reducing the inflammation. It should be kept there for hours or until the inflammation subsides.

Lemons.—The sipping of sweetened lemon juice or strong lemonade is also good to cleanse the mouth and throat.

If there are abscess formations on the tonsils as in quinsy, it is best to have a physician treat the case. It may also be necessary to lance the tonsils.

If the tonsils remain enlarged and give much trouble, they may have to be removed. It is a well known fact that enlarged or inflamed tonsils induce rheumatism and for this reason they should be removed if giving much trouble. Weakly anaemic people are more subject to the disease. So to avoid trouble of this kind, build up the general health.

TOOTHACHE.

No one should suffer long with the toothache, they should go to a dentist as soon as possible and have the cause removed.

It is said that to press the nerve just below the temple in front of the middle of the ear, will stop the ache.

To prevent the toothache wash mouth every morning with warm salt water and a good tooth powder. Milk of magnesia is a splendid tooth and mouth wash.

First Aid and Home Treatment.

Oil of Peppermint.—After cleaning the cavity well, dip a small piece of cotton in some oil of peppermint or creosote and pack the cavity.

Ammonia.—Dip some cotton in ammonia and pack cavity.

Oil of Sassafras.—Rub the gum with oil of sassafras.

Kerosene.—Dip cotton in kerosene and insert in cavity of the tooth.

Alum and Salt.—Powder equal parts of alum and salt and mix. Dip some wet cotton in the powder and insert in the cavity.

TUBERCULOSIS.

DESCRIPTION.—This disease is caused by a specific germ called the bacillus tuberculosis. These germs are found in the lesions and discharges from the seat of infection. In adults this is generally the lungs, while in children it usually affects the bones, joints, and lymph glands. The most common form is that affecting the lungs and is of two kinds, acute and chronic.

SYMPTOMS.—The acute form is similar to pneumonia, beginning with a chill, rise in temperature, night sweats, difficult breathing, short, hacking cough, the sputum being rust colored at first, later becoming purulent. There is general emaciation and weakness which increases with the rapid development of the above symptoms. This is known as "quick consumption," the patient often dying in a few weeks.

The symptoms of the chronic form are practically the same as those of the acute, however, they do not develop so rapidly, the patient often lingering for years. The temperature is characteristic of the disease, being low in the morning and rising toward evening, the cheeks often having a peculiar, hectic flush. There is usually absence of fever in the morning, however it develops toward evening. the pulse being soft and rapid. The symptoms may be very mild at the beginning, the patient apparently being in good health. If the disease is recognized in the early stages and taken in hand at once, there is every hope for recovery. However, it must not be neglected, as neglect may mean years of suffering and death.

NURSING.—This very fatal disease is wholly preventable by the proper mode of living. One having tuberculosis tendencies should follow carefully the instructions given in the "How to Keep Well" department on the nature and prevention of the disease.

In the nursing and treatment of this disease, there are four essential elements

—rest; pure air; plenty of good, wholesome, easily digested food; cheerful and comfortable surroundings.

Rest in the open air is necessary. The patient should spend much time in a hammock or on a bamboo couch out-of-doors, a bed on the porch or in a room with at least two large windows, all of which must be wide open. Do not be afraid of night air. All out-of-door air is good, however avoid draughts or becoming too cool. In very cold weather, woolen bed slippers, a soft warm cap, heavy flannel night clothes and a hot water bottle may be needed. Take as much thorough rest as possible—rest from manual and mental labor and from all sports. Stay in bed as many hours of the twenty-four as possible and take complete rest on Sunday. Strict temperance should also be enforced.

In the nursing of the disease both patient and nurse must be exceedingly careful that the infection is not spread to others. The patient should sleep alone and be furnished with a sputum cup. The cup should be emptied and disinfected at least three times a day. The sputum should be burned. If the patient is able to be about he should either carry a sputum cup with him, or expectorate in cloths which may be burned. He should not be allowed to kiss others. Both he and the nurse or other members of the family should take the greatest care that none of the infections be transmitted to cuts, scratches or wounds on the hands, as germs may easily enter the body in this way.

Steam inhalations sometimes relieve the coughing for a time. These may be given by wrapping a towel around the head and holding the head over a vessel containing boiling water.

There is no drug known, however rare or expensive, that is a cure for this disease and all drugs advertised as such should be avoided for they are generally harmful in some way. A hospital not only offers the most favorable conditions for a cure, but also does away with danger of infecting members of the family.

Change of climate is rarely necessary. The money which would be spent in sending a patient to different states can generally be spent to better advantage in constructing a place for open-air sleeping or providing good milk, eggs and other nourishing foods, and also for woolen clothes.

Diet.—The diet for a consumptive should consist of an abundance of raw eggs, milk, soup made from such nutritious foods as beans, peas, rice, barley, oysters, also beef tea and chicken broth. Cream, butter, olive oil, and fat meats are good if the patient can digest them. Fresh fish, vegetables and fruits may be given. In case of indigestion liquid foods should be served. The meals should be very daintily and tastily prepared and served under the most inviting conditions. A person affected with tuberculosis should be encouraged to eat freely of the most nutritious foods, even between meals.

TUMORS.

A tumor is an abnormal growth similar to that of cancer and may occur in practically the same parts of the body. There are also tumors of the brain which may be caused by blows on the head or severe emotional shocks, in which case the patient should be operated upon as soon as possible, otherwise bags of ice should be applied to the head driving the blood from the head.

There are many kinds of tumors such as, fibrous, fatty, muscular, and nerve tumors. If located on the surface as on the jaw or face, an operation may be a permanent cure, but if in the deeper parts of the body, a return after being removed is probable.

In case of tumors and cancers a competent surgeon should be consulted and the trouble removed in its earliest stages.

TYPHOID FEVER.

DESCRIPTION.—This is a continued fever caused by a specific micro-organism known as the bacillus typhus, or poison from this germ entering blood.

These little germs generally enter the system through the alimentary canal in the water or milk we drink or in the food we eat. Serious epidemics of the disease have resulted from infected drinking water and from milk infection. Water from shallow wells which receive the surface drainage or seepage from a near-by cess pool, or from stagnant ponds is very likely to be infected with the germs. Also water used from rivers which receive the sewage from cities is very likely to contain the germs. The disease has often been contracted by eating raw oysters or clams, or food which has been infected by germ carrying flies. The excreta and urine from a patient suffering with the disease is laden with the germs and should be promptly and thoroughly disinfected. Flies from this may infect food or water. It may also be contracted from the bedding and clothing worn by the patient. The ways of preventing the disease as given in the "How to Keep Well" department should be carefully observed.

All ages and both sexes are liable to contract it, however, it is more prevalent between the ages of 15 to 25 years. It occurs more in the fall, October and November, than other seasons of the year and generally after a very hot summer.

INCUBATION.—This is generally about 10 to 12 days, however, as it is often very hard to tell just where the germs came from and when they entered the body, it is hard to determine this period.

SYMPTOMS.—The Onset of the disease may be very gradual, it being four or five days, perhaps, or a week after the disease really sets in, before the patient takes to his bed. The first symptom which is usually recognized as the beginning, is feverishness, although this may be preceded by languor, weakness, headache, aching pains in the back and limbs and a general "all in" feeling. The temperature rises gradually, step by step for four or five days till it reaches 103 or 104 degrees F. and occasionally it runs as high as 105 degrees. The pulse is rapid, there is headache varying in intensity, nose bleed, diarrhea, tenderness and discomfort in the stomach and bowels and often a gurgling in the lower right side of the abdomen.

Instead of setting in gradually it may come on suddenly with a severe chill, high fever, headache, nausea, vomiting, pain in abdomen, sweats and sore throat.

The symptoms of the **Established Disease** depend largely on the complications which may arise. As a general rule the symptoms of the first period of the disease continue. The tongue which is moist and slightly coated at first becomes covered with a thick coat, is dry and baked, often becoming cracked and bleeding. The breath is foul with a characteristic odor. The thirst is intense during the fever. Nausea and vomiting may occur after the disease is established as well as at the onset. Rose colored spots appear on the chest, back and abdomen. Each spot lasts about three days and then disappears. A few fresh ones come on every day or two till about the third week when they disappear. The stomach and intestines become bloated and drum like. The "bell sound" may occur and when general over the abdomen it indicates perforation of the intestines. The diarrhea may be very bad, the bowels moving as often as twenty times in a day. This is generally the case where there is much ulceration of the bowels. The stools are dark at first, however, they soon become yellow, watery and very offensive. There is often blood mixed with them.

The nervous symptoms vary much with the severity of the attack and with the peculiarities of the patient. One of the first of these is the headache which generally lasts about ten days. There is also sleeplessness and often extreme restlessness. Although the mental condition may remain clear throughout the disease, there is often delirium varying in degree from lightheadedness to that of the most violent nature. This generally comes on about the 10th or 12th day. If the case is typical and the disease runs its usual course, the third week is the most critical period. The symptoms are usually at their worst and the patient's strength is very low. As a rule the disease runs its course in from 20 to 30 days, however, it may be of much shorter duration or it may continue much longer, the period depending largely on the complications and the nursing.

COMPLICATIONS and SEQUELAE.—There are a host of these which may occur. The severity and duration of the fever so debilitates and weakens the body, that it is subject to most any disease or derangement. Statistics show that about 35 percent of the deaths are due to these complications and sequelæ. The most common and dangerous of these are: peritonitis, appendicitis, chronic diarrhea, perforation of the bowels, diseases of the heart, lobar-pneumonia, bronchopneumonia, bronchitis, pleurisy and meningitis. In case any of these develop they must have special attention.

NURSING.—In practically no other disease does the nursing and diet play such an important part as in Typhoid Fever. The patient should be put to bed as early as possible and kept there until the disease is broken up. In a clean, cheerful room, well lighted, plenty of pure fresh air and a temperature of 65 degrees F. It is absolutely necessary that the patient be kept perfectly quiet, not rising for anything, be the case ever so mild, as by so doing he may cause perforation or hemorrhage of the bowels, which is a very serious complication. It is not well to give purgatives, unless ordered by the attending physician, as these often irritate the bowels and may cause perforation. All excreta, including the urine, discharges from the body, should be immediately and thoroughly disinfected. This may be done by mixing each passage with chloride of lime. Making a solution by mixing one pound of the lime with 4 gallons of water. A pint or quart of this should be stirred in with each passage. Whitewash or a carbolic acid solution may be used instead. Or if there are no disinfectants at hand, boiling water may be thrown over the excreta, or it may be mixed with sawdust and burned. It should not be thrown out or deposited where it will likely contaminate the water supply. All soiled bed linen or body linen should be boiled. The nurse must be exceedingly careful in this respect as the smallest portion of the excreta is loaded with germs, and can produce the disease in another person.

The patient's mouth should be kept clean so as to prevent the formation of dark brown accumulations called sordes, on the teeth, gums, lips and tongue. The nurse or mother should report to the physician any cough, nosebleed, character of expectoration, pain in the ear, deafness, or any other extraordinary symptom which may develop. If there is delirium, this should also be reported, and the patient should not be left alone for a single moment. The nurse must be kind, gentle but firm, cheerful and equal to any emergency. She must not let the patient know by word or look that there is anything wrong.

Hemorrhage.—In case of hemorrhage, the foot of the bed should be raised as high as possible or the patient's head lowered. Ice or ice cold cloths may also be applied to the abdomen and the patient must be kept perfectly quiet on his back so that the blood may coagulate and prevent further hemorrhage.

Perforation.—This is caused by the breaking of an ulcer of the intestines which permits the contents of the bowels to escape into the peritoneal cavity. There will be sudden and sharp pain in the abdomen, which will be bloated and tender, rapid pulse, fall of temperature, vomiting, and signs of collapse. In a case of this kind, the nurse may apply hot fomentations to the abdomen and down the limbs, give stimulants and keep the patient absolutely quiet.

Bloating.—This is due to the accumulation of gas in the bowels. Apply turpentine fomentations or a flaxseed meal poultice to the abdomen. Some apply ice poultices.

Temperature.—The temperature may be reduced by means of the tepid sponge bath. This not only reduces the temperature but soothes the patient, stimulates the nervous, circulatory and respiratory systems.

Bed Sores.—These may be prevented by keeping the sheets dry, smooth and free from wrinkles. The back may also be rubbed with olive oil or vaseline in order to keep the moisture from being absorbed. Rub the back with alcohol or dust it over with powdered starch, corn-starch or borax. The patient's position should also be changed often. If the skin breaks, apply the white of an egg to the parts.

Diet.—The diet should be such as will be easily digested, leave as little residue as possible and at the same time nourish the patient to the greatest extent. Milk is one of the best foods which can be given and as much as two pints may be taken by the patient in 24 hours. It can be diluted with lime-water or barley water and may be taken warm or cold as the patient desires. It may also be peptonized. Whey, buttermilk, albumin of eggs in water, koumiss, beef tea, clear and free from fat, may be given. The milk may be flavored with cocoa, coffee or tea if the patient so desires. Oysters are very nourishing, easily digested and are often retained by the patient when all else fails. In all cases the food should be taken in little sips and a small amount at a time. It should be remembered that the patient's mouth and lips are most always dry and parched and should be moistened before feeding. If the patient is asleep, he should be awakened for feeding during the day.

Do not feed any solid foods until the patient is well on the road to complete recovery. By feeding solid food too early the patient may have a serious relapse. As soon as the bowels are in good condition bread and milk, fish, vegetables, etc., may be added to the diet, however, the taking of solid foods should be very gradual. It is better to begin with such foods as custards, soft-boiled eggs, puddings, cream toast, etc.

Thirst.—To relieve the thirst the patient may be given plenty of good, pure, cool water, lemonade, orangeade, etc. These will flush out the kidneys and help to carry off the poisons from the body.

Treatment.—As stated above, the nursing and diet are practically all important in handling this disease. A competent physician should be called early and all treatments that are used should be prescribed by him.

Convalescence.—During convalescence the same watchful care must be exercised as during the disease, or some of the serious after-effects may result. The patient should be given as strengthening diet as he can stand and be allowed to sit up or get up when his strength permits, and when he can do so without getting tired. If there is a return of the fever or diarrhea he must go back to bed and return to the simple diet. The patient must follow the instructions of the attending physician to the letter.

ULCERS.

DESCRIPTION.—An ulcer is a sore, discharging purulent matter. It may be acute or chronic. Acute inflammation usually accompanies an acute or spreading ulcer. Chronic ulcers are difficult to heal, since they must be stimulated before being treated.

Ulcers must be kept thoroughly clean and soothing applications used.

First Aid and Home Treatment.

Chickweed.—Chickweed chopped and boiled in lard will relieve pain.

Spirits of Turpentine and Mutton Tallow.—One teaspoonful of spirits of turpentine with melted mutton or beef tallow makes a good salve.

Peroxide of Hydrogen or Salt Water.—Wash with peroxide of hydrogen one part to four parts water, or a hot saline solution.

Mutton Tallow.—Apply hot mutton tallow to the ulcer after being washed with water colored with blue stone.

Charcoal and Raw Potato.—Powdered charcoal and grated raw potatoes is very good.

Lard, Sweet Oil and Carrots.—Lard or sweet oil added to carrots, boiled and mashed fine, is a good soothing and healing poultice.

Wood Sage and Chickweed.—Wood sage and chickweed mashed together make a fine poultice for chronic ulcers.

Carrots.—Clean the parts well, grate a carrot and apply as poultice three times a day.

Carbolic Acid.—Wash with pure water containing a few drops of carbolic acid.

VARICOSE VEINS.

DESCRIPTION.—This is an enlarged, knotty, congested condition of the veins, usually those of the legs and arms being more commonly affected. Where it occurs in the veins of the anus or lower bowel, it is called piles. It occurs more often in women than in men and is very common during or soon after pregnancy.

The cause is an obstruction to the free return of the blood to the heart. This may be due to diseases of the heart and lungs, pregnancy, tight garters, occupation which requires much standing or anything which may obstruct the free return of the blood.

NURSING.—Those having a tendency in this way should keep off their feet as much as possible, especially keep from standing. The veins should be supported by well-fitting elastic or silk stocking, or a bandage applied from below upwards. The bandage may be made of cheese cloth or elastic webbing and should not be applied too firmly. The figure eight method of bandaging is the most suitable and should be applied before the patient gets out of bed in the morning and kept on until he returns to bed in the evening. It is well for the patient to sleep with the feet slightly elevated so as to relieve the blood pressure. It is also well to massage the affected parts as this not only relieves the tired, aching feeling but also the congestion. In severe cases it may be necessary to remove the affected veins by operation. In case this is done the operation must be performed under thoroughly sanitary conditions.

WARTS.

DESCRIPTION.—A wart is a small, usually hard tumor of the skin, often hard to remove, but nothing serious.

First Aid and Home Treatment.

Nitric Acid.—Take nitric acid in a small vessel with half as much water as you have acid and apply to the wart with a little piece of wood or a toothpick, taking care not to allow a drop to fall. Just wet the stick and place on top of the wart until a burning sensation begins. Repeat daily and the wart will disappear in a week or two.

Acetic Acid.—Cover the end of a toothpick with absorbent cotton and dip into acetic acid, apply to the wart after the surface around it has been greased with vaseline. Allow the acid to dry by evaporation. The wart usually disappears within several days.

Milkweed.—Bruised milkweed applied to warts many times a day is good.

Iodine.—Apply tincture of iodine to remove warts.

Nitrate of Silver.—Nitrate of silver will destroy warts.

Alum.—A friend was very successful in removing a large seed wart from underneath the fingernail and on the end of the finger, by applying burnt alum.

WENS.

DESCRIPTION.—The sebaceous or oil glands located just beneath the skin open into the hair follicles by means of ducts. When one of these ducts is closed, by some injury or strain, the gland secretion accumulates and forces the skin up into a tough mound. The growth may vary from the size of a pea to that of a marble.

First Aid and Home Treatment.

The removal of a wen by the knife is easy and effective, but should be done by a physician.

Equal parts of fine salt and the yolk of an egg beaten together and freely applied many times a day, will open the skin when the mass can be taken out.

WHOOPING-COUGH.

DESCRIPTION.—This is a very common, infectious, contagious disease caused by a specific micro-organism. It affects children of all ages, but young babies are especially liable to have it. It is contagious throughout its course which generally continues for a period of six or eight weeks. It is characterized by catarrhal conditions of the air passages and spasmodic, convulsive coughing accompanied by the well-known "whoop." Although one attack generally confers immunity, other members of the family often have a cough very similar which might be termed a "sympathetic" cough. The disease is not often fatal, however, aside from the deaths which result directly from it, there are very many which are indirectly traceable to it, owing to the complications and after-effects.

INCUBATION.—The incubation period is generally from seven to sixteen days after exposure.

SYMPTOMS.—The first symptoms, extending over a period of five or six days, are those of an ordinary cold, with cough, slight fever, etc. This is known as the first period of the disease. The second period of the disease is known as the spasmodic period. The cough gradually increases in severity from the first period till there are paroxysms of coughing, in which the child becomes blue in the face and apparently on the verge of suffocating, when a long drawn noisy, whooping inspiration occurs. Although in cases of young babies no whoop may be present at all, simply the severe paroxysms of coughing. During a severe fit of coughing the child often holds to something for support, thick stringy mucus is expectorated, vomiting occurs and sometimes hemorrhages from the nose and lungs. These fits of coughing occur more frequently at night, and often extend over a period of several weeks gradually becoming less frequent and less violent till they stop altogether. After these paroxysms have ceased the coughing may last for some time in a mild form, especially if the disease is contracted during the winter. This last period is known as the period of decline.

COMPLICATIONS.—If the case is a very severe one, such complications may occur as hemorrhages, pneumonia, convulsions, diarrhea and vomiting.

SEQUELAE.—If the child is allowed to take cold or is not properly nourished during the disease, the system may be so weakened that he will readily contract such diseases as pneumonia, consumption, bronchitis, etc. Although the attack is not severe, these after-effects should be well guarded against.

NURSING.—Except in very severe cases, with complications, it is unnecessary to keep the child confined to the bed or house. The chief thing is to keep the child well nourished and be sure to give him plenty of pure fresh air day and night. He should spend much time in the open air during the day and sleep in a well ventilated room at night. As a rule the child should be fed more often than usual, with good nourishing, easily digested food, as on account of the vomiting he often loses much of the food taken. The child should be kept from other children, and mothers should not wilfully expose their children to this disease, as it is capable of causing death and serious after-effects.

First Aid and Home Treatment.

No cure for the disease has been found.

Drugs should not be given as they usually do more harm by upsetting the stomach, than they do good by relieving the cough. This is especially the case with very small children. The following will help shorten the period of duration:

Great care should be taken to avoid taking cold.

Chestnut Leaf Syrup.—Take one ounce of the dry leaves, put in one quart of water and boil down one-third. Strain this, add one pound of dark brown sugar, and boil till one pint remains. Give one teaspoonful every hour. A tea made from the leaves is also good.

Garlic Syrup.—Make a syrup from garlic and give about five drops several times a day. This will relieve the cough.

Onions or Mustard.—If there is a tendency to bronchitis, a mustard paste or onion poultice may be applied till the skin is red.

Peach Leaf Tea.—Make a tea with one ounce of dry peach leaves to a quart of boiling water. Let the patient drink freely of this.

Flaxseed Tea is good.

Castor Oil and Molasses.—Mix four tablespoonfuls of castor oil and eight tablespoonfuls of molasses and give one tablespoonful several times a day.

Peony Root.—Make a tea by boiling two tablespoonfuls of powdered peony root in one pint of water. This is very good for whooping cough.

Clover Blossoms.—Steep 2 ounces of dried red clover blossoms in a pint of boiling water for 4 hours. Give a glassful every little while through the day.

Alum and Honey.—Use two grains of alum dissolved in honey.

Cough Syrup.—Mix one lemon, sliced, one-half pint of flaxseed, one quart water, two tablespoonfuls of pulverized rock candy and two ounces of honey. Simmer for several hours, but do not boil. If less than a pint add enough water to make a pint. Strain and keep cool. Give one tablespoonful three times a day and after each coughing spell. Start to do this when the cough first starts and it will help very materially.

Cough Remedy.—Boil three lemons pared and sliced, five cents worth of flaxseed and three pints of rain water, to one half the quantity and strain. Dissolve three-fourth pound of rock candy, one stick licorice and two tablespoonfuls of goose grease in a little hot water and add to first part. Add five cents worth of glycerine. Keep cool. Shake well before using. Take one teaspoonful every two or three hours. Give babies one half teaspoonful.

WORMS.

DESCRIPTION.—Worms are intestinal parasites usually found in children. Babies are generally free from them. The Tapeworm is found in adults. There are three kinds of worms—tape, round and pinworms.

SYMPTOMS.—The symptoms are not very definite, as they might apply to several diseases. They are such as bad breath, headache, dizziness, loss of appetite, colic, etc. The only reliable symptom is their presence in the stools.

THREADWORM.—Threadworm is about one-half inch long and looks very much like thread. It sometimes causes intense itching in the rectum, at night especially. Give a good dose of castor oil followed by an injection of warm water, then another of about 3 drams of quassia chips to one pint of water. Another very effective remedy is santonin ½ grain, calomel ½ grain, sugar four grains. This will make two doses, take one morning and evening for three days. Follow with saline laxative. Give a dose of castor oil and an injection of warm salt water daily.

ROUNDWORM.—Roundworm is about four to ten inches long and looks like an earth worm, except in color and it is stiffer in structure. It may be found singly or in numbers. Give santonin and calomel as for threadworm, followed by a saline laxative. If not effective, repeat.

TAPEWORM.—Tapeworm is from ten to thirty feet long and about one-third of an inch wide, is composed of many small segments and is flat, from which quality it gets its name. This worm is taken into the body either in food or drink. Generally through raw meat, beef or pork. There is sometimes a twitching of the face or limbs and this disease is a common cause of convulsions. For the expulsion of a tapeworm you better see a physician.

First Aid and Home Treatment.

Pumpkin Seeds.—Soak four ounces of pumpkin seeds in water for twelve hours and then take the solution.

Pumpkin Seed and Veal.—Cook four ounces of powdered pumpkin seeds and one ounce of veal together till substance is all out of veal. Do not eat anything for twenty-four hours, then eat one-half of the soup, after one hour eat the other half of the soup. Take a good cathartic.

Santonin.—Mix santonin two grains, castor oil one ounce. Give one teaspoonful three or four times a day.

Oil of Male Fern.—Give one or two drams of oil of male fern, two hours after this give a good dose of castor oil. Give a very light diet for a day, just a glass of milk and toast, so that the worms will be hungry enough to take the drugs. Give a good cathartic, then use the following remedy: 2 or 3 ounces of pumpkin seeds, oleoresin aspidium 1 or 2 drams, pomegranate 1 dram. After 12 hours give a good dose of castor oil.

The head of the worm must be passed or it will grow another body. Be sure to prepare well before taking any medicines, as preparation is the principal item whatever remedy is used.

FOR YOUNG MEN

It is the desire of every young man to be successful in his life work, regardless of what that may be. To be successful in a large way, means the utilization to the fullest extent of all his powers, physical, mental and moral. It is the survival of the fittest in the great game of life. It is the man who is "fit," who has a strong, sound body in which is housed a strong, keen mind, coupled with a clear sense of his moral obligations to himself and society, that takes a large part, not only in the shaping of the world's affairs, but who is successful in the true sense of the word, even in the common every-day tasks.

The chain is only as strong as its weakest link. You may think you are "fit," however, the unusual moment comes, requiring unusual effort, unusual strength in every way. It may be the crisis in your life, when you most want to prove your ability and strength, and then if you have squandered your powers, physically, mentally or morally, this may be your Waterloo. If you have retained your full manly powers, you will rejoice as a strong man, for the opportunity of testing your strength and be successful.

Few young men realize the great effect the sex nature has upon the life. We wish to quote here from an article written by M. J. Exner, M. D., secretary The International Committee of Young Men's Christian Associations. Doctor Exner states: "One of the most interesting and significant discoveries in recent years has been the fact that the development of the essential characteristics of manhood and womanhood is dependent upon a product which the sex glands furnish to the blood. In the male the rugged form, the powerful muscles, the qualities of will, of initiative, of courage, the social instinct, love, and the spiritual sense are dependent upon the reproductive glands for their development. If these glands are destroyed in boyhood, the normal male qualities either do not develop or are greatly modified. The sex organs hold the key to the normal development of the individual in body, in mind, and in spirit." Stop! young man, to consider whether you can afford it or not, before you begin to sow the "wild oats." Any activity or practice or habit of mind which precociously stimulates sexual activity during the growing years of boyhood and young manhood is harmful to the finest development of the individual. It must also become plain that a young man's ideals of sex and of love have more to do with determining the character and the richness of his life in any human relationship than any other influence.

It is the man of strong noble character that the times demand and who is winning today and will win in the future. The man of questionable weak character has no place in the big things of life. The first necessity in the formation of a strong character, a life of rich experience and self-mastery, is the choice of an adequate ideal. Every young man should have an ideal, an aim, an object,

272

a purpose in life. It is the all absorbing purpose, the great ideal, that takes possession of the young man, keeps his mind busy, his life occupied, that makes him efficient and successful.

Every young man should master his impulses and refrain from all forms of sexual indulgence. For that is the only life which permits of the development of a fine character. A noble character must be forged out of first quality material. Pure imagination, right thinking, unselfish desires and manly conduct, are the materials out of which it must be builded.

The life of self-mastery is the only one consistent from the standpoint of life's efficiency, for high efficiency demands full mastery of all our powers, will, initiative, concentration, sustained application and singleness of purpose. The unchaste life is one of the greatest destroyers of personal efficiency.

The pure life is the only one that permits of a full and fine development of love and this is the biggest thing in a man's life. Out of this grow the things that make life worth while. The chaste life on the part of the young man is the only standard that is fair to woman, that assures the safety of the home and good parenthood.

Every young man should know these facts regarding his sex nature and the great danger in the abuse of his sex powers. He should know that his sex nature plays an important part in his life and has a profound effect on his success, physically, mentally and morally. Few realize this and know that when they abuse these powers, they are tearing away the very foundation of success, or that on which success is builded. They do not wake up to the fact until they have undermined health, their physical life, until they have weakened their mental powers and developed a perverted imagination, and until they have dulled their moral perceptions, losing that clearness of moral vision which should be a guide to them in their home life and their relations with society at large.

The object of this article is only to give a bit of advice and warning. It is the duty of every father to talk these things over with his son when he comes to the right age and give him a clear understanding of their importance in his life.

VENEREAL DISEASES.

Gonorrhea and syphilis, which are known as the venereal diseases, are contracted and spread through promiscuous sex relations. They are very rarely contracted in any other way. They are most loathsome and serious and it is not the intention to suggest any treatment here but to strongly advise the unfortunate victim to go to the best physician he can find and remain under his care until he is pronounced safe. Any attempt at home treatment may mean a life of invalidism and misery. Do not go to a "quack" doctor, one who advertises. The best is the cheapest in the end.

Prevention is always the best. Choose a high ideal, keep the mind well occupied, uncompromisingly avoid evil influences, conquer evil suggestions the instant they come into the mind by turning the thoughts to the big worth-while things of life. Remember, "What a man thinketh in his heart so is he."

PRESCRIPTION DEPARTMENT

This department will be found very valuable in every home, as we have only given the prescriptions which can be made up in the home and those that have been proven reliable through years of use. According to law, no druggist is allowed to fill prescriptions which contain narcotics such as opium, laudanum, morphia, etc., so all such prescriptions have been eliminated from the list. The patent prescriptions which have been used, have been carefully selected and analyzed by the best chemists, and while we do not claim them to be exactly the same as the originals, the analysis has been as exact as it is possible to obtain, and we claim the prescriptions given will produce preparations as good in uses and action as the originals. These prescriptions can be made up for but a fraction of what they cost ready-made—and in this way this department will also prove a money saver for the purchaser.

In the preparation of these medicines, we urge that the directions be followed carefully. Measure every ingredient exactly and mix as directed, as only in so doing can the best results be obtained. In the administering and storing of medicines, note carefully the cautions as given below.

CAUTIONS.

Shake all bottles before using, as frequently the most important part of the remedy is in the form of a sediment.

Carefully place the cork in the bottle after using, as many remedies contain substances which evaporate.

Measure exactly. Never guess at doses. A regular graduate glass and dropper should be used, as spoons vary in size and are not reliable. Hold the glass on a level with the eye when measuring.

It is well to give medicine containing iron or acids through a tube or straw as iron discolors the teeth and acids corrode the enamel of the teeth. If a straw or tube is not obtainable after taking the medicine, the patient should brush the teeth with a solution of baking soda and water.

A small piece of ice placed in the mouth before taking a disagreeable dose will make it less disagreeable.

Never use drugs from unlabeled bottles. Read the label twice.

Never give medicine in the dark or in a dim light. Many accidents happen this way.

Hold the bottle with label side up to avoid defacing the label and wipe the rim of the bottle with a piece of gauze.

Never give tablets or pills which have been accidentally left outside of their container nor medicine which has been left in a glass unlabeled. Keep your mind on what you are doing.

HOW TO RECKON A CHILD'S DOSE.

A good rule by which to reckon a child's dose is as follows: Make a fraction by using the child's age for the numerator and the child's age plus 12 for the denominator. The result will be the part of an adult's dose which should be given the child for the age specified. For example $\dfrac{6 \text{ years}}{6+12} = 6/18$ or $1/3$. A child six years old should be given one-third the dose of an adult.

THE WAY TO TAKE OILS.

In taking oils, the disagreeable taste may be lessened in the following ways: Pour a little orange juice into a glass, drop the oil in the center and add more orange juice, then swallow quickly. The oil will be surrounded by the juice like an egg in its shell. Lemonade or grape juice may be used instead of orange juice.

If the spoon is first dipped in sweet milk the oil will not adhere to it. This is well to remember in giving oils with a spoon.

Turpentine or Croton oil may be given on sugar from a spoon.

LINIMENTS.

Pain Killer.—1 quart witch hazel; ½ ounce caynore tincture; 2 ounces gum camphor; 2 ounces tincture of ammonia; ¼ ounce chloroform. Mix this and let stand a day before using.

Arnica Liniment.—1 quart witch hazel; 2 ounces tincture arnica; 1 ounce oil of spike and 1 ounce oil of hemlock. Let stand well stirred for a whole day. Fine for any kind of ache, burn, or sprain.

All Around Liniment.—2 ounces chloroform; ½ ounce tincture aconite; 5 ounces liquid soap.

Sweeny Liniment.—8 ounces witch hazel; 1 dram tincture aconite; 4 ounces turpentine; 2 ounces spirits of camphor; 1 ounce tincture cantharides; 1 dram red pepper; and oil of spike 2 ounces. While applying this rub briskly.

Rheumatism Liniment.—2 tablespoonfuls of extract of belladonna; 1 ounce olive oil; ½ ounce turpentine. Stir together and apply.

Camphor Liniment.—Dissolve ½ ounce of camphor gum in 2 fluid ounces of olive oil. This is fine for neuralgia and rheumatism.

Liniment for Chapped Hands, Etc.—1 dram camphor gum; ½ dram peruvian balsam; 1 fluid ounce oil of almonds, all of which can be dissolved slowly over a fire. Add ½ fluid ounce glycerine, and 15 drops oil nutmeg. Shake well. This will give excellent results.

All Ache Liniment.—2 ounces oil cajeput; 1 ounce each oils of sassafras, spike, cloves, origanum; 1½ ounces oil of mustard; 1 ounce tincture of capsicum; gum camphor 2 ounces; 2 quarts of alcohol. This when well shaken together will make a fine liniment for any pain, ache, or inflammation. A cloth can be saturated with the liniment and laid on the throat for soreness or hoarseness.

Egg Liniment.—Take 1 pint vinegar; 1 pint of turpentine and add five fresh eggs. Beat and stir this together. It will be yellow in color because of the eggs, however, this is known by many farmers to be the best liniment they have ever used. Many know it by the name of White Liniment. Adding ammonia will make it white as well as give it quicker drying and cooling properties. Many farmers have been glad of an opportunity to pay from five to ten dollars for this prescription.

Golden Oil.—Mix thoroughly two ounces each of liquid iodine and ammonia, and four ounces each of linseed oil and turpentine. This is strong but will be very good for rheumatism.

Mustang Liniment.—To 2 ounces each of spirits of hartshorn and olive oil, add 8 ounces of crude petroleum and 1 ounce of vinegar. This is excellent for sprains or lameness in man or beast.

Hamlin's Wizard Oil.—Mix one ounce of spirits of camphor, one-half ounce each of oil of sassafras and ammonia, two drams oil of cloves, four drams of chloroform and six drams spirits of turpentine. To this add ten drams of witch hazel. Very good, used externally.

Kerosene Liniment.—Dissolve one ounce camphor gum in one-half pint of kerosene. This is very penetrating and good for the joints.

Limewater Liniment.—Mix 4 ounces limewater, 2 ounces camphor and 4 ounces olive oil. Shake well before using and apply for sunburn, scalds, burns or bruises.

Cough Liniment.—Take 2 ounces rectified oil of amber, 2 ounce oil of stillingia, four ounces olive oil and six drams lobelia. Mix thoroughly and apply externally for whooping cough, rheumatism, sciatica and asthma.

Nerve Liniment.—Mix 1 ounce sulphuric ether, 1 ounce spirits of hartshorn, one-half ounce spirits of turpentine, one ounce sweet oil, one-half ounce chloroform and one-half oil of cloves. Apply this to any external location for twitching of the muscles or nerves.

Lemon Liniment.—Take 1 ounce oil of lemon, 1 ounce strong vinegar, 2 ounces rose water, 3 ounces turpentine and 1 egg yolk. These must be beaten and mixed well together. Always shake before using. When using, rub on the stomach, chest, back or throat for pneumonia, asthma or sprains.

Witch Hazel Liniment.—Mix 1 ounce fine cut tobacco with 4 ounces tincture arnica, 4 ounces soap liniment and 4 ounces extract of witch hazel. Let this stand several days keeping it stirred and then strain it. It will be found to be a fine application for any aches or pains.

Mustard Liniment.—Mix 2 fluid drams each of oil of mustard, turpentine and chloroform and add one pint of witch hazel. Shake well before using.

Lightning Liniment.—Take 1 grain aconite, 1 dram oil of mustard, 1 dram chloroform, ½ ounce strong ether, and 1 pint of witch hazel. This is very good for rheumatism, neuralgia, nervous pains and headaches when used externally.

Rheumatic Liniment.—Mix 2 ounces each of oil of cedar, oil of cajeput, oil of cloves and oil of sassafras. Shake and apply to parts several times daily.

Home Liniment.—Mix ½ pint good vinegar, ½ spirits of camphor, ½ ounce muriate of ammonia and 1 pint of clean rain water. Soak cloths in this and apply. This is very good for inflammatory rheumatism.

Olive Oil Liniment.—Mix with ½ pint of olive oil a small sized cake of camphor gum, one good tablespoonful of kerosene and 15 drops of carbolic acid. Set this on a stove and bring it to a boil. Cool and use for sprains and lameness.

Man and Beast Liniment.—To a pint of clean spirits of turpentine add one-half ounce each of oil of sassafras, origanum, and oil of amber. Shake until well mixed together. Many people have used this for sprains, sore throat, bruises, rheumatism and as an application to relieve a horse of thistloe or poll evil.

OINTMENT AND SALVES.

Ringworm Ointment.—2 drams iodine; 1 dram iodide of potassium; 6 fluid drams alcohol and 3 drams of water. Mix well together and apply.

Household Salve.—Mix 1 ounce of crystal carbolic acid; 2 ounces white wax and 16 ounces of petrolatum. The petrolatum and wax should be carefully melted on a stove. Then take it to a window and stir in the acid crystals. Good for sores, bruises, and roughness.

Good Arnica Salve.—Dissolve 2 drams solid extract of arnica in hot water. Melt 14 ounces lard and 2 ounces of good wax and stir in the arnica. If too thick add more lard. This will be found good for bruises and bunches on people or animals.

Zinc and Camphor Salve.—Melt 20 ounces petrolatum and 2 ounces good paraffin together and into this drop 5 drams of gum camphor and 4 ounces zinc oxide. Be sure this is all mixed together in every part. Very good for healing.

Stick Salve.—Pine pitch, 6 ounces; resin, 4 ounces; turpentine gum, 2 ounces; beeswax, 2 ounces; balsam of fir, 2 ounces; Venice turpentine, 1 ounce. Melt these solid substances together on a stove or in a very hot water bath. Do not let them burn. They must be stirred thoroughly. Add the liquids. Let cool, pour on cold slab and roll into sticks. When applying heat the end over a lamp or stove. Excellent for healing.

Ointment for Felons.—Soften a little strong soap and add plenty of salt. Apply this to the end of the finger affected by a felon and it will be quickly drawn to a head.

Lard and Tar Ointment.—Take 1 cup of melted lard; 1 cup strong tar; 1 tablespoonful of turpentine and stir together. This has been used effectively in keeping flies from wounds on animals as well as helping to heal quickly.

Kerosene Salve.—Melt 2 tablespoonfuls of pure beeswax; ½ cup of lard; 1 tablespoonful of salted butter and add 4 tablespoonfuls of kerosene oil, the juice of a small onion and a half teaspoonful of camphor. This has the combined qualities of keeping out the air, keeping away flies, healing a wound from the inner surface and draws to a head or brings out the pus in a wound.

Salve for Sores and Bruises.—Arnica, 5 cents worth; glycerine, 5 cents worth; beeswax, 5 cents worth; rosin, the size of a small hazelnut; 5 cents worth of fresh suet, rendered. Put all into a clean vessel and melt over a slow fire. Then set out to cool.

Lip Salve.—1½ ounces of spermaceti, ½ ounce of white wax, 6 drachms camphor, 4 tablespoonfuls of lard. Mix well.

Home-Made Salve.—Take 1 cup of elderberry bark, shave fine, fry in 1½ cups of fresh lard till the bark becomes black. Strain while hot. Fine for burns and skin disease.

Carbolic Salve.—Mix 1 teaspoonful of vaseline and 4 drops of carbolic acid.

Home Salve.—Take 1 ounce each of resin, lard and beeswax and melt slowly over a fire. Let it cool a little and add one ounce of oil of spikenard. This is very good for curing old sores and keeping them clean.

Frostbite Salve.—Mix lard and black gunpowder. Keep away from a fire. This has been used by many men caught in snowstorms while hunting.

Garden Salve.—Cut up a good strong onion and heat it for some time in melted lard. After straining add several drops of lemon juice. Apply several times a day. It is very good for reducing the inflammation in wounds.

Itch Ointment.—Mix 2 ounces of sulphur with 1 cup lard. This is very good for skin diseases.

Catarrh Ointment.—Melt 1 good tablespoonful of tar and 2 tablespoonfuls of fresh unsalted butter together. Let cool and apply inside the nostrils several times daily with the tip of the finger.

Glycerine Ointment.—Add 1 teaspoonful of carbolic acid to 15 teaspoonfuls of glycerine. This is fine for wounds or cuts.

Pile Ointment.—Mix 40 grains iron persulphite with 1 ounce pure lard. Add a couple drops of the oil of bitter almond. Apply several times daily.

Toothache Wax.—Melt together 1 dram oil of cloves, ½ ounce crystal carbolic acid and one and one-half ounce yellow wax. Soak thin layers of absorbent cotton in the liquid before it cools. After cooling cut and roll it into tubes. When needed for a hollow tooth, clip off the desired quantity and place in tooth. This is very effective.

Boil Ointment.—Mix with 1 ounce of cold cream 5 drops of carbolic acid, one and one-half drams fluid extract of ergot, two teaspoonfuls of starch, two teaspoonfuls of zinc oxide and apply by placing on a piece of gauze or cotton which can be laid over the boil.

Eye Salve.—Melt together 2 teaspoonfuls of white wax and 6 teaspoonfuls of fresh lard. When nearly cool, add one grain of camphor gum, five grains zinc oxide and a little oil of rose. This is good if rubbed on the eye for inflammation and sore eyes.

Butter Ointment.—Add a few drops of camphor to a small amount of butter.

PLASTERS AND POULTICES.

Nature's Plaster.—Pine pitch, 6 teaspoonfuls; resin, 8 teaspoonfuls; beeswax, 3 teaspoonfuls; lard, 7 teaspoonfuls; and 1 teaspoonful each of turpentine, palm oil and olive oil. These should be melted together and thoroughly mixed. This will make plenty of material for a number of plasters. It can be kept in a good iron or enamel pot and when needed it has to be rewarmed. Fine for inflammation or sprains. Can be applied to bare skin.

Linseed Poultice.—Pour linseed meal into ½ pint of boiling water. Pour gradually stirring all the time so it will not lump. Add enough to make a reasonably thick poultice. This will aid in suppuration or bringing to a head, boils, tumors, inflammation, etc. A little warm lard added will prevent the poultice hardening. Apply between clean pads of cotton.

Bread and Milk Poultice.—One of the finest poultices is made by soaking stale bread in good milk until it is well softened. Drain off enough milk to leave a well dampened quantity of bread. Put this between clean cloths and apply. Fine for inflamed eyes, swellings, or bruises.

Horseradish Poultice.—Grate plenty of horseradish and apply to a joint or bunch. This is very good for rheumatism or sciatica or neuralgia.

Potato Poultice.—Grate fresh potatoes. These are very cooling in effect and are good for burns, scalds and weak eyes when applied as a poultice.

Mustard Plaster.—Mix dry mustard and three parts flour with warm water to a satisfactory thickness. If it is too strong when applied add a little more flour to it.

Poultice for Suppurating Wounds.—Bind freshly bruised garlic or onions on a wound. It is used by the great surgeons in Europe to cleanse a wound quickly. Elderly French women who were acting as nurses got extraordinary results in healing wounds of all wounded soldiers and upon investigations by the heads of the surgical department, they found garlic and onions were being used. It is use of the simple ingredients which often get the best and most surprising results.

Mullein Weed Poultice.—Bruise a number of the leaves and tie on a bruise or swelling. They are fine for reducing swellings on people or cattle.

Smartweed Poultice.—This plant grows in fence corners and around damp places in the barnyard. When it is pulled up and pounded with a round stick it makes one of the very finest applications for stings, bruises, sprains and cuts. It can be folded in a bandage and put on any part of the body.

Slippery Elm Poultice.—Add hot water to a quantity of powdered slippery elm bark and apply. This is very soothing.

Cranberry Poultice.—Crush cranberries and use as a poultice. This will be found very good for erysipelas.

Flaxseed Poultice.—Add flaxseed to boiling water and allow to boil until it becomes thick. Spread on a clean cloth and apply. Cover well to retain heat.

Onion Poultice.—Onions sliced and fried in lard make a fine poultice to relieve congestion of the lungs, croup, etc.

Charcoal Poultice.—Take equal parts of flaxseed meal and animal charcoal and add these to boiling water. Spread on a cloth and apply. This will be found fine for carbuncles or boils.

PATENT PRESCRIPTIONS
Arabian Balsam.

Oleum gossypium ....15 oz.
Oleum origani .... 1 oz.
Oleum terebinth .... 4 dr.
Mix together.
Dose.—Four drops.

Aseptin.

Alum .... 1 part
Borax .... 2 parts
This is a preservative for milk and meats, etc.

Atomizer's Solution.

Menthol .... 1 gr.
Camphor .... 1 gr.
Liquid albolene (American mineral oil), enough to
    make .... 1 oz.
This is good for nose trouble.

Ayer's Hair Vigor.

Acetate of lead.................................. ¾ oz.
Flowers of sulphur.............................. ½ oz.
Glycerine .... 3½ oz.
Water .... 20 oz.

Ayer's Sarsaparilla.

Fluid extract sarsaparilla........................ 3 oz.
Fluid extract may apple.......................... 2 oz.
Fluid extract yellow dock........................ 2 oz.
Fluid extract stillingia .... 3 oz.
Iodide potassium .... 90 gr.
Iodide iron .... 10 gr.
Sugar .... 1 oz.
Mix together.
Blood purifier.
Dose.—One teaspoonful before meals.

Bareel's Indian Liniment.

Tincture capsicum .... 1 dr.
Oil origanum .... ½ oz.
Oil sassafras .... ½ oz.
Oil pennyroyal .... ½ oz.
Oil hemlock .... ½ oz.
Alcohol .... 1 qt.
Mix together.
This makes a good liniment for general purposes.

Barker's Bone and Nerve Liniment.

Oil of turpentine 1   oz.
Oil of thyme .... ½ oz.
Oil of tar .... ¼ oz.
Camphor 4   dr.
Franklin oil (black oil, lubricating oil), sufficient to
     make ½ pt.

This liniment is good for man or beast and is excellent for rheumatism, sprains, bruises, etc.

Bay Rum.

Alcohol .... ½ pt.
Extract of bay rum........................... 6 dr.
Water .... ½ pt.

This makes a good hair dressing.

B. B. B.—Blood Purifier.

Burdock fl. ex. .... 2 oz.
Yellow dock fl. ex................................ 2 oz.
Sarsaparilla fl. ex................................. 2 oz.
Senna fl. ex. .... 2 oz.
Alcohol .... 4 oz.
Simple syrup .... 16 oz.

Brown's Bronchial Troches.

Gum arabic, powdered .... 2 oz.
Cubebs, powdered .... 2 oz.
Sugar, powdered .... 12 oz.
Extract licorice, powdered .... 8 oz.
Extract conium .... ½ oz.

Mix together and add just enough water so that the mixture may be rolled out and cut into little squares. This is good for irritated throat, colds, coughs, etc.

Bucklen's Arnica Salve.

Extract arnica .... ½ oz.
Raisins, seedless .... 4 oz.
Tobacco, fine cut .... ¼ oz.
Resin cerate .... 4 oz.
Vaseline .... 1 oz.
Water .... sufficient

Boil the raisins and tobacco in one-half pint of water till the strength is extracted; press out the liquid and boil down to two ounces. Soften the extract of arnica with a little hot water and mix the liquid with it; then mix this thoroughly with the resin cerate and vaseline which have been previously warmed.

Camphor Ice.

Spermaceti .... 1½ oz.
Sweet almonds, oil of............................. ½ oz.
Gum camphor .... ¾ oz.

Put in an earthen vessel and heat just enough to dissolve it, then pour into a little jar.

Castoria.

Rochelle salts 1   oz.
Manna 1   oz.
Senna 4   dr.
Fennel, bruised .... 1½ dr.
Sugar 8   oz.
Boiling water .... 8 fl. oz.

Oil of wintergreen enough to flavor. Pour the water on the ingredients. Cover and let stand till cool. Strain, add the sugar, stir till dissolved and flavor with wintergreen.

Dose.—Two to four teaspoonfuls.

Chamberlain's Colic, Cholera and Diarrhea Remedy.

Tinct. capsicum .... 2½ oz.
Tinct. camphor 2   oz.
Tinct. guaiacum .... 1½ oz.

Dose.—Five to ten drops on sugar every hour until relieved.

Cough Remedy.

Ammonium chloride .... 40 oz.
Syrup of squills, comp. .... 1 oz.
Syrup of ipecac .... 1 oz.
Syrup of wild cherry........................... 1 oz.
Syrup of tar .... 1 oz.

Dose.—One teaspoonful every three hours.

Cough Remedy.

Menthol .... ½ gr.
Ammonium chloride .... 40 gr.
Elixir potassium bromide....................... 1 oz.
Syrup of licorice .... 1 oz.
Water .... 1 oz.

Dose.—One teaspoonful every three hours.

Cuticura Ointment.

This ointment consists of a base of petroleum jelly, colored green, perfumed with oil of bergamont and containing about 9 drops of carbolic acid to the ounce.

Cuticura Resolvent.

Rhubarb, powdered .... 1 dr.
Aloes, socot .... 1 dr.
Iodide potass. .... 36 gr.
Whisky .... 1 pt.
Dose.—One teaspoonful before each meal.

Dandruff Cure.

Benzine .... 8 fl. dr.
Oil of cade .... 2 fl. dr.
Coal tar .... 2 fl. dr.
Green soap .... 2 fl. dr.
Oil of turpentine .... 2 fl. dr.
Rub soap and tar together. Add the oil of cade and then incorporate the other ingredients.
Directions.—Rub a little into the scalp and then wash well with soap.

Earache Remedy.

Two percent solution of carbolic acid in glycerine.
Place drop or two on cotton and insert in ear.

Ely's Cream Balm.

Vaseline .... 1 oz.
Thymol .... 3 gr.
Carbonate bismuth .... 15 gr.
Oil wintergreen .... 2 dp.
Mix well. Good for catarrh and is used by dipping the finger in the balm and inserting in the nostrils.

Frost Bites and Chilblains.

Powdered camphor .... 30 gr.
Ichthyol .... 2 dr.
Ointment of lead subacitate.................... 4 dr.
Apply twice daily.

Frostilla.

Grain alcohol .... 2½ oz.
Glycerine .... 3 oz.
Quince seeds .... 30 gr.
Hot water .... 10½ oz.
Pour hot water on the quince seeds and steep till a mucilage is formed and then strain through muslin. To this add the glycerine and shake thoroughly. The desired perfume should be mixed with the alcohol and then this should be mixed with the mucilage, and all shaken well.
This is a fine preparation for chapped hands.

Gargling Oil.

Crude petroleum .... 3¼ oz.
Ammonia water .... 1½ oz.
Soft soap 4   oz.
Benzine 4   oz.
Crude oil amber .... ½ oz.
Tincture of iodine .... ¼ oz.
Water .... 1¼ pt.

Mix the petroleum and soap, add the ammonia water, oil of amber and tincture of iodine, and mix thoroughly. Then add the benzine and finally the water.

Genuine White Oil Liniment.

Oil turpentine .... 21 parts
Oil origanum .... 20 parts
Camphor .... 20 parts
Ammonia carbonate .... 19 parts
Castile soap .... 19 parts

Water enough to make 300 parts by weight.

Giles's Iodide of Ammonia Liniment.

Camphor .... ½ oz.
Aqua ammonia 2   oz.
Oil of lavender .... ¼ oz.
Oil of rosemary .... ¼ oz.
Iodine .... ½ dr.
Alcohol 1   pt.

Dissolve the iodine in the alcohol; add the camphor and then the oils; then add enough water of ammonia to remove the dark color of the mixture.

Gombault's Caustic Balsam.

Oil of camphor .... 1 fl. dr.
Cottonseed oil .... 2 fl. oz.
Croton oil .... 4 fl. dr.
Oil turpentine .... 2 fl. dr.
Oil thyme .... ½ fl. dr.
Kerosene .... 4 fl. dr.
Sulphuric acid .... 20 minims

First mix the croton and cottonseed oils and then add the sulphuric acid, stirring continually, then add the other ingredients.

Green Mountain Salve.

Mutton tallow	1½ oz. troy
Beeswax	1½ oz. troy
Burgundy pitch	1½ oz. troy
Resin	2½ lb. troy
Venice turpentine	½ fl. oz.
Balsam fir	½ fl. oz.
Oil hemlock	½ fl. oz.
Oil red cedar	½ fl. oz.
Oil origanum	½ fl. oz.
Oil wormwood	¼ fl. oz.
Powdered verdigris	½ oz.

Melt together the first four ingredients and then add the oils. Rub up the verdigris with a little oil and put it in with the other ingredients, stirring well Then put the mixture in cold water and work into rolls.

Hall's Hair Renewer.

Salt	1 dr.
Lead acetate	½ dr.
Sulphur precipitated	½ dr.
Bay rum	1 fl. oz.
Jamaica rum	2 fl. oz.
Glycerine	4 fl. oz.
Water	8 fl. oz.

Mix well and rub into the roots of the hair once a day.

Hamburg Breast Tea.

Anise seed	2 oz.
Orris root	1 oz.
Mullein flowers	2 oz.
Licorice root	3 oz.
Coltsfoot	4 oz.
Marshmallow flowers	8 oz.

Mix all together and use by putting two teaspoonfuls in a glass of boiling water. When cool pour off the water carefully and drink it.

Good for colds on the chest.

Hamburg Tea.

Senna	8 parts
Manna	3 parts
Coriander	1 part

Good for biliousness and headaches, also constipation.

Dose.—One teaspoonful to a cup of hot water. Drink when cool.

Hamlin's Wizard Oil.

Tinct. capsicum .... ½ oz.
Tinct. myrrh .... ½ oz.
Oil sassafras .... ½ oz.
Chloroform .... ½ oz.
Gum camphor .... 1 oz.
Alcohol .... 1 pt.

Harlem Oil.

Linseed oil .... 1 lb.
Flowers of sulphur .... 2 oz.
Oil of amber .... 2 oz.
Oil of turpentine ....Sufficient

Mix sulphur and linseed oil and boil slowly till sulphur is dissolved. Then take off the fire and when somewhat cooled add the oil of amber and enough oil of turpentine to make preparation about as thick as molasses.

Dose.—Ten drops taken with sugar before meals.

Good for bladder and kidney troubles.

Holloway's Ointment.

Yellow wax .... 10 parts
White wax .... 10 parts
Turpentine .... 25 parts
Lard .... 50 parts
Sweet oil .... 75 parts

Melt the ingredients together over a slow fire and stir till cool. This makes a fine ointment for general purposes.

Hop Bitters.

Tinct. of hops .... ½ oz.
Tinct. of senega .... 3 dr.
Tinct. of buchu .... 3 dr.
Podophyllin (dissolved in spirits of wine)........ 10 gr.
Tinct. of cochineal .... 20 dr.

Distilled water sufficient to make 1 pint.

Mix all together.

Dose.—One to two teaspoonfuls before meals.

Hostetter's Bitters.

Sugar 6   oz.
Gentian root 6   oz.
Columbo root 6   oz.
Orange peel 6   oz.
Calamus root 6   oz.
Peruvian bark 6   oz.
Cloves .... ½ oz.
Cinnamon 1   oz.
Rhubarb 2   oz.

Diluted alcohol enough to make one gallon.
Grind the solids and mix the alcohol.
Dose.—One tablespoonful three times a day.

Kendall's Spavin Cure.

Camphor .... ½ oz.
Turpentine 1   fl. oz.
Alcohol 2   fl. oz.
Petroleum oil (heavy) .... ½ fl. dr.
Oil of rosemary 1   fl. dr.
Iodine 25   gr.

Mix the oils without filtering and dissolve the camphor and iodine in them.

Kickapoo Indian Oil.

Camphor .... ½ oz. tr.
Tinct. capsicum .... ½ fl. oz.
Oil turpentine 1   fl. dr.
Oil peppermint .... ½ fl. dr.
Oil wintergreen .... ½ fl. dr.
Alcohol sufficient to make........................ 1   pt.

Mix all together. Good for rheumatism and as a general liniment.

Liniment for Man and Beast.

Balsam fir .... 1 oz. tr.
Myrrh, powdered .... 1 oz.
Aloes, powdered .... 1 oz.
Alcohol .... 8 fl. oz.

Lydia Pinkham's Compound.

Beth root .... 1½ oz.
Cassia 2   oz.
Unicorn root 2   oz.
Poplar bark 2   oz.
Partridgeberry vine 4   oz.
Cramp bark 4   oz.
Sugar .... 1½ lb.
Alcohol 1   pt.
Water ....sufficient quantity

The first six drugs should be reduced to a moderately coarse powder. Pour boiling water on these and let stand cold, and then percolate with water until five pints are obtained, add the sugar, bring to a boil, remove from fire and when cold add alcohol and strain.

Dose.—One teaspoonful before meals.

Magnetic Liniment.

Muriate ammonia .... 2 dr.
Tinct. cantharides .... 2 dr.
Sulphuric ether .... 1 oz.
Oil of origanum .... 1 oz.
Alcohol .... 1 pt.

Mexican Mustang Liniment.

Kerosene oil 3   dr.
Black oil 1   dr.
Oil of thyme .... ½ dr.
Oil of amber, crude .... ½ dr.
Oil of turpentine................................. ½ dr.
Soap .... 35 gr.
Caustic potash 3   gr.
Water ....3 oz. 2 dr.

The soap and caustic potash should be placed together in a bottle or flask and then dissolve in two ounces of hot water; this mixture should be shaken vigorously as the mixed oils are added in small quantities at a time When the mixture has once assumed a creamy consistency, the oils may be added more rapidly. Water (quite warm) should be added till a full pint is made. Much care should be used in adding the water and mixing the ingredients. If the oils do not emulsify readily, it will be necessary to begin over again as either too much oil was added at first or the water was not warm enough. Much care must be observed in order to insure success.

Nerve and Bone Liniment.

Oil of hemlock	1 oz.
Oil of origanum	1 oz.
Oil of amber	1 oz.
Oil of rosemary	1 oz.
Turpentine	1 pt.
Linseed oil	1½ pt.

Mix all together and use externally.

Oil of Joy.

Oil of sassafras	½ oz.
Oil of cedar	½ oz.
Tinct. of guaiac	½ oz.
Gum camphor	¼ oz.
Water of ammonia	2 oz.
Tinct. of capsicum	1 oz.
Chloroform	1½ oz.
Alcohol	2 pt.

Mix thoroughly and shake well before using.

Paine's Celery Compound.

Lemon peel	¼ oz.
Orange peel	¼ oz.
Coriander seed	¼ oz.
Red cinchona	1 oz.
Celery seed	2 oz.
Hydrochloric acid	15 minims
Glycerine	3 fl. oz.
Syrup	4 fl. oz.
Water	4 fl. oz.
Alcohol	5 fl. oz.

Grind all the solids into a moderately coarse powder, mix the acid and water, add the glycerine and alcohol, and in the mixture so prepared macerate the powder for twenty-four hours; then percolate, adding enough alcohol and water in the proportion given to make 12 fl. oz. Then add the syrup filter if necessary.

This makes a very good tonic.

Dose.—One teaspoonful before meals.

Radway's Ready Relief.

Alcohol	½ oz.
Ammonia, water of	½ oz.
Capsicum, tinct. of	½ oz.
Soap liniment	1½ oz.

Mix thoroughly. This makes a good counter irritant.

Robberts' Camphor-Tar Ointment.

Liquid tar .... 1 oz.
Camphor .... 1 oz.
Lard .... 8 oz.

Mix well together.

Royal Catarrh Cure.

Common salt .... 98.00 parts
Muriate of berberine .... .65 parts
Carbolic acid .... 1.35 parts
Total (parts by weight) 100.00

Seven Sutherland Sisters' Hair Grower.

Common salt 1   dr.
Bay rum 7   fl. oz.
Dist. ext. of witch hazel 9   fl. oz.
Hydrochloric acid (5 percent)............. 1   dr.
Magnesia .... ½ oz.

Mix the bay rum and witch hazel, then add the magnesia and shake well; filter and dissolve the salt in the filtrate, then add the hydrochloric acid. This makes a good hair tonic.

Skinner's Dandruff Mixture.

Bay rum .... 1 pt.
Glycerine .... 4 oz.
Chloral hydrate .... 1 oz.

Sore Throat.

Iron chloride, tinct. of .... 1½ dr.
Glycerine ....2½ dr.
Simple syrup enough to make................... 2   oz.

Dose.—One teaspoonful every four hours.

Syrup of Figs.

Figs 6   oz.
Prunes 3   oz.
Senna leaves .... 3½ oz.
Cassia pulp .... 4½ oz
Tamarind .... 4½ oz.
Coriander seed .... 1½ oz.
Ext. licorice 3   dr.
Ess. peppermint 3   dr.
Simple syrup 1   qt.

Make a water extract of the drugs so as to measure one pint and dissolve in this two pounds of sugar to make the syrup.

Dose.—One teaspoonful every two hours until relief is obtained.

Tapeworm Remedy.

Male fern .... 2 dr.
Gum arabic .... 2 dr.
Kamala .... 1 dr.
Fennel water .... 2½ oz.
Distilled water .... 2½ oz.
Syrup of orange .... 1 oz.
Spirits of chloroform .... ½ dr.

Directions.—The above is to be taken in three doses within three hours on an empty stomach, followed by large dose of epsom salts.

Tonsilitis Remedy.

Crystal iodine .... 1 gr.
Potassium iodide .... 3 gr.
Glycerine to make................................ 4 oz.

Dose.—One teaspoonful in glass of warm water used as a gargle.

Trask's Magnetic Ointment.

Lard .... 3 oz.
Raisins .... 3 oz.
Fine cut tobacco .... 3 oz.

Simmer well together. Then strain, pressing out all from the drugs. This makes an excellent ointment for skin diseases.

HANDY TABLES OF WEIGHTS AND MEASURES.

1 Minim usually equals............................1 drop
60 Minims equal.............1 fluid dram or 1 teaspoonful
8 fluid drams equal ....1 fluid ounce or 2 tablespoonfuls
16 fluid ounces equal................................1 pint

1 fluid dram equals ....1 teaspoonful
1 fluid ounce equals.....................2 tablespoonfuls
2 fluid ounces equal ....A wineglassful
4 fluid ounces equal ....A teacupful
6 fluid ounces equal ....A coffeecupful

1 drop usually equals..............................1 grain
20 grains equal ....1 scruple or 1-3 teaspoonful
3 scruples equal....................1 dram or 1 teaspoonful
8 drams equal.................1 ounce or 2 tablespoonfuls

BEAUTY HINTS

Hands.

For Perspiration of the Hands.—Glycerin, 1 ounce; salicylic acid, 75 grains; borax, 60 grains; boracic acid, 40 grains. Wash hands and dry thoroughly before applying the lotion. Rub on the hands four or five times a day.

If the hands perspire while sewing simply wash them in alum water.

To Make Hands Plump.—Wash hands in warm water, then rub in cocoa butter or any good skin food for five minutes, after which hold the hands for an instant in ice cold water. Wipe dry. The cold water closes the pores while they are filled with cream.

To Whiten the Hands.—Lanolin, 100 grains; paraffin (liquid), 25 grains; extract of vanilla, 10 drops; oil of roses, 1 drop. Mix and apply after washing the hands.

Glycerin, 2 ounces; water, 2 ounces; lemon, 4 tablespoonfuls; add a few drops of carbolic acid. Shake well and apply after washing the hands. This will soften as well as whiten them.

To Avoid Chapping.—After they have been in water or soapsuds, a very good remedy is to wash them in vinegar. This will keep them soft and white as well as keep them from chapping.

Remedy.—Quince seed, ½ ounce; alcohol, ½ pint; glycerin, 2 gills; rosewater, 4 ounces; tincture of benzoin, 2 ounces. Soak the quince seed in a quart of lukewarm soft water, let stand for twenty-four hours, shaking occasionally. Then strain through cloth and add glycerin, alcohol, and the rosewater. Last of all add the two ounces of benzoin. Mix these thoroughly and let stand twenty-four hours before using.

Bleach.—Lemon juice is an excellent bleach for the hands and also for the finger nails. Lemon juice should be a part of every woman's toilet.

Honey Bleach.—White honey, 5 ounces; glycerine, 2 drams; alcohol, 2 ounces; perfume as desired. Use often.

Rose Bleach.—Benzoin tincture, ¼ ounce; rosewater, 6 ounces. Use after washing.

To Soften.—Soak 1 ounce of quince seeds in a quart of soft water over night. Strain them in the morning and add 2 ounces of rosewater, 2 ounces glycerine, one ounce alcohol and three drops carbolic acid. Mix thoroughly and apply to chapped or cracked hands.

For the Nails.—To supply the oil which has been removed by too frequent washing, the following should be used, oil of bergamot, 3 drops; petroleum, 1 ounce; white castile soap (powdered), 60 grains.

To break the habit of biting the nails apply bitter aloes. With this on the nails, the person is not likely to try to bite them the second time.

To dip the fingers in strong alum solution or powdered quinine is good to break the habit of biting the nails.

Feet.

Callouses or Corns.—For painful callouses or corns, place several layers of adhesive plaster in a kind of cushion over the corn. This relieves the callous or corn from friction, and it will gradually disappear.

For Swollen or Aching Feet.—Bathing in vinegar relieves them greatly.

Witch hazel is good. Use one or two teaspoonfuls of camphor to four ounces of witch hazel. After bathing, rub the feet well with this solution. It is very soothing as well as healing.

Olive oil is very good for the feet. Rub thoroughly after bathing.

Bunions are the result of great friction or pressure. The large joint of the big toe is usually the one afflicted. The joint should be relieved of all pressure. If possible a loose slipper should be worn so as to give the toe plenty of room to spread to its natural position. Then take a piece of adhesive plaster and bandage the place affected. This will relieve the inflammation and the bunion will gradually disappear.

To paint the bunion with iodine, 2 drams; carbolic acid, 2 drams mixed with glycerin is good.

Walking pigeon toed often relieves the friction and pressure on a bunion.

Red Nose.—Solution—Powdered calamine, 1 dram; glycerin, ½ dram; zinc oxide, 30 grains; cherry laurel water, 4 ounces. Shake the lotion well before applying to the nose. It may be used both morning and night.

To Reduce a Double Chin, the following exercise should be used daily: with the open hand press firmly downward from the point of the chin to the neck, throwing the head back at the same time. Also bathe the chin frequently with cold water; ice water is best.

For wrinkles about the eyes stroke with the finger tips over and below the eyes, from the nose toward the temples. Unless you are an expert, do not try to massage both sides of the face at the same time, for that is liable to cause the skin to become flabby in time by stretching it in contrary directions.

For Perspiration.—Frequent bathing is one of the best cures for perspiration. Bathe in warm water to which has been added enough of tincture of benzoin to make it creamy. Immediately after drying the body dust with the following powder: camphor, 2½ drams; orris root, 4 ounces; starch, 16 ounces.

Powder for Perspiration.—Oxide of zinc, 4 drams; boracic acid, 4 drams; lycopodium, 8 drams; powdered starch, 2 ounces; powdered orris root, 1 ounce. Mix the ingredients and sift a number of times through a fine sifter. The powder is slightly astringent, and highly recommended for excessive perspiration.

Orris Root Powder for Perspiration.—Phenic acid, 3 drams; alcohol, 5½ drams; starch 6¼ ounces; florentine orris root, 5½ ounces; essence of violet, 32 minims. Dissolve the acid in the alcohol, add the violet essence, then the starch and orris root. This powder can be used for the hands or any other part of the body.

After the bath bathe the parts with a solution composed of the following: salicylic acid, ½ ounce; alcohol, 4 ounces. This is a most excellent remedy for the feet.

Face.

For Sunburn.—The following formulas are very good for destroying the ravages of summer wind and sun: Cut a cucumber into rather small pieces without peeling, crush this thoroughly until it is a pulp-like mass, then strain through cloth, squeezing out as much of the juice as possible, then put the refuse and juice into an enameled saucepan and let simmer for ten minutes, but do not boil.

A cream of the following is good: glycerin, 1-3 ounce; oil of roses, 4 drops; rosewater, 1-3 ounce; white wax, 2-3 ounce; spermaceti, 1 ounce; oil of almonds, 4 ounces.

To relieve inflammation caused by cold wind: spermaceti, ½ ounce; oil of almonds, ½ gill; white wax, ½ ounce; rose water, 1 ounce; witch hazel, 1 ounce.

Benzoic acid, 3 grains; anhyderous lanolin, 5 drams; oil of sweet almonds, 16 drops; oil of cacao, 16 grains.

Glycerin, 6 ounces; Florentine orris root, 1 ounce; pulverized borax, 1 ounce; pulverized tragacanth, ½ ounce; extract of cassia, ½ ounce; oil of roses, 12 drops.

Arrowroot, ¼ ounce; orange flower water, ¼ ounce; glycerin, 5½ ounces; oil of roses, 4 drops; oil of orange, 4 drops.

Powder to Protect the Skin.—Cream is not enough to protect the skin against rough cold winds. Powder should also be dusted over the cream. The following is a good protecting powder: pulverized orris root, 2 ounces; well pulverized rice, 7 ounces; oil of rose geranium, 20 drops. After thoroughly mixing, sift through cloth.

For Removing Tan.—Lemon juice is one of the safest remedies for removing tan and whitening the skin. Rub a slice of lemon over face or tanned spots, let juice remain on for two or three hours or over night. After washing off with warm water and a mild soap, massage the face well with some good cream. Continue this lemon treatment every night until the tan is removed or the dark skin peels off. If it proves painful, stop for a day or so and use cold cream. Be careful not to get the second coat of tan before this is healed as the second will be harder to remove than the first.

Chapped Lips.—To prevent chapped or withered looking lips, the following is a splendid remedy—cold cream, 4 drams; lanolin, 4 drams; bor-glycerin (50 percent solution), 3 drams. Press the mixture gently on the lips at night and before going out into the cold wind.

Cleansing Creams.—Plain olive oil or melted cocoa butter will cleanse, soften and nourish dry skin.

White wax, 1 ounce; spermaceti, 1 ounce; sweet almond oil, 6 ounces; distilled water, 1 ounce; glycerin, 1 ounce; salicylic acid, 15 grains. The skin should be thoroughly cleansed every night, so that the dust accumulated during the day does not clog the pores.

White wax, 2 ounces; white glycerin, 2 ounces; sweet almond oil, 4 ounces; oil of violets, 10 drops. Apply to the face with finger tips and then dry with a soft towel, use just before retiring. In the morning instead of using soap and water, pour a little toilet water on a soft towel to cleanse the face. You will find that this will not only cleanse the skin, but will also reduce the pores in a short time.

For Coarse Pores.—When the texture of the skin is coarse and pitted with enlarged pores, the following lotion will prove very beneficial—alum, 70 grains; almond milk (thick), 1½ ounces; rosewater, 6 ounces. Dissolve the alum in the rosewater, then pour slowly into the almond milk, stirring constantly. Apply with a soft linen cloth before retiring.

Skin Bleach.—Apply to the skin morning and evening the following lotion: tincture of benzoin, 30 drops; glycerin, 2 ounces; rosewater, 3 ounces.

To whiten the skin bathe in milk daily. Occasionally add a little lemon juice. This will make the skin soft as well as white.

Massage Cream.—Spermaceti, 2½ drams; white wax, 2½ drams; oil of bitter almonds, ½ dram; almond oil, 1½ ounces; lanolin, ½ ounce; elder flower water, 1½ ounces; witch hazel, ½ ounce. Melt the spermaceti and wax, in an earthen dish, set in a basin of boiling water, all the lanolin, then beat the oils in slowly. Remove the vessel from the heat and add the elder flower water and witch hazel. Apply as you would any other cold cream, always stroking the face upward.

Cucumber Lotion.—Blanched almonds, 1¾ drams; shaving cream, or melted castile soap, 1 dram; sweet almond oil, 3½ ounces; juice of cucumber. ½ pint; deodorized alcohol, 1½ ounces. This is a splendid lotion for whitening, softening, and cleansing.

To Clear the Complexion.—Apply a lotion made of one quart of milk and the juice of one apple. Apply night and morning.

Freckles.—Lemon juice is one of the simplest and yet most effective remedy for freckles. Use either the pure juice of the lemon rubbed from a slice, or equal parts of lemon juice and glycerin may be used very effectively.

Freckles that are persistent may be treated with a lotion composed of the following: lactic acid, 4 ounces; glycerin, 4 ounces; rosewater, 1 ounce. Apply several times a day and at night rub cold cream well into the skin.

Freckles and Sunburn.—Glycerin, 1 ounce; citric acid (lemon), 3 drams; borax, 2 drams; hot water, 11 ounces; red rose petals, 1 ounce. Dissolve the acid and borax in the water; infuse the petals for an hour; then strain through a cloth. After twenty-four hours take the clear portion which is obtained by pouring from one vessel to another, add to this the glycerin. Apply as often as agreeable.

Pimples.—The following lotion is good: oxide of zinc, 2 scruples; lanolin, 75 grains; sulphur percipitate, 75 grains; sweet almond oil, 1¼ drams; extract of violet, 10 drops. Apply after bathing the skin in warm water.

The following is excellent for banishing pimples and blackheads in addition to general cleanliness; one ounce of green soap tincture and thirty drops of peroxide of hydrogen make an excellent blackhead and pimple eradicator. Mix and apply with absorbent cotton, rubbing thoroughly. Allow to remain for a half hour then wash off with cold water. Do this three or four times a day.

To Remove Warts.—Make a poultice of scraped potato, tie this on the wart at bedtime. Do this twice a week for three or four weeks and the wart will disappear and leave no mark.

Neck.—Cucumber cream is excellent to whiten the neck. Use essence of cucumber, 1 dram; blanched almonds, ¼ pound; juice of cucumbers, 1 pint; refined spirits of wine, ½ gill; spermaceti, ½ ounce; white wax, ½ ounce.

One ounce of lanolin to which has been added 5 to 10 drops of any desired perfume is an excellent cream for the neck.

Green Bath for Neck.—Lavender water, 1 ounce; olive oil, 7 ounces.

Never use hot water on the neck as it tends to relax the tissues. When the neck is washed with warm water it should be thoroughly rinsed with cold water, or better, ice water. This cold application in itself is a splendid tonic, and it is really astonishing how quickly the neck responds to this daily ice rub.

To Whiten the Neck.—Mix pulverized magnesia, 1 ounce; boracic acid, 1 ounce, with sufficient lemon juice to make a soft paste. Spread this over the throat and neck for one hour every day until the skin whitens. Should the bleach irritate the skin, apply cold cream.

Horseradish for Lame Neck.—Fresh horseradish root, 1 ounce; buttermilk, 1 pint, or in place of the buttermilk you may use 2 ounces of vinegar. Grate the horseradish and steep it for four hours, then add the buttermilk or the vinegar. This is good in extreme cases, but is too strong to use often.

Cream for Developing.—Glycerin, 1 ounce; lemon juice, 1 ounce, or rosewater, 1 ounce, and ten drops of benzoin is very good.

Dip the finger tips in some good cold cream, then place the finger tips so that they will meet on the upper part of the breastbone, then massage lightly upward in a rotary motion to the neck from the breastbone to the chin.

Exercise for the Neck.—Bend the head forward, backward, and sideways as far as possible, then roll the head in a semicircle. Practice this exercise ten minutes night and morning. This exercise should not be used if there is any tendency to goiter.

Proper exercise is one of the very best ways to develop the neck. Thorough cleanliness is one of the first requisites to a well developed and beautiful neck. Wash with warm water in which ten drops of benzoin has been added. Then give the following exercise: stand perfectly erect, the right foot in front of the left, the knees straight, place the thumbs at the side and base of the neck. Interlace the fingers at the back of the head, so as to steady it. Then move the head as far to the left as possible, then to the right until you can feel the strain of the muscles in the neck. Then move it backward and forward as far as possible. A few minutes of these exercises three times a day will develop the neck in a few months.

Try to make the head reach the collar band at the back. Never try to draw the head in but let it fall easily.

Hair.

Hair on Arms.—Wet the hair with pure peroxide of hydrogen to which has been added a few drops of ammonia. This will bleach the hair so that it will be less conspicuous and the ammonia is to kill the roots. The treatment should be repeated several times to get the required result.

Shampoo.—Orris root and corn meal makes a good dry shampoo. Rub well through the hair and then brush thoroughly.

Orris root rubbed well through the hair and then thoroughly brushed out will make the hair fluffy and clean. Try to keep the powder off of the scalp as much as possible.

Vermin in Hair.—Rub tincture of larkspur, diluted into the scalp, tie up the hair in a cloth and after twenty-four hours give a thorough shampoo with castile soap. If necessary repeat the treatment until cured. This is harmless and effective.

Tonic for Falling Hair.—Massage and brush the scalp well to remove all dandruff, then apply the following: cantharides, ¼ ounce; cologne, ½ ounce; witch hazel, 2 ounces; rosewater, 8 ounces. Separate the hair into parts and apply this mixture to the scalp with a tooth brush, then massage in order to loosen the scalp. Cantharides is a powerful stimulant and should not be used on an oily scalp.

For hair that is too dry castor oil applied to the scalp with a medicine dropper, or with the finger tips will be found effective. Divide the hair in strands and rub the oil into the scalp. Try to keep the oil from the hair as much as possible.

To give dead looking hair lustre use brilliantine. Put a few drops in the palm of the hand and rub on the brush, then brush the hair thoroughly. This gives it the gloss of healthy hair.

To Darken Switches.—Use the following: pure olive oil, 4 ounces; green walnut shells, 2 ounces; alum, ¼ ounce. Heat together in a double boiler. Then filter and add perfume.

Sage Tea Is Good to Darken Hair.—Make a strong tea of dried leaves, strain carefully, then add two teaspoonfuls of alcohol. Rub well into the hair.

To Keep the Hair from Turning Grey.—Pure lard, 2 ounces; spermacetti, 2 drams; iodide of bismuth, 2 drams; oil of orange, 5 drops. The spermaceti and lard should be melted together and while cooling add the bismuth and oil of orange. Rub well into the scalp before retiring.

To prevent grey hair cleanliness is a great aid. The following is a good preparation to cleanse the scalp: rosewater, ½ pint; rum, ½ pint; whites of two eggs.

For Dry Hair.—Separate the hair into strands, and apply olive oil with a tooth brush, being careful to wet the scalp and not the hair.

Hair Tonic.—Witch hazel rubbed into the scalp at night on a piece of cotton or soft cloth, will clean the head and make it feel refreshed.

Split Hair.—This is usually due to a poor condition of the hair, or may be caused by too frequent shampooing, the hair becoming too dry. The ends of the hair should be carefully clipped. Massage the scalp well and get rid of dandruff. This will usually remove the trouble. If the hair is too dry apply a little castor oil to the hair.

Curling Fluids.—A good curling fluid is made by steeping one tablespoonful of bruised quince seed to a pint of hot water. Pour the water over the seeds and allow it to stand for several hours. If too thick, thin it with a few drops of toilet water. Moisten the hair with the fluid before curling.

Thirty grains of gum arabic, six drams of spirits of camphor, one ounce of powdered borax, and one pint of warm water. Dissolve solids in warm water and when cool add camphor. Wet hair with this solution then roll on kid curlers or arrange in any way desired.

Dampen the little hairs about the face with bay rum or alcohol before curling; this will keep them in curl during damp weather.

For Eyebrows.—To darken light brows, use a mixture of Chinese ink and rose water. Do not allow any of this to get into the eyes.

For scanty eyebrows and lashes use plain yellow vaseline. Apply with a tiny brush or with the finger tips. This is good to darken, and it makes them grow long and thick.

Oil of roses for scanty eyebrows will promote the growth. Apply with brush or finger tips.

Lanolin is good for the growth of the brows and lashes.

Petrolatum oil applied with a tiny brush will improve the growth of the eyebrows.

To massage with olive oil is good for the eyebrows and lashes. This should be done every night.

Scalp.

Dry salt rubbed well into the roots of the hair both cleans and stimulates the scalp.

Salt water rubbed well into the roots of the hair is a good stimulant and keeps the hair from falling out.

Bay rum is good to make the hair fluffy and is cooling to the scalp.

Rubbing the scalp with the finger tips will stimulate the circulation, giving the roots of the hair vitality and life. It is also good to rub the hair with the hands to give it gloss.

Oily Scalp.—For a very oily scalp, use one tablespoonful of limewater to each egg well beaten together and rubbed into the scalp and hair, then rinse with tepid water and lastly with cold water to close the pores. For dark hair use tar or sulphur soap instead of the egg shampoo.

Common Coal Oil for Scalp.—Common coal oil when applied properly is the best of remedies for dandruff and to restore hair. Many say that it works like magic, and beats any other hair tonic. Apply to the scalp with a cloth, then comb off the dandruff with a fine toothed comb. Follow this by washing in warm soapy water, to which a tablespoonful of borax has been added. The borax will soften the water and make the hair soft and fluffy. If the scalp is extremely tender put the oil in a little melted lard. To remove the odor a little toilet water or perfume may be placed in the last rinsing water. All odor soon evaporates in the open air.

Dandruff.—Glover's "Mange Cure" for dandruff. Apply the liquid to the scalp once a week, rubbing in well with the finger tips. Allow to remain on the scalp for an hour or so, then wash well with good soap and hot water, and rinse thoroughly.

The causes of dandruff are so many that it is useless to try to mention them all. Some of the most frequent are: unclean combs and brushes, too frequent shampoos with cheap soaps and powders, and improper ventilation of the scalp. Dandruff may be caused by indigestion, poor circulation, anemia, constipation, etc. The very best external remedy for dandruff is to brush the hair thoroughly every morning and night with a stiff, clean brush.

Sulphur Remedy for Dandruff.—To one quart of soft water add one ounce of sulphur, shake three or four times thoroughly during an interval of several days. After the sulphur has settled to the bottom of the receptacle, use the clear liquid. Apply liberally to the scalp every day. This will not only remove the dandruff, but will make the hair soft and glossy. This sulphur remedy will darken light hair.

MEMORANDA

INDEX

HEALTH

A

	PAGE.
Abortion	95
Abscess	189
Aching of the Feet	215
Acid Burns	152
Aconite, Poisoning by	162
Acute Articular Rheumatism	249
Acute Gastritis	230
Acute Peritonitis	240
Adenoids	8, 189
Ailments of Baby, Common	137
Ailments of Teething	128
Alcohol	16
Alcohol and Listerine, Gargle	91
Alcohol as an Antiseptic	90
Alcohol Bath	80
Alcohol Gargle	90
Alcohol, Mouth Wash	90
Alcohol, Poisoning by	163
Alkaline Bath	6
Alkali Burns	152
Alum as an Emetic	161
Ammonia as a Stimulant	162
Anemia, Diet for	73
Antimony, Poisoning by	163
Antiseptics	90
Apoplexy	141
Appendicitis	190
Apple Cup Custard	77
Arabian Balsam	280
Arm, Hemorrhage of	181
Arm Sling	145
Arnica Salve	277
Aromatic Cascara, Laxative	91
Arsenic, Poisoning by	163
Arterial Hemorrhage	180
Articles, Necessary for Confinement	101
Articles, Needed for the Expectant Mother	101
Artificial Feeding of the Baby	118
Artificial Respiration in Drowning	160
Artificial Respiration in Electrical Injuries	171
Aseptic Wounds	187
Aseptin	280
Asthma	191
Atomizer's Solution	280
Ayer's Hair Vigor	280
Ayer's Sarsaparilla	280

B

	PAGE.
Babies, Chafing of the Skin in	139
Babies, Eczema in	139
Babies, Milk Crust in	140
Baby, Artificial Feeding of	118
Baby, Bad Habits of	133
Baby, Care of Genital Organs	113
Baby, Care of Ears	113
Baby, Care of Eyes	113
Baby, Care of Milk for	119
Baby, Care of Mouth	113
Baby, Care of Nose	113
Baby, Caution in the Care of	136
Baby, Cold in the Head	139
Baby, Colic in	138
Baby, Common Ailments of	137
Baby, Constipation of	138
Baby Department	99
Baby, Development of	127
Baby, Diarrhea	137
Baby, Discipline of	132
Baby, Drinking Water for	125
Baby, Early Training of	134
Baby, Feeding of	114
Baby, General Care of	130
Baby, Habits of	132
Baby, Heating or Cooking Milk for	119
Baby, Hiccough in	138
Baby, How to Feed	120
Baby, How to Give Bottle to	123
Baby, How to Keep Well	134
Baby, How to Lift	113
Baby, Milk for	119
Baby, Modification of Milk for	122
Baby, Equipment for	105
Baby, Overfeeding of	125
Baby Pacifiers	133
Baby, Preparation of Food for	122
Baby, Prickly Heat in	139
Baby, Punishment of	134
Baby's Bed	103
Making the Bed	105
Pillow for	104
Baby's Clothing	106
Bands	107
Diapers	108
Nightgowns	107
Caps	109
Cloaks	109
Pads	109
Petticoats	107

	PAGE.
Shirts	107
Shoes	109
Slips	107
Stockings	109
Wrappers	107
Baby's Room	103
Cleaning	103
Heating	103
Lighting	103
Ventilating	103
Baby's Sleep, Things That Disturb	132
Baby's Teeth	127
Baby's Teeth, Care of	127
Baby's Teeth, Growth of	127
Baby, Toys for	137
Baby, Training of	132
Baby, Underfeeding of	125
Baby, Vehicles for	135
Baby, Weaning of	128
Baby, When Not to Take Out	136
Baby, What to Feed	120
Baby, When to Feed	118
Baby, When to Wean	129
Back Rest, Use of	70
Bad Habits of the Baby	133
Baked Oysters	77
Bandage, Cravat	146
Bandage, Eye	147
Bandage, Figure Eight	143
Bandage, Foot	145
Bandage, Palm of Hand	147
Bandage, Hand	145
Bandage, Head	146
Bandage, Jaw	147
Bandage, Neck	147
Bandage, Roller	141
Bandage, Spiral	143
Bandage, Spiral Reverse	143
Bandage, Triangular	144
Bandage, Triangular, Application of	145
Bandaging	141
Bands for Baby	107
Bareel's Indian Liniment	280
Barker's Bone and Nerve Liniment	281
Bath, Alcohol	80
Bath, Cleansing	5
Bath, Cold	5
Bath, Daily	65
Bath, Foot	81
Bath, Hot	6
Bath, Hot for Convulsions	78
Bathing	110
Bathing for Nursing Mother	115
Bath, Mustard	82
Bath, Salt or Saline	5, 82
Bath, Sitz	80
Bath, Soda or Alkaline	6, 81
Bath, Sponge for Reducing Temperature	79
Bath, Starch	81
Bath, Sulphur	82

	PAGE.
Bath to Induce Perspiration	78
Baths for Therapeutic Purposes, Methods of Giving	78
Baths, Soothing	8
Bay Rum	281
B. B. B. Blood Purifier	281
Beauty Hints	292
Bed for Sick Room	60
Bed, To Make for Patient	62
Bed Wetting	133
Bed with Patient in It, To Change	62
Bedding for Sick Room	61
Bedsores	68
Bee Sting	151
Beef Juice	76
Beef Steak, Invalid's	77
Beef Tea	76
Belladonna	164
Bichloride of Mercury	31
Bichloride of Mercury, Poisoning by	164
Bichloride of Mercury, an Antiseptic	90
Biliousness	192
Birth Registration	101
Bites	150
Bites, Cat	150
Bites, Dog	150
Bites, Mad Dog	183
Bites or Stings of Insects	150
Bites of Snakes	183
Blackheads	242
Bladder, Inflammation of	193
Bleach, Skin	295
Bleeding of Nose	183
Blister Beetle	165
Blood Poison	254
Blue Vitriol, Poisoning by	164
Body Hygiene	1
Boil Ointment	278
Boils	193
Bones in the Throat	174
Boracic Acid (Boric), an Antiseptic	90
Borax, Gargle	91
Borax, Mouthwash	90
Borin, Mouthwash	90
Bottle, How to Give to the Baby	123
Bottle, Weaning from	130
Bottles, Nursing	122
Bowels, Care of	12
Brain, Compression of	156
Brain, Concussion	157
Bread and Milk Poultice	279
Breast Feeding	114
Breasts, Changes in	94
Bright's Disease	194
Broiled White Fish	77
Bronchial Catarrh	198
Bronchitis	195
Brown's Bronchial Troches	281
Bruises	151
Bucklin's Arnica Salve	281
Bullet Wounds	152

PAGE.

Bunions 196
Burning of the Feet.................215
Burns 152
Burns, Acid 152
Burns, Alkali 152
Burns, Carbolic 153
Burns, Electrical 171
Burns, Severe 153
Burns, Slight 153
Butter Ointment 278

C

Callouses 293
Calomel, Laxative 91
Camphor 164
Camphor Ice 282
Cancer 196
Cankers 257
Cantharides 165
Cap for Baby................109
Capillary Hemorrhage 181
Carbolic Acid, Poisoning by.........165
Carbolic Acid, Used as Antiseptic..... 90
Carbolic Burns 153
Carbolic Salve 277
Carbuncles 197
Cardiac Diseases, Diet for........... 73
Care of Baby, Cautions...........136
Care of the Baby, General..........130
Care of Baby's Teeth...............127
Care of Bowels 12
Care of Ears..................... 7
Care of Eyes..................... 6
Care of Feet.................... 12
Care of Hands.................... 11
Care of Milk for the Baby..........119
Care of Mouth.................... 9
Care of Mouth of Patient............. 66
Care of Nipples..................123
Care of Nose.................... 7
Care of Patient................... 64
Care of Patient at Night.............. 71
Care of Patients Hair.............. 66
Care of Scalp.................... 6
Care of Sick Room................. 58
Care of Sick Room Supplies.......... 60
Care of Skin.................... 4
Care of Teeth.................... 9
Care of Teeth of Patient............. 66
Care of Teeth of the Expectant
  Mother.......................101
Care of Throat................... 11
Carrying Human Filth to Human
  Mouths—Various Ways of......... 41
Carrying the Patient in a Sitting
  Posture 69
Castor Oil, Laxative 91
Castoria 282
Cat Bites 150
Catarrh 198
Catarrh, Bronchial 198

PAGE.

Catarrh, Gastric 198
Catarrhal Headache 221
Catarrh Ointment 278
Causation and Prevention of Typhoid
  Fever 38
Caution in the Care of the Baby......136
Caution in Use of Drugs.............162
Cautions in Filling Prescriptions......274
Cellar, The Hygiene of.............. 18
Certified Milk for Baby.............119
Cessation of Menstruation........... 94
Chafing of Skin in Babies...........139
Chamberlain's Colic, Cholera and
  Diarrhea Remedy 282
Change of Life.................... 93
Changes in the Breasts............. 94
Changing the Diaper................109
Changing the Nightgown of Patient... 67
Chapping 199
Chapping of Hands, To Avoid........292
Chapped Lips 295
Charcoal Poultice 219
Chemical Disinfectants 30
Child's Dose, How to Reckon........275
Chin, Double, to Reduce............293
Chicken Pox 199
Chilblains 200
Chloral Hydrate, Poisoning by.......165
Chloral, Poisoning by..............165
Chloroform, Poisoning by...........165
Choice and Preparation of Bed....... 60
Choking 154
Chronic Constipation, Diet for........ 74
Chronic Rheumatism 248
Cleaning Baby's Room...............103
Cleanliness of Sick Room............ 58
Cleansing Bath 5
Cleansing Creams 295
Cloaks for Baby...................109
Clothing 15
Clothing for Baby..................109
Clothing for Expectant Mother.......100
Clothing for the Patient............ 71
Clothing, To Extinguish Fire from......174
Cocoa and Chocolate................ 76
Coffee 76
Cold Bath 5
Cold Compresses 158
Cold Compress for the Eye........... 87
Cold Pack Complete................. 86
Cold Pack for the Chest Only........ 86
Cold Sores 257
Colds 201
Colds, Nature and Prevention........ 35
Colic 203
Colic in Babies...................138
Collapse 154
Common Ailments of Baby...........137
Complete Cold Pack................. 86
Complete Hot Pack................. 85
Complexion, To Clear...............295

PAGE.

Compound Licorice Powder, Laxative. 91
Compress 154
Compress, Cold, for the Eye......... 87
Compress, Hot 87
Compress, Hot, for the Eye......... 87
Compresses, Cold 158
Compression of the Brain............156
Concussion of the Brain.............157
Confinement, Necessary Articles for..100
Congestion of the Kidneys...........233
Conjunctivitis 204
Constipation 204
Constipation of Babies...............138
Constipation, How to Prevent........ 12
Convulsions 157
Convulsions, Hot Bath for.......... 78
Corns 207, 293
Corrosive Sublimate, Poisoning by...164
Corrosives, Poisoning by............161
Cough, Whooping 269
Cough Remedy 282
Coughs 206
Counter Irritants 83
Cradle, Use of...................... 71
Cramps 88
Cramps, Treatment of...............157
Cranberry Poultice 279
Cravat Bandage 146
Cream for Developing...............296
Cream Massage 295
Cream of Tomato Soup.............. 77
Creamed Celery 77
Creamed Egg 77
Creams, Cleansing 295
Croton Oil, Poisoning by............166
Croup, Membraneous 209
Croup, Spasmodic 207
Curling, Fluids 298
Cuticura Ointment 282
Cuticura Resolvent 283
Cuts 158

D

Daily Bath 65
Dandruff 299
Dandruff Cure 283
Deadly Nightshade 164
Death 158
Developing, Cream for..............296
Development of the Baby............127
Diabetes 208
Diaper, Changing 109
Diaper, To Put on..................109
Diapers for Baby...................108
Diarrhea 209
Diarrhea of Babies.................137
Diarrhea, Summer 89
Diet for Nursing Mother............115
Diet of Patient.................... 72
Diets for Special Diseases.......... 73

PAGE.

Digestion, Process of...............114
Digitalis, Poisoning by..............166
Diphtheria 209
Diphtheria, Laryngeal 210
Discipline of Baby..................132
Diseased Eyes 214
Disinfectants 29
Disinfectants, Chemical 30
Disinfectants, How to Use.......... 31
Disinfectants, Natural.............. 29
Dislocation 159
Dislocation of Finger 160
Dislocation of Jaw.................159
Dislocation of Shoulder.............159
Disposal of Excreta, Soiled Linen, etc.. 59
Disposal of Human Excreta.......... 22
Disturbances in the Urine.......... 94
Dobell's Solution, Gargle............ 91
Dog Bites 150
"Don'ts" 48
Dose, How to Reckon a Child's.......275
Double Chin, To Reduce.............293
Douche, Giving a................... 83
Drink for Expectant Mothers........100
Drinking Water for the Baby........125
Drowning 160
Drugging 15
Drugs and Drugging................ 15
Drugs, Poisoning by................ 160
Dry Shampoo 297
Duration of Pregnancy............. 95
Dysentery 212
Dyspepsia 226

E

Ear, Foreign Bodies in..............175
Earache 213
Earache Remedy 283
Early Training of Baby..............134
Ears, Care of...................... 7
Eczema 214
Eczema in Babies...................139
Egg Lemonade 78
Eggs in Milk...................... 77
Electrical Burns 171
Electrical Injuries 171
Ely's Cream Balm...................283
Emergency Department 141
Emetic, Alum as....................161
Emetic, Mustard as.................161
Emetic, Salt as....................161
Emetics 161
Enema, Giving an.................. 82
Enlarged Tonsils 260
Epilepsy 173
Epsom Salts, Laxative.............. 91
Erysipelas 214
Ether, Poisoning by................165
Excessive Menstruation 92
Excreta, Human, Disposal of........ 22

PAGE.

Excreta of Patient, Disposal........ 59
Exercise 4
Exercise for Expectant Mothers.......100
Exercise for Neck...................297
Exercise for Nursing Mother........115
Exhaustion, Heat 179
Expectant Mother, Articles Needed for.101
Eye Bandage 147
Eye, Cold Compress for............. 87
Eye, Foreign Bodies in.............176
Eye, Hot Compress for............. 87
Eyebrows, To Darken...............298
Eyelids, Granular 204
Eye Salve 278
Eyes, Care of...................... 6
Eyes, Diseased 215
Eyes, Weak 215

F

Face, Care of......................294
Face, Hemorrhage 181
Fainting 173
Falling Hair, Tonic for............297
Feeding, Artificial, Baby..........118
Feeding, Breast 114
Feeding, Normal 124
Feeding of the Baby................114
Feet, Aching 216
Feet, Burning of...................216
Feet, Care of...................12, 293
Feet, Swollen 293
Feet, To Keep from Tiring Quickly...216
Felons 216
Fever, Diet for.................... 75
Fever, Intermittent 233
Fever, Malaria 234
Fever, Pernicious 233
Fever, Remittent 233
Fever, Rheumatic 249
Fever, Scarlet 251
Fever, Typhoid 254
Figure Eight Bandage...............143
Finger, Dislocation of.............160
Finger Sucking 133
Fire 174
Fish Bones in the Throat...........174
Fish Hooks 174
Fits 174
Flax Meal Poultice.............84, 279
Flies as Germ Carriers............. 28
Fluids, Curling 298
Food for Expectant Mothers.........100
Food, Preparation of for Baby......122
Foods 13
Foot Bandage 145
Foot Bath 81
Foot Bath in Bed, to Give.......... 81
Foot, Hemorrhage of................182
Foot, Nail in..................183, 188
Forearm, Hemorrhage of.............182

PAGE.

Foreign Bodies in Ear..............175
Foreign Bodies in Eye..............176
Foreign Bodies in Nose.............177
Foreign Bodies in Throat...........175
Formaldehyde, Disinfectant......... 30
Foxglove, Poisoning by.............166
Fractures 177
Freckles 295
Freckles and Sunburn...............296
Freezing 178
Frost Bite Salve...................278
Frost Bites 178, 200
Frostilla 283
Fungus 168
Furniture of Sick Room............. 57

G

Gallstones 217
Gangrene 218
Garden Salve 278
Gargles 90
Gargling Oil 284
Gas Poisoning 178
Gastric Catarrh 198
Gastritis, Acute 230
General Nursing 54
General Treatments 88
Genuine White Oil Liniment.........284
German Measles 236
Germs and Their Carriers.......... 28
"Get the Habit"................... 51
Getting Patient Up in a Chair...... 69
Giles' Iodide of Ammonia Liniment...284
Glycerine Ointment 278
Goitre 219
Gombault's Caustic Balsam..........284
Gout 219
Granular Eyelids 220
Green Mountain Salve...............285
Grippe 220
Gum, Hemorrhage of.................181
Gunshot Wounds 178, 187

H

Habits of Baby.....................132
Hair 297
Hair, Dry Remedy for...............298
Hair, Falling, Tonic for...........297
Hair of Patient, Care of........... 66
Hair on Arms.......................297
Hair, Split........................298
Hair, To Darken....................298
Hair, To Keep from Turning Gray....298
Hair Tonic 298
Hair, Vermin in....................297
Hall's Hair Renewer................285
Hamburg Breast Tea.................285
Hamburg Tea 285
Hamlin's Wizard Oil................286
Hand Bandage 145
Hand, Hemorrhage of................182

PAGE.

Hands, Care of...................... 11
Hands, Chapping to Avoid.............292
Hands, Perspiration of...............292
Hands, To Bleach... 292
Hands, To Make Plump.............292
Hands, To Soften....................292
Hands, To Whiten....................292
Handy Table of Weights and
  Measures 291
Harlem Oil 286
Hay Fever 221
Head Bandage 146
Head Lice 89
Headaches 88, 222
Headache, Catarrhal 222
Headache, Nervous 223
Headache, Neuralgic 223
Headache, Sick 223
Heat Exhaustion 179
Heat Stroke 185
Heating Baby's Room.................103
Heating or Cooking Milk for Baby....119
Hemorrhage 179
Hemorrhage, Arterial 180
Hemorrhage, Capillary 181
Hemorrhage, Nature's Treatment of.179
Hemorrhage of Arms..................181
Hemorrhage of Face..................181
Hemorrhage of Forearm...............182
Hemorrhage of Foot..................182
Hemorrhage of Gum...................181
Hemorrhage of Hand..................182
Hemorrhage of Leg...................182
Hemorrhage of Lungs.................182
Hemorrhage of Nose..................181
Hemorrhage of Stomach...........182
Hemorrhage of Neck..................181
Hemorrhage of Scalp.................181
Hemorrhage of Thigh.................182
Hemorrhage of Varicose Veins......182
Hemorrhage, Venous.................180
Hernia 224
Hiccough in Babies 138
High Calorie Typhoid Diet.......... 76
Hives 225
Holloway's Ointment 286
Holly Berries, Poisoning by.........166
Home Hygiene 17
Home-made Salve 278
Home Salve 278
Home Nursing 54
Hoarseness 206
Hop Bitters 286
Horseradish Poultice 279
Hostetter's Bitters 287
Hot Bath for Convulsions............ 78
Hot Compress 87
Hot Compress for the Eye 87
Hot Pack Complete 85
Hot Pack, Patrial 86
Hornet Sting 151

PAGE.

House, The Hyginene of 19
Household Salve 277
"How To Keep Well" 1
"How To Keep Well" Baby.......... 42
  Baby's Rights 42
  Bathing 44
  Bottle Feeding 43
  Clothing 45
  Development 46
  Sleep 46
Human Excreta, Disposal of 22
Human Filth, Various Ways of Carry-
  ing to Human Mouth 41
Human Mouths 41
Hydrochloric Acid, Poisoning by.....166
Hydrogen Peroxide, Gargle 91
Hydrophobia 225
Hygiene, Body 1
Hygiene, Home 17
Hysteria 182

I

Incised Wounds 187
Indigestion 226
Infant Stools 125
Infant Paralysis 227
Ingrown Toenails 230
Infection of Wounds 188
Inflammation of Bladder.............193
Inflammation of Large Intestines........228
Inflammation of Small Intestines........229
Inflammation of Stomach.............230
Inflammatory Rheumatism.............249
Influenza 220
Injuries, Electrical 171
Insect Bites and Stings.............150, 183
Insomnia 231
Instructions to Expectant Mothers.... 99
Intermitent Fever 233
Intestines, Large, Inflammation of.......228
Intestines, Small, Inflammation of....229
Invalid's Beef Steak 77
Iodine, Poisoning by................166
Iodoform, Poisoning by 167
Irritants, Poisoning by.............161
Irritants, Counter 83
Itch 231
Itch Ointment 278
Ivy Poison 167, 232

J

Jaundice 233
Junket 76
Jaw Bandage 147
Jaw, Dislocation of 159

K

Kendall's Spavin Cure 287
Kerosene Salve 277

PAGE.

Kickapoo Indian Oil......................287
Kidneys, Congestion of 233
Knee Rest, Use of 70

L

Labor 96
Labor, Emergency Care of 97
Lacerated Wounds 189
Lacerations 158
Lard and Tar Ointment 277
Large Intestines, Inflammation of... 228
Laryngeal Diphtheria 209
Laudanum, Poisoning by 167
Laxatives 91
Lead, Poisoning by....................167
Leg, Hemorrhage of...................182
Lemon Juice, Mouth Wash.......... 90
Leucorrhea (Whites) 93
Lice 234
Lice, Head 89
Lifting Patient from the Chair........ 68
Light and Sunshine 3
Lighting Baby's Room 103
Lighting of Sick Room.............. 57
Lime 31
Liniment for Man and Beast 287
Liniments 275
    All Ache Liniment 275
    All Around Liniment 275
    Arnica Liniment 275
    Camphor Liniment 275
    Cough Liniment 276
    Egg Liniment 275
    Golden Oil 276
    Hamlin's Wizard Oil 276
    Home Liniment 276
    Kerosene Liniment 276
    Lemon Liniment 276
    Lightning Liniment 276
    Lime Water Liniment 276
    Liniment for Chapped Hands 275
    Man and Beast Liniment..........277
    Mustard Liniment 276
    Mustang Liniment 276
    Nerve Liniment 276
    Olive Oil Liniment 277
    Pain Killer 275
    Rheumatic Liniment 276
    Rheumatism Liniment 275
    Sweeney Liniment 275
    Witch Hazel Liniment 276
Linseed Meal Poultice 84-279
Lip Salve 277
Lips, Chapped 295
Listerine, Mouth Wash 90
Liver, Functional Disorders, Diet for. 74
Location of Sick Room 56
Lock Jaw 183-260
Lunar Caustic, Poisoning by 167-169
Lungs, Hemorrhage of 182

PAGE.

Lydia Pinkham's Compound 288
Lye, Poisoning by 167

M

Mad Dog and Cat Bites 183
Magnetic Liniment 288
Malaria Fever 234
Management and Routine of Sick
    Room 59
Massage Cream 295
Masturbation 133
Mattress, How to Protect 62
Measles 235
Measles, German 237
Medicines to Induce Sleep, Not to
    be Given 132
Membraneous Croup 209
Menopause (Change of Life)......... 93
Menstruation 92
Menstruation, Cessation of...........94
Menstruation, Excessive 92
Menstruation, Painful 92
Menstruation, Suppression of 93
Methods of Giving Bath for
    Therapeutic Purposes 78
Mexican Mustang Liniment 288
Milk and Albumen 78
Milk, Certified for Baby 119
Milk Crust in Babies 140
Milk for the Baby 119
Milk, Heating or Cooking for Baby..119
Milk, Method of Modification 122
Milk, Modification of, for Baby........122
Milk, Pasteurization of 122
Milk Supply 27
Milk, Utensils Necessary for Modi-
    fication of 122
Miscarriage 96
Modification of Milk for Baby 122
Modification of Milk, Method of......122
Modification of Milk, Utensils Nec-
    essary 122
Monk's Hood, Poisoning by 162
Morning Sickness 94
Mosquitoes, as Germ Carriers 29
Mother, Nursing 115
Mother, Nursing, Bathing for 45
Mother, Nursing, Diet for 115
Mother, Nursing, Exercise for.......115
Mother, Nursing, Recreation for.....115
Mothers, Expectant, Bathing 100
Mothers, Expectant, Care of Bowels.100
Mothers, Expectant, Care of Teeth....101
Mothers, Expectant, Cleanliness of...100
Mothers, Expectant, Clothing of.....100
Mothers, Expectant, Exercise for....100
Mothers, Expectant, Food and Drink.100
Mothers, Expectant, Instructions to.. 99
Mothers, Expectant, Care of Kidneys.100
Mothers, Expectant, Medicine for.....100
Mothers, Expectant, Rest for 100

PAGE.

Mothers, Expectant, Care of Skin....100
Mothers, Expectant, Sleep for 100
Mouth, Care of 9
Mouth, Sore 257
Mouth Washes 90
Mullen Weed Poultice 279
Mumps 238
Muscular Rheumatism 247
Mushrooms 168
Mustard, as Emetic 161
Mustard Bath 82
Mustard Paste or Plaster............84, 279
Mustard Poultice 84

N

Nails in Foot 183-188
Nails, to Supply Oil of 293
Narcotics, Poisoning by 161
Nasal Wash 89
Natural Disinfectants 29
Nature's Plaster 279
Necessary Articles for Confinement..101
Neck Bandage 147
Neck, Exercise for 297
Neck, Green Bath for 296
Neck, Hemorrhage of 181
Neck, Lame, Horseradish for 296
Neck, to Whiten 296
Nerve and Bone Liniment 289
Nervous Headache 223
Neuralgia 239
Neuralgic Headache 223
Nicotine 170
Nightgown, Changing the 67
Nightgowns for Baby..............107
Nipples, Rubber, Best Kind........123
Nipples, Rubber, Care of 123
Nitric Acid, Poisoning by 166-168
Normal Salt Solution, Antiseptic..... 90
Normal Feeding 124
Nose Bleed 183
Nose, Care of 7
Nose, Foreign Bodies in 177
Nose, Hemorrhage of 181
Nose, Red 293
Nurse, the 55
Nursing Bottles 122
Nursing, General 54
Nursing, Home 54
Nursing, Mother 115
Nursing Mother, Bathing for 115
Nursing Mother, Diet for 115
Nursing Mother, Exercise for 115
Nursing Mother, Recreation 115
Nursing Mother, Sleep for 116
Nursing, Regularity in............118
Nursing, Technique of 117

O

Oatmeal Gruel 78
Oil of Joy 289

PAGE.

Oily Scalp 299
Ointments and Salves 277
  Boil Ointment 278
  Butter Ointment 278
  Carbolic Salve 278
  Catarrh Ointment 278
  Eye Salve 278
  Frostbite Salve 278
  Garden Salve 278
  Glycerine Ointment 278
  Good Arnica Salve 277
  Home Made Salve 278
  Home Salve 278
  Household Salve 277
  Itch Ointment 278
  Kerosene Salve 277
  Lard and Tar Ointment 277
  Lip Salve 277
  Ointment for Felons 277
  Pile Ointment 278
  Ringworm Ointment 277
  Salve for Sores and Bruises........277
  Stick Salve 277
  Toothache Wax 277
Ointment for Felons 277
Omelet for the Sick 78
Onion Poultice 279
Opium, Poisoning by 168
Orange Jelly for the Sick 77
Other Equipment for the Baby 105
Overfeeding of the Baby 125
Oxalic Acid, Poisoning by 168
Oxygen, Value of 1

P

Pacifiers 133
Pads for Baby 109
Paine's Celery Compound 289
Painful Menstruation 92
Paralysis, Infantile 228
Paregoric, Poisoning by 169
Paris Green, Poisoning by 169
Partial Hot Pack.................. 86
Partial Temperature of Bath........ 80
Pasteurization of Milk 122
Patent Prescriptions 280
  Arabic Balsam 280
  Aseptic 280
  Atomizer's Solution 280
  Ayer's Hair Vigor 280
  Ayer's Sarsaparilla 280
  Bareel's Indian Liniment 280
  Barker's Bone and Nerve Liniment.281
  Bay Rum 281
  B. B. B. Blood Purifier 281
  Brown's Bronchial Troches 281
  Bucklin's Arnica Salve 281
  Camphorice 281
  Castoria 282

PAGE.

Chamberlain's Colic, Cholera and
    Diarrhea Remedy 282
Oils, Way to Take....................275
    Cough Remedy 282
    Cuticura Ointment 282
    Cuticura Resolvent 283
    Dandruff Cure 283
    Earache Remedy 283
Ely's Cream Balm....................283
    Frostilla 283
    Frostbites and Chilblains...........283
    Gargling Oil 284
    Genuine White Oil Liniment......284
    Gile's Iodide of Ammonia Liniment.284
    Gombault's Caustic Balsam 284
    Green Mountain Salve..............285
    Hall's Hair Renewer...............285
    Hamburg Breast Tea 285
    Hamlin's Wizard Oil 286
    Harlem Oil 286
    Holloway Ointment 286
    Hop Bitters 286
    Hostetter's Bitters 287
    Kendall's Spavin Cure 287
    Kickapoo Indian Oil 287
    Liniment for Man and Beast.......287
    Lydia Pinkham's Compound..........288
    Magnetic Liniment 288
    Mexican Mustang Liniment 288
    Nerve and Bone Liniment 289
    Oil of Joy 289
    Paine's Celery Compound 289
    Radway's Ready Relief 289
    Robert's Camphor Tar Ointment...290
    Royal Catarrh Cure...............290
    Seven Sutherland Sister's Hair
        Grower 290
    Skinner's Dandruff Mixture 290
    Sore Throat 290
    Syrup of Figs 290
    Tapeworm Remedy 291
    Tonsilitis Remedy 291
    Trask's Magnetic Ointment 291
Patient, Care and Teatment of.......64
Patient, How to Help into Bed........68
Patient, Making the Bed for..........62
Patient, to Make Comfortable in Bed. 67
Patient, Weak or Helpless, to Raise... 68
Peritonitis, Acute 240
Pernicious Fever 233
Perspiration, Bath to Induce 78
Perspiration of Feet 293
Perspiring Feet 215
Petticoats for Baby 107
Phenol, Poisoning by................165
Phosphorus, Poisoning by 168
Pile Ointment 278
Piles 241
Pimples 242, 296

PAGE.

Pink Eye 204
Plaster, Mustard 84
Plasters and Poultices................279
    Bread and Milk Poultice 279
    Charcoal Poultice 279
    Cranberry Poultice 279
    Flaxseed Poultice 279
    Horseradish Poultice 279
    Linseed Poultice 279
    Mullein Weed Poultice 279
    Mustard Plaster 279
    Nature's Plaster 279
    Onion Poultice 279
    Potato Poultice 279
    Poultice for Suppurating Wounds...279
    Slippery Elm Poultice 279
    Smartweed Poultice 279
Pleurisy 242
Pneumonia 243
Pneumonia, Nature and Prevention... 36
Poisoning, Ptomaine 245
Poisons 160-183
Poisons and Drugs...................160
Poisoning, Gas 178
Poke Berries, Poisoning by............169
Pores, Coarse, What to do...........295
Posture 13
Potato Poultice 279
Potato Soup 77
Poultice, Flaxseed Meal 84
Poultice for Suppurating Wounds....279
Poultice, Linseed Meal............... 84
Poultice, Mustard 84
Poultices 84
Pregnancy, Duration of 95
Pregnancy and Emergency Care...... 94
Pregnancy, Signs of 94
Preparation of Food for the Baby....122
Prescription Department 274
Prescriptions, Cautions in Filling.....274
Preventive Measures for Typhoid Fever.. 41
Prevention of Colds 35
Prevention of Miscarriage 96
Prevention of Pneumonia 36
Prevention of Tuberculosis........... 37
Prickly Heat in Babies 139
Process in Digestion.................114
Proud Flesh 187
Provision for Care of the Sick....... 56
Prune Whip 78
Prussic Acid, Poisoning by..........169
Ptomaine Poisoning 169, 246
Puberty 91
Pulse, The 64
Punctured Wounds 187
Punishment of Baby 134

Q

Quickening, The 95
Quiet and Privacy of the Sick Room... 58

R

PAGE.

Rabies 225
Radway's Ready Relief 289
Rawness Between Toes 215
Recipes for the Sick Patient......... 76
Recreation 4
Recreation for Nursing Mother.......115
Regularity in Nursing 118
Remittent Fever 233
Respiration 65
Respiration, Artificial, During
    Electrical Injuries 171
Respiration, Artificial, in Case of
    Drowning 160
Rest 4
Rest for Expectant Mothers 60
Rheumatic Fever 249
Rheumatism 247
Rheumatism, Acute, Articular 249
Rheumatism, Chronic 248
Rheumatism, Diet for 74
Rheumatism, Inflammatory 249
Rheumatism, Muscular 247
Rheumatism, Sciatic 248
Rhubarb, Laxative 91
Ringworm 250
Ringworm Ointment 277
Robbert's Camphor-Tar Ointment....290
Rochelle Salts, Laxative 91
Royal Catarrh Cure 290
Rub, Salt 82
Rupture 224

S

"Safety First" 47
Saline Bath 5
Salt as Emetic....................161
Salt Bath 5-82
Salt, Gargle 91
Salt, Mouthwash 90
Salt of Lemon 171
Salt Rheum 214
Salt Rub 82
Salve for Sores and Bruises 277
Scalp, Care of 6
Scalp, Oily 299
Scarlet Fever 251
Sciatic Rheumatism 248
Seidlitz Powder, Laxative 91
Septic or Poisonous Wounds 187
Septicemia 254
Seven Sutherland Sisters' Hair Growe..r290
Severe Burns 153
Shampoo, Dry 297
Shirred Eggs 77
Shrits for Baby 107
Shock 183
Shoes for Baby 109
Shot Wounds 178
Shoulder, Dislocation of...........159

PAGE.

Sick Headache 223
Sickness, Morning 94
Sick Room, The 56
Sick Room, Care and Cleanliness..... 58
Sick Room, Furniture of 57
Sick Room, Lighting of 57
Sick Room, Location of............ 56
Sick Room, Management and
    Routine of 59
Sick Room, Quiet and Privacy of...... 58
Sick Room Supplies, Care of 60
Sick Room, Temperature 58
Sick Room, Ventilation of.......... 57
Signs of Pregnacy 94
Silver Nitrate, Poisoning by 169
Siphonage 161
Sippets 77
Sitz Bath 80
Skin Bleach 295
Skin, Care of 4
Skin of Face to Protect 294
Skinner's Dandruff Mixture 290
Sleep 4
Sleep, Baby's Things That Disturb....132
Sleep for Expectant Mothers 100
Sleep for the Baby, Amount of........130
Sleep for Nursing Mother 116
Slight Burns 153
Sling, The 149
Sling, Arm 145
Slippery Elm Poultice 279
Slips for Baby 107
Small Intestines, Inflammation of....229
Smallpox 255
Smartweed Poultice 279
Snake Bites 183
Soda Bath 6, 81
Soda Bicarbonate Solution, Antiseptic. 90
Soiled Linen 59
Sore Mouth 257
Sore Throat 89, 258
Soothing Baths 81
Sorrel, Poisoning by...............171
Spanish Fly, Poisoning by 165
Spasmodic Croup 207
Special Exercise 32
    Back, for 33
    Breathing, for 32
    Chest Development, for 33
    Constipation, for 33
    Hands, for 34
    Kidneys, for 33
    Legs, for 34
    Liver for 33
    Neck, for 34
    Spine, for 33
    Stationary run 33
Spiral Bandage 143
Spiral Reverse Bandage 143
Splinters 184
Splints 184

PAGE.

Split Hair 298
Sponge Bath for Reducing
  Temperature 79
Sprains 185
Starch Bath 81
Stick Salve 277
Stimulant, Ammonia as 162
Stimulant, Strong Coffee as..........162
Stimulant, Strychnine as.............162
Stimulants 162
Sting, Bee 151
Sting, Hornet 151
Stings or Bites of Insects 150
Stockings for Baby 109
Stomach, Hemorrhage of 182
Stomach, Inflammation of 230
Stools, Infant 125
Strong Coffee as Stimulant............162
Strychnine, Poisoning by...........170
Strychnine as Stimulant 162
Stupes, Turpentine 88
Stye 259
Sucking Thumb or Finger 133
Suffocation 185
Sugar of Lead, Poisoning by........170
Sulphate of Copper, Poisoning by.....164
Sulphur Bath 82
Sulphuric Acid, Poisoning by 166
Summer Diarrhea 89
Sunburn 294, 296
Sunshine, Value of 3
Sunstroke 185
Suppression of Menstruation 93
Suppression of the Urine 259
Surroundings, Hygiene of 21
Switches, to Darken 297
Syncope 173
Syrup of Figs 290

T

Taking the Temperature 64
Tan, for Removing 294
Tapeworm Remedy 291
Tartar Emetic 170
Tartaric Acid, Poisoning by 170
Tea for the Sick Patient 76
Technique of Nursing 117
Teeth, Baby's 127
Teeth, Baby's, Growth of 127
Teeth, Care of 9
Teeth and Mouth of Patient, Care of 66
Teething, Ailments of 128
Temperature Bath, Partial 80
Temperature of Sick Room 58
Temperature, Sponge Bath for
  Reducing 79
Temperature, Taking the 64
Tetanus 185, 260
Tetter 214
Thigh, Hemorrhage of 182

PAGE.

Throat, Care of........................ 11
Throat, Fish Bones in 174
Throat, Foreign Bodies in 175
Throat, Sore 89-258
Thumb or Finger Sucking 133
Tincture of Iodine, Antiseptic 90
Tincture of Myrrh, Mouthwash 90
Tobacco 16
Tobacco, Poisoning by 170
Toenails, Ingrown 230
Toes, Rawness Between 215
Tomato Soup, Cream of 77
Tonic, Hair 298
Tonsils 8
Tonsils, Enlargement of 260
Tonsilitis Remedy 291
Toothache 90, 262
Toothache Wax 278
Tourniquets 186
Toys for the Baby 137
Training of Baby..................132, 134
Trask's Magnetic Ointment 291
Treatment of Patient 64
Treatments, General 88
Triangular Bandage 144
Triangular Bandage, Application of..145
Tuberculosis 262
Tuberculosis, Diet for 75
Tuberculosis, Nature and Prevention. 37
Tumors 263
Turpentine Stupes 88
Typhoid Diet, High Calorie 75
Typhoid Fever 264
Typhoid Fever, Causation and Pre-
  vention 38
Typhoid Fever, Diet for 75

U

Ulcers 267
Underfeeding the Baby 125
Urination, Disturbances of............ 94
Urine, Suppression of 259
Utensils Necessary for Modification
  of Milk 122

V

Vaccination 255
Varicose Veins 267
Varicose Veins, Hemorrhage of 182
Varioloid 254
Vehicles for the Baby 135
Veins, Varicose 267
Veneral Diseases 273
Venous Hemorrhage 180
Ventilating Baby's Room 103
Ventilation 2
Ventilation of Sick Room............ 57
Vermin as Germ Carriers 29
Vermin in Hair 297
Vegetables Acids, Poisoning by......170

W

PAGE.

Warts 268
Wars to Remove 296
Wash, Nasal 89
Water Supply 21
Water, Drinking for Baby 125
Weak Eyes 214
Weak or Diseased Eyes 214
Weaning from the Bottle 130
Weaning the Baby 128
Wens 268
Wetting Bed 133
Whites 93
"Who Am I" 47
Whooping Cough 269
Wolf's Bane 162
Worms 271
Wounds 186

PAGE.

Wounds, Aseptic 187
Wounds, Bullet 152
Wounds, Gunshot 187
Wounds, Incised 187
Wounds, Infection of 188
Wounds, Lacerated 187
Wounds, Septic or Poisonous 187
Wounds, Punctured 187
Wrappers for the Baby 107

Y

Young Men 272

Z

Zinc and Camphor Salve 277

www.ingramcontent.com/pod-product-compliance
Lightning Source LLC
Chambersburg PA
CBHW081715220526
45468CB00008B/1859

9781974095032